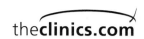

HEMATOLOGY/ ONCOLOGY CLINICS OF NORTH AMERICA

Sickle Cell Disease

GUEST EDITOR
Cage S. Johnson, MD

October 2005 • Volume 19 • Number 5

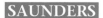

An Imprint of Elsevier, Inc.
PHILADELPHIA   LONDON   TORONTO   MONTREAL   SYDNEY   TOKYO

W.B. SAUNDERS COMPANY
A Division of Elsevier Inc.

Elsevier, Inc. · 1600 John F. Kennedy Boulevard · Suite 1800 · Philadelphia, Pennsylvania 19103-2899

http:/www.hemonc.theclinics.com

**HEMATOLOGY/ONCOLOGY CLINICS
OF NORTH AMERICA**
October 2005
Editor: Kerry Holland

Volume 19, Number 5
ISSN 0889-8588
ISBN 1-4160-2777-7

Reprints. For copies of 100 or more, of articles in this publication, please contact the Commercial Reprints Department, Elsevier Inc., 360 Park Avenue South, New York, New York 10010-1710. Tel. (212) 633-3813 Fax: (212) 462-1935 email: reprints@elsevier.com

The ideas and opinions expressed in *Hematology/Oncology Clinics of North America* do not necessarily reflect those of the Publisher. The Publisher does not assume any responsibility for any injury and/or damage to persons or property arising out of or related to any use of the material contained in this periodical. The reader is advised to check the appropriate medical literature and the product information currently provided by the manufacturer of each drug to be administered to verify the dosage, the method and duration of administration, or contraindications. It is the responsibility of the treating physician or other health care professional, relying on independent experience and knowledge of the patient, to determine drug dosages and the best treatment for the patient. Mention of any product in this issue should not be construed as endorsement by the contributors, editors, or the Publisher of the product or manufacturers' claims.

Hematology/Oncology Clinics of North America (ISSN 0889-8588) is published bi-monthly by W.B. Saunders Company. Corporate and editorial offices: Elsevier, Inc., 1600 John F. Kennedy Boulevard, Suite 1800, Philadelphia, PA 19103-2899. Accounting and circulation offices: 6277 Sea Harbor Drive, Orlando, FL 32887-4800. Periodicals postage paid at Orlando, FL 32862, and additional mailing offices. Subscription prices are $210.00 per year (US individuals), $315.00 per year (US institutions), $270.00 per year (foreign individuals), $380.00 per year (foreign institutions), $240.00 per year (Canadian individuals), and $380.00 per year (Canadian institutions). Foreign air speed delivery is included in all *Clinics* subscription prices. All prices are subject to change without notice. POSTMASTER: Send address changes to *Hematology/Oncology Clinics of North America*, W.B. Saunders Company, Periodicals Fulfillment, Orlando, FL 32887-4800. **Customer Service: 1-800-654-2452 (US). From outside the US, call 407-345-4000.** E-mail: hhspcs@harcourt.com

Hematology/Oncology Clinics of North America is covered in *Index Medicus, EMBASE/Excerpta Medica, and BIOSIS.*

Printed in the United States of America.

ELSEVIER
SAUNDERS

HEMATOLOGY/ONCOLOGY CLINICS
OF NORTH AMERICA

Sickle Cell Disease

GUEST EDITOR

CAGE S. JOHNSON, MD, Professor of Medicine and of Physiology and Biophysics; and Director, Comprehensive Sickle Cell Center, Keck School of Medicine, University of Southern California, Los Angeles, California

CONTRIBUTORS

CHRISTINE AGUILAR, MD, Director of Pediatric Rehabilitation, Children's Hospital & Research Center, Oakland, California

SAMIR K. BALLAS, MD, Professor of Medicine and Pediatrics, Cardeza Foundation for Hematologic Research; and Department of Medicine, Jefferson Medical College, Thomas Jefferson University, Philadelphia, Pennsylvania

JACKIE BUCK, RGN, BSc Hons, MSc, Nurse Research Fellow, John Walls Renal Unit, Leicester General Hospital, Leicester, England, United Kingdom

OSWALDO CASTRO, MD, Professor Emeritus of Medicine, Howard University College of Medicine, Center for Sickle Cell Disease, Washington, District of Columbia; and Critical Care Medicine Department, National Institutes of Health, Bethesda, Maryland

ELAINE Y. CHIANG, MD, Fellow, Department of Medicine, Mount Sinai School of Medicine, New York, New York

ANDREA CLARE, MD, Dermatologist, former MRC Laboratories, University of the West Indies, Kingston, Jamaica, West Indies

SALLY C. DAVIES, MBBS, PhD, FRCP, FRCPCh, FMedSci, Professor, Imperial College Faculty of Medicine, Central Middlesex Hospital, London, England, United Kingdom

GEOFFREY G. EMERSON, MD, Clinical Instructor, Casey Eye Institute, Portland, Oregon

PAUL S. FRENETTE, MD, Associate Professor, Department of Medicine; and Immunobiology Center, Mount Sinai School of Medicine, New York, New York

MARK T. GLADWIN, MD, Head, Vascular Therapeutics Section, Cardiovascular Branch, National Heart, Lung, and Blood Institute; and Critical Care Medicine Department, National Institutes of Health, Bethesda, Maryland

KATHRYN HASSELL, MD, Associate Professor of Medicine; and Director, Colorado Sickle Cell Treatment and Research Center, University of Colorado Health Sciences Center, Denver, Colorado

CAGE S. JOHNSON, MD, Professor of Medicine and of Physiology and Biophysics; and Director, Comprehensive Sickle Cell Center, Keck School of Medicine, University of Southern California, Los Angeles, California

GERARD A. LUTTY, PhD, Professor of Opthalmology, Wilmer Ophthalmological Institute, Johns Hopkins Hospital, Baltimore, Maryland

JUNETTE S. MOHAN, PhD, Physiologist, former MRC Laboratories, University of the West Indies, Kingston, Jamaica, West Indies

LYNNE NEUMAYR, MD, Children's Hospital & Research Center, Oakland, California

IHEANYI E. OKPALA, MBBS (Hons), MSc, FRCPath, FWACP, Hematology Department, St. Thomas' Hospital, London, England, United Kingdom

DARLEEN R. POWARS, MD, Professor of Pediatrics, Department of Pediatrics, Division of Hematology/Oncology, Women's & Children's Hospital, Keck School of Medicine at the University of Southern California, Los Angeles, California

ZORA R. ROGERS, MD, Associate Professor of Pediatrics, Division of Pediatric Hematology/Oncology, The University of Texas Southwestern Medical Center at Dallas; and Director of the Clinical Core, Southwestern Comprehensive Sickle Cell Center, Dallas, Texas

BERYL E. SERJEANT, FIMLS, Chief Technologist, former MRC Laboratories, University of the West Indies; and Sickle Cell Trust (Jamaica), Kingston, Jamaica, West Indies

GRAHAM R. SERJEANT, MD, FRCP, Professor Emeritus, University of the West Indies; Director, former MRC Laboratories, University of the West Indies; and Sickle Cell Trust (Jamaica), Kingston, Jamaica, West Indies

MARILYN J. TELEN, MD, Wellcome Professor of Medicine; Chief, Division of Hematology; Director, Duke-UNC Comprehensive Sickle Cell Center; and Co-Director, Duke Hospital Transfusion Service, Duke University Medical Center, Durham, North Carolina

ELLIOTT VICHINSKY, MD, Director of Hematology/Oncology, Children's Hospital & Research Center, Oakland, California

SAM O. WANKO, MD, Fellow, Divisions of Hematology, Oncology, and Bone Marrow Transplant, Duke University Medical Center, Durham, North Carolina

WING-YEN WONG, MD, Associate Professor of Pediatrics, Department of Pediatrics, Division of Hematology/Oncology, Children's Hospital Los Angeles, Keck School of Medicine at the University of Southern California, Los Angeles, California

HEMATOLOGY/ONCOLOGY CLINICS
OF NORTH AMERICA

Sickle Cell Disease

CONTENTS   VOLUME 19 · NUMBER 5 · OCTOBER 2005

> The vaso-occlusion model has evolved impressively over the past several decades from polymerization-based concepts to a complex, wide-ranging schema that involves multistep, heterogeneous, and interdependent interactions among sickle erythrocytes (SSRBCs), adherent leukocytes, endothelial cells, plasma proteins, and other factors. Endothelial activation, induced directly or indirectly by the proinflammatory behavior of SSRBCs, is the most likely initiating step toward vaso-occlusion. Given the complexity and dynamic relationships of the potential mechanisms leading to vaso-occlusion, further in vivo studies in relevant sickle cell animal models will most likely yield the greatest advances and promote the development of novel, more effective therapeutic strategies.

> Management of sickle cell disease continues to be primarily palliative, including supportive, symptomatic, and preventative approaches to therapy. There are three major types of sickle cell pain: acute, chronic, and neuropathic pain. The acute painful episode is the insignia of the disease and the most common cause of hospitalization. Its management entails the use of nonpharmacologic and pharmacologic modalities. Pain management should follow certain principles that include an assessment stage, treatment stage, reassessment stage, and adjustment stage. Chronic sickle cell pain may also be due to certain complications of the disease, such as leg ulcers and avascular necrosis; intractable chronic pain may be due to central sensitization. Management of chronic pain should take a multidisciplinary approach.

> Sickle cell disease (SCD) is the most commonly inherited hemoglobinopathy in the United States. Blood transfusion is a critical part of the multidisciplinary approach necessary in the management of SCD; however, blood transfusions are not without complications. The successful

use of transfusion as a treatment strategy in SCD requires the critical review and knowledge of transfusion methods, generally accepted indications, clinical situations in which transfusion generally is not considered, the selection of blood products, and strategies to prevent transfusion-related complications.

Abnormal rheologic behavior of sickle cells is the result of increased viscosity of the blood caused by the polymerization of hemoglobin S and the resultant production of dense, dehydrated sickle erythrocytes. As the viscosity of sickle cells increases, there is a negative impact on blood flow, which contributes to the vascular occlusion process, the hallmark of the sickling disorders. Blood flow is directly proportional to the blood pressure and inversely proportional to the blood viscosity. Blood flow has important implications for the diagnosis and management of hypertension in sickle cell patients and for transfusion therapy for the acute and chronic complications of this disease.

Regional complete infarctions in children with sickle cell anemia (HbSS) are often associated with stenosis of the large intracranial arteries and result in lifetime disability. Incomplete infarction occurs more frequently than previously recognized and has far-reaching effects on neurocognitive development and the risk for overt secondary strokes into adulthood. Clinical and neuroimaging modalities have been highlighted in an algorithmic approach, with the studies giving the highest yield in results and most likely to be available listed in sequential order. The recognition of an emerging "second peak" incidence in the third decade of life is worrisome and warrants more intense scrutiny and diagnosis of subtle findings of stroke in this young adult population.

Recent large clinical studies of the acute chest syndrome (ACS) have improved our understanding of its pathophysiology and epidemiology. However, there is still a need for better methods of distinguishing vaso-occlusion from fibrin or fat embolism, for rapid diagnostic tests to make positive identifications of microbial infection, for adjunctive therapies that would affect prognosis, and for identification of factors that influence prognosis. The difference in clinical course and severity between children and adults supports the results of current studies indicating multiple causes for ACS. The mainstay of successful treatment remains high-quality supportive care. The judicious use of transfusion therapy has a major role in preventing mortality in the absence of a specific therapy that consistently improves the clinical course.

Pulmonary hypertension affects nearly one-third of adults with sickle cell disease and is related to hemolysis. Although pulmonary pressures are not as high as in other forms of pulmonary hypertension, sickle cell patients poorly tolerate even moderate elevations of pulmonary pressures, because this complication predicts short survival. Tricuspid regurgitant jet velocity measured noninvasively by echocardiography is an adequate tool to screen for pulmonary hypertension. Because patients with pulmonary hypertension are older and often severely affected by other vaso-occlusive complications, optimizing their treatment with hydroxyurea or transfusions is important. Newer agents such as sildenafil and bosentan have demonstrated efficacy in other forms of pulmonary hypertension, and future clinical trials may prove them helpful in sickle cell patients.

Persons with sickle cell disease (SCD) are more likely to undergo surgery than are the general population during their lifetime. For example, cholecystectomy as a consequence of gallstones is more frequent in persons with SCD, as is hip arthroplasty in younger people as a result of avascular necrosis of the femoral head. Because surgery exposes patients to many of the factors that are known to precipitate red blood cell sickling, persons with SCD undergoing surgery require meticulous clinical care to prevent perioperative sickle cell–related complications. Even with meticulous care, approximately 25% to 30% of patients will have a postoperative complication. This article provides readers with information about the role of surgery in SCD and the measures that should be taken to ensure patients are well cared for in the perioperative period.

With advances in management, men and women with sickle cell disease are enjoying an improved quality of life well into adulthood, when they may elect to plan a family. Pregnancy has been associated with exacerbation of sickle cell disease and may place women, especially those with sickle cell anemia (HbSS), at an additional risk for obstetric complications. Appropriate management by health care providers familiar with sickle cell diseases and high-risk obstetric care can result in a successful pregnancy for most women with sickle cell disease.

Priapism in Sickle Cell Disease 917
Zora R. Rogers

Priapism, an unwanted painful prolonged erection of the penis, is a little discussed but common complication of sickle cell disease. What is known about the prevalence of priapism, efficacy of management approaches, and outcome is drawn primarily from retrospective and single-center reports. Priapism occurs in two patterns: prolonged and stuttering (ie, recurrent brief episodes that resolve spontaneously). If priapism persists for 4 hours or more without detumescence, the patient is at risk for irreversible ischemic penile injury, which may terminate in fibrosis and impotence. Large multicenter studies examining the epidemiology and current treatments and well-organized trials of novel therapies are urgently needed for patients who have sickle cell disease and priapism.

Bone and Joint Disease in Sickle Cell Disease 929
Christine Aguilar, Elliott Vichinsky, and Lynne Neumayr

Bone and joint disorders are the most common cause of chronic pain in patients who have sickle cell disease. The femoral head is the most common area of bone destruction in sickle cell patients, although other disease-related problems include avascular necrosis of the humeral head, changes in the thoracic and lumbar spine, infection with encapsulated organisms (*Salmonella* and *Staphylococcus aureus* are the most common), bone marrow disturbances, and dental effects. Complications can occur at any location: epiphyseal, metaphyseal, or diaphyseal. The location and the extensiveness of the problems determine the pain and structural damage. The hip joint is particularly vulnerable in sickle cell disease. This article highlights aspects of sickle cell disease that affect healthy bone and joint function and discusses treatment options.

Leg Ulceration in Sickle Cell Disease: Medieval Medicine in a Modern World 943
Graham R. Serjeant, Beryl E. Serjeant, Junette S. Mohan, and Andrea Clare

Leg ulceration is now recognized as an important complication of sickle cell disease, especially of the SS genotype. Since there is no convincing evidence of delayed healing of operation scars or of wounds elsewhere in the body, it must be concluded that factors specific to the lower leg render patients prone to delayed healing at this site. Many lesions are traumatic in origin and since there is considerable variation in healing rates among the normal population, it is useful to define chronic leg ulceration on the basis of a minimal duration, which in Jamaican studies has required at least 3 months and sometimes 6 months before healing. This minimal duration avoids the difficulties of interpreting the significance of briefer lesions since the moment of final healing may be poorly defined (patients may conclude that a scab represents healing whereas small lesions persist beneath) and often goes undocumented as patients may not report and medical attendants may not enquire, the date of final healing.

HEMATOLOGY/ONCOLOGY CLINICS
OF NORTH AMERICA

Hematol Oncol Clin N Am 19 (2005) xi–xiii

HEMATOLOGY/ONCOLOGY CLINICS
OF NORTH AMERICA

PREFACE

Sickle Cell Disease

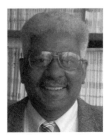

Cage S. Johnson, MD

Guest Editor

Nearly 10 years ago, Sam Charache and I were asked to edit an issue for the *Hematology/Oncology Clinics of North America* on sickle cell disease [1]. In the intervening years, Dr. Charache has retired from Johns Hopkins University but remains active at national meetings and with other academic activities. Unfortunately, he declined the invitation to coedit this issue. Consequently, I have made my best attempt to follow the path he illuminated with his wisdom and scientific judgement. As in the prior issue, I have asked the individual authors to provide clinicians with practical guidelines and advice on the diagnosis and management of some of the important treatment issues in this complex disease. We tried to limit therapeutic choices to discussion of agents that had some clinical experience, rather than cast our eyes too far into the future. Finally, as in the 1996 issue, these articles reflect the recommendations of a single voice, in contrast to a consensus opinion, as in the monograph published by the National Heart, Lung, and Blood Institute. That monograph, *The Management of Sickle Cell Disease* (4th edition) [2], can be found at http://www.nhlbi.nih.gov/health/prof/blood/sickle/index.htm and is a valuable resource for complications not covered in this issue, as well as for additional information on the disorders covered herein.

During the years since the prior issue, data from large clinical studies has better defined the clinical course of sickle cell disease (see the review by Bonds [3]). At the same time, considerable progress has been made in our overall understanding of the pathophysiologic basis for the disease and its complications. These data provide stronger support for the therapeutic recommendations made by the authors, in the absence of data from controlled trials.

0889-8588/05/$ – see front matter
doi:10.1016/j.hoc.2005.09.001

The field is rapidly moving from the bench to the bedside as our understanding of the pathophysiology increases at the molecular and cellular levels. In the next 10 years, I fully expect that the foundation for therapeutic recommendations will be even stronger as the results of ongoing and planned controlled clinical trials become available. By then we should have answers to questions such as:

- Will transfusion prevent silent cerebral infarcts and alleviate its effect on quality of life for these patients?
- Can patients with cerebrovascular disease be transitioned to agents such as hydroxyurea with efficacy equal to or better than transfusion?
- Do other hemoglobin F–modulating agents, such as decitabine, have equal or better clinical efficacy?
- Will early treatment with hemoglobin F modulators ameliorate the end-organ damage of this disease with reasonable toxicity?
- Will erythrocyte-hydrating agents, such as Gardos-channel inhibitors, improve the efficacy of hydroxyurea?
- Will treatment of pulmonary hypertension, for which a number of agents are under study, improve survival and quality of life?
- Will treatment with angiotensin-converting enzyme inhibitors or angiotensin receptor blockers alter the course of sickle nephropathy?
- What is the best management strategy for acute priapism, as well as its prophylaxis?
- What is the role, if any, of glucocorticoids in the management of acute vaso-occlusive pain or in acute chest syndrome?

These and other issues are in active investigation, and results will be available in the near future.

Finally, there are studies of molecules that block adhesion receptors and could favorably impact vaso-occlusion, an important addition to our therapeutic armamentarium, such as the development of a recombinant P-selectin glycoprotein ligand that binds to P-selectin and, to a lesser degree, E-and L-selectin. Recent studies using monoclonal antibodies and knockout mice have shown that P-selectin mediates the initial interaction of sickle erythrocytes and leucocytes with activated endothelial cells [3–5]. Thus blockade of P-selectin using this fusion protein could provide clinical benefit through inhibition of the adhesion of leucocytes and sickle erythrocytes to endothelium in the vaso-occlusive process. Additional agents that inhibit other adehesogenic proteins involved in the vaso-occlusive process, such as the integrin $\alpha_V \beta_{3,}$ are being studied [6–8].

On the horizon remains the promise of gene therapy, whose continued progress is eagerly monitored by all of us who care for these patients [9]. Thus there is reason for cautious optimism, because patients currently receive much better care than in past decades, and there is every indication that progress is being made more rapidly than before.

Cage S. Johnson, MD
Comprehensive Sickle Cell Center
Keck School of Medicine
University of Southern California
RMR 304, 2025 Zonal Avenue
Los Angeles, CA 90033, USA
E-mail address: cagejohn@email.usc.edu

References

[1] Charache S, Johnson CS, editors. Sickle cell disease. Hematol Oncol Clin North Am 1996; 10(6).

[2] National Institutes of Health. The management of sickle cell disease. 4th edition. NIH Publication No. 02–2117. Available at: http://www.nhlbi.nih.gov/health/prof/blood/sickle/index.htm.

[3] Bonds DR. Three decades of innovation in the management of sickle cell disease: the road to understanding the sickle cell disease clinical phenotype. Blood Rev 2005;19:99–110.

[4] Matsui NM, Borsig L, Rosen SD, et al. P-selectin mediates the adhesion of sickle erythrocytes to the endothelium. Blood 2001;98:1955–62.

[5] Hicks AER, Nolan SL, Ridger VC, et al. Recombinant P-selectin glycoprotein ligand-1 directly inhibits leucocyte rolling by all 3 selectins in vivo: complete inhibition of rolling is not required for anti-inflammatory effect. Blood 2003;101:3249–56.

[6] Kaul DK, Tsai HM, Liu XD, et al. Monoclonal antibodies to $\alpha_v\beta_3$ (7E3 and LM609) inhibit sickle red blood cell-endothelium interactions induced by platelet-activating factor. Blood 2000;95:368–74.

[7] Lutty GA, Taomoto M, Cao J, et al. Inhibition of TNF-alpha-induced sickle RBC retention in retina by a VLA-4 antagonist. Invest Ophthalmol Vis Sci 2001;42:1349–55.

[8] Tilley JW, Chen L, Sidduri A, et al. The discovery of VLA-4 antagonists. Curr Top Med Chem 2004;4:1509–23.

[9] Puthenveetil G, Malik P. Gene therapy for hemoglobinopathies: are we there yet? Curr Hematol Rep 2004;3:298–305.

Hematol Oncol Clin N Am 19 (2005) 771–784

HEMATOLOGY/ONCOLOGY CLINICS
OF NORTH AMERICA

Sickle Cell Vaso-Occlusion

Elaine Y. Chiang, MD[a], Paul S. Frenette, MD[a,b,*]

[a]*Department of Medicine, Mount Sinai School of Medicine, One Gustave L. Levy Place, Box 1079, New York, NY 10029, USA*
[b]*Immunobiology Center, Mount Sinai School of Medicine, New York, NY 10029, USA*

The last century has seen a flourishing of intensive study into the origin of sickle cell disease and the pathophysiology underlying vaso-occlusion. Sickle cell anemia was first described in a dental student from Grenada in 1910 by James Herrick [1], who hypothesized that his symptoms arose from the sickle-shaped erythrocytes in the blood. Two decades later, it was discovered that sickle-shaped erythrocytes were more prominently found in the relatively deoxygenated venous circulation and that these erythrocytes regained their normal shape after reoxygenation [2–4]. In their landmark paper of 1949, Linus Pauling and colleagues [5] verified the abnormal electrophoretic mobility of the mutated hemoglobin molecule in the erythrocytes of patients with sickle cell disease. The differentiating characteristic of sickle hemoglobin (HbS) was later discovered to be a single amino acid substitution on the β-globin chain of HbS [6], which leads to the abnormal susceptibility of HbS to polymerization in the presence of decreased pH or oxygen tension. From these early observations, sickle cell vaso-occlusion appeared to result from the passive physical obstruction of small blood vessels with deoxygenated, rigid, sickle-shaped erythrocytes. However, it became increasingly recognized that HbS polymerization alone was not sufficient to produce vaso-occlusion.

Conceptualization of sickle cell vaso-occlusion grew beyond the hemoglobin molecule when it was recognized that sickle erythrocytes had a striking propensity to adhere to cultured vascular endothelial cells [7,8]. In addition, in vitro adhesiveness of sickle erythrocytes (SSRBCs) was shown to correlate with clinical disease severity [9]. The adherence of SSRBCs to the endothelium has since been well characterized in various in vitro and ex vivo models [10,11]. It is now recognized that SSRBCs actively participate in vaso-occlusion through multiple overlapping cell and matrix adhesion molecules. Both dense, sickle-shaped erythrocytes and immature reticulocytes may participate in adhesion

The authors recognize the tremendous contributions made by their colleagues in the field of sickle cell disease and regret that they cannot include all work within the scope of this article.
* Corresponding author. Department of Medicine, Mount Sinai School of Medicine, One Gustave L. Levy Place, Box 1079, New York, NY 10029. *E-mail address:* paul.frenette@mssm.edu (P.S. Frenette).

to the vascular endothelium. Reticulocytes appear to be more adherent than mature erythrocytes to cultured endothelium in vitro [12–14]; however, it may be that older erythrocytes subjected to repetitive cycles of deoxygenation can regain or maintain their adhesiveness [15]. These findings led to a proposed model in which reticulocytes initiated vaso-occlusion by first adhering to the endothelium, then secondarily adhering to and trapping circulating dense SSRBCs. However, recent evidence from clinical observations and animal models suggests that vaso-occlusion most likely results from a complex inter-play of several processes, involving SSRBCs, endothelial cells, leukocytes, and platelets, along with coagulative factors and other plasma proteins. This article focuses on the contributions of the cellular elements and selected plasma pro-teins, which demonstrate the significant advances made in our current under-standing of sickle cell vaso-occlusion.

CONTRIBUTIONS OF SICKLE HEMOGLOBIN POLYMERIZATION AND ERYTHROCYTE SICKLING

Repetitive cycles of SSRBC sickling and unsickling may lead to severe erythro-cyte membrane injury, generating damaging oxygen radicals. This process may also lead to abnormal erythrocyte cation homeostasis, resulting in dehydrated, dense cells and irreversibly sickled cells; these cell forms most likely exacerbate the underlying hemolytic anemia and vascular obstructions (see further discus-sion). Dehydration of erythrocytes may occur by means of each of three cation transporters expressed in the plasma membrane, including the Ca^{2+}–sensitive Gardos channels, the K^+Cl^- cotransporter, and the Na^+ pump [16]. Deoxygen-ation, HbS polymerization, and subsequent membrane permeabilization have been hypothesized to permit passive Na^+ and Ca^{2+} cation entry and activation of the Gardos channels, resulting in the net loss of KCl and cell dehydration [16]. The promising therapeutic potential of the Gardos channel inhibitor clotri-mazole, which decreased the numbers of dense and irreversibly sickled cells in addition to lowering the rate of hemolysis, encouraged the development of the more potent and specific inhibitor ICA-17043 and the channel activity–lowering L-arginine, both of which are currently under clinical investigation [17,18].

MECHANISMS OF ERYTHROCYTE ADHESION

The molecular mediators of SSRBC adhesion to the vascular endothelium have been characterized in great detail over the past 20 years, in both in vitro and animal models. This interaction has been shown to be largely mediated by cell surface receptors on both erythrocytes and endothelial cells. Adhe-sion molecules on erythrocytes that mediate interactions with endothelial cells include α4β1 integrin, Lutheran blood group antigen, cluster designation 36 (CD36), putative selectin ligands, and sulfated glycolipids. α4β1 binds to fibronectin and vascular cell adhesion molecule–1 (VCAM-1), which is expressed in response to inflammatory stimulants. The Lutheran blood group antigen binds laminin [19,20], a cyclic adenosine monophosphate-dependent interaction that may be mediated by the small guanine triphosphatase Rap1

[21] and enhanced by the presence of epinephrine [22]. Interestingly, further studies of the effects of epinephrine on the adhesive function of SSRBCs demonstrated that epinephrine also promotes SSRBC adhesion to the endothelial integrin $\alpha V \beta 3$ by means of intercellular adhesion molecule–4 (ICAM-4) [23]. This finding suggests that adrenergic hormones may contribute to the association between vaso-occlusive episodes and physiologic stress.

Significantly, the soluble ligands thrombospondin (TSP) and von Willebrand factor (vWF), elevated levels of which have been found in the blood of sickle cell patients [24], have well-described roles as bridging molecules mediating additional adhesion pathways between erythrocytes and endothelial cells. TSP has been shown to facilitate erythrocyte CD36 binding to several endothelial cell receptors, including endothelial CD36, cell surface heparin sulfate, and $\alpha V \beta 3$ integrin [25]. In addition, TSP immobilized on the endothelial surface binds to erythrocytes; this pathway may be mediated by $\alpha 4 \beta 1$ on CD47-stimulated erythrocytes [26]. Both TSP and vWF bind to $\alpha V \beta 3$; monoclonal antibodies to $\alpha V \beta 3$ integrin were shown to prevent SSRBC adhesion to the endothelium in a rat ex vivo model [27]. In this study, platelet-activating factor (PAF) was used to enhance SSRBC adherence to the endothelium and was also found to increase endothelial expression of vWF. This evidence suggests that vWF may contribute to the observed erythrocyte binding to endothelial $\alpha V \beta 3$. The unusually large multimeric forms of vWF greatly increased SSRBC binding to the endothelium in an in vitro flow model [28,29], and this interaction was suggested to result from glycoprotein Ib (GPIb)–like receptors on endothelial cells and GPIb- or GPIIb/IIIa–like receptors on erythrocytes [29]. In addition to erythrocyte receptors, other surface-anchored lipids, such as phosphatidylserine and sulfated glycolipids, may contribute to erythrocyte adhesiveness. Interestingly, phosphatidylserine is restricted to the inner leaflet of the intact erythrocyte bilayer membrane; however, this normal phospholipid asymmetry is lost in sickle cell disease, possibly because of membrane damage from recurrent sickling. Phosphatidylserine-exposing SSRBCs demonstrate greater in vitro adhesiveness to endothelial cells, which is also mediated by TSP [30,31].

SICKLE CELL DISEASE AS A SYNDROME OF CHRONIC VASCULAR INFLAMMATION

The adhesion of SSRBCs to the endothelium is not self-limited, because it may in turn induce signals that trigger oxygen radical formation and activation of the transcription factor NF-κB in endothelial cells. NF-κB contributes to chronic vascular activation by upregulating endothelial adhesion molecules, including E-selectin, VCAM-1, and ICAM-1, potentially allowing further interactions with SSRBCs as well as the recruitment of circulating leukocytes. Endothelial P-selectin, which is expressed in the early phases of inflammation and in increased levels in transgenic sickle cell mice, may also participate in the vaso-occlusive process by decreasing blood flow dynamics [32]. This phenomenon is not observed in P-selectin knockout animals and is abrogated in sickle cell mice pretreated with P-selectin monoclonal antibody. The proinflammatory phenotype of endothelial cells in the cerebral venules of sickle cell mice was also demonstrated by increased white blood cell recruitment in mice treated with or without hypoxic stimulation; this effect was attenuated in endothelial P-selectin knockout animals [33].

Vascular inflammation is further evidenced by the elevated plasma levels of soluble VCAM-1 in patients during vaso-occlusive sickle crises and by the presence of circulating endothelial cells bearing an activated phenotype during both steady and crisis states [34,35]. Notably, the inflammatory stimulus of hypoxia and reoxygenation, which induced endothelial oxidant production and an exaggerated inflammatory response in a transgenic sickle mouse model, was significantly attenuated by the administration of the NF-κB inhibitor sulfasalazine [36]. In addition, sulfasalazine administration resulted in a reduction of ICAM-1 and VCAM-1 expression on the circulating endothelial cells of three patients in a small pilot study, as well as in the tissues of sickle mice [37].

Another anti-inflammatory agent, dexamethasone, was found to inhibit NF-κB, VCAM-1, and ICAM-1 expression in the liver, lungs, and skin of transgenic sickle mice after hypoxia and reoxygenation [38]. Dexamethasone additionally preserved blood flow, reduced leukocyte recruitment to the endothelium, and prevented vascular occlusion in these animals. Endothelial cell activation and adhesion molecule expression, therefore, appear to be critical factors in the vaso-occlusive process. In addition, the significance of nitric oxide (NO), which maintains vasoregulatory homeostasis, has begun to be explored in detail in recent years. Local, constitutive production of NO by endothelial cell nitric oxide synthase results in vasorelaxation as well as in antioxidant and anti-inflammatory activity, such as the reduction of VCAM-1 expression [39]. In addition, NO limits platelet aggregation, inhibits leukocyte adhesion, and modulates endothelial proliferation [39]. Reduced bioavailability of NO in sickle cell disease may lead to vasoconstriction and the reduction of blood flow, potentially contributing to vaso-occlusion. Currently, a number of NO-based therapies are under investigation, including inhaled NO and oral arginine supplementation. Notably, a potential role exists for subendothelial matrix molecules in vaso-occlusion; certain inflammatory stimuli, such as thrombin, may cause contraction of endothelial cells such that the profound adhesion of SSRBCs to thrombin-stimulated endothelial cells also occurs with exposed matrix in interendothelial gaps [40].

The chronic proinflammatory environment is propagated by elevated levels of circulating cytokines, including interleukin-1 (IL-1), tumor necrosis factor–α (TNF-α), endothelin-1, and granulocyte-macrophage colony stimulating factor (GM-CSF), which are most likely secreted by both activated endothelial cells and monocytes [41,42]. Placenta growth factor (PlGF) has been shown to activate monocytes and increase their mRNA levels of IL-1, TNF-α, and various chemokines (eg, monocyte chemoattractant protein–1, IL-8, and macrophage inflammatory protein–1β) [43]. Elevated plasma levels of PlGF have been found in sickle patients and were shown to correlate with disease severity [44]. Monocytes, in turn, can then further activate endothelial cells, as evidenced by the expression of endothelial adhesion molecules, tissue factor, and the activation of NF-κB following incubation with monocytes in vitro [45]. In addition, vascular inflammation has been demonstrated in transgenic sickle mouse models; these animals all displayed elevated blood levels of the acute phase proteins serum amyloid-P component and IL-6, as well as upregulated expression of ICAM-1, VCAM-1, platelet–endothelial cell adhesion molecule, and NF-κB in lung tissues [34].

LEUKOCYTE ADHESION: A PREREQUISITE TO VASO-OCCLUSION

Clinical observations have suggested a role for leukocytes (WBCs) in the pathophysiology of sickle cell disease [46]. Elevated WBC counts have been correlated with poor outcome in patients [47]. In particular, elevated steady-state WBC counts were shown to be a risk factor for stroke and acute chest syndrome in children who have sickle cell disease [48,49]. The clinical benefit of hydroxyurea treatment was observed to follow a reduction in the peripheral blood neutrophil (PMN) counts, even without the anticipated increase in protective fetal hemoglobin [50]. Furthermore, case reports of severe sickle pain crises triggered by the administration of myeloid growth factors G-CSF or GM-CSF have resulted in a relative contraindication of the use of these drugs in patients with sickle cell disease [51–53]. In vitro, SSRBCs have been shown to bind to PMNs in a static adhesion assay [54], suggesting the direct participation of leukocytes in vaso-occlusion. It is intriguing that the PMN count is notably lower in individuals of African descent, and one may speculate that lower PMN counts hold an evolutionary advantage in a population with a high prevalence of the HbS mutation in regions where malaria is endemic.

Like endothelial cells, circulating WBCs display an activated phenotype, as evidenced by the expression of activated β2 integrin adhesion molecules [55] and cytokine-inducible CD64 (FcγRI) [56], by increased release of leukocyte elastase, and by increased shedding of L-selectin and CD16 (FcγRIII) [57] from WBCs of patients who have sickle cell disease. In transgenic sickle mice, WBC activation was also demonstrated in vivo by an increased number of adherent WBCs recruited to the endothelium compared with nonsickle control animals, following either hypoxia and reoxygenation or TNF-α as an inflammatory stimulus [58,59].

The role of leukocytes in the vaso-occlusive process may be multifactorial. It is likely that the recruitment of large-diameter, less deformable, adherent WBCs to the endothelium can impair blood flow. For example, it has been estimated that as few as six adherent WBCs per 100 μm of venular length can increase vascular resistance twofold [60]. Therefore, WBC adhesion may promote erythrocyte sickling and vascular occlusion by increasing SSRBC transit time in the microcirculation. In the authors' laboratory, intravital microscopic observations of the cremaster muscle microcirculation in sickle cell mice have revealed that circulating erythrocytes interact directly with adherent WBCs in the postcapillary venules of the cremaster muscle. In fact, although circulating SSRBCs did have occasional direct interactions with the endothelium, most

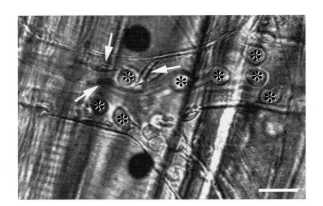

Fig. 1. Circulating SSRBCs interact predominantly with adherent WBCs. Approximately 65 minutes after surgical preparation of the cremaster muscle of sickle cell mice, a procedure that generates moderate local inflammation, adherent WBCs (*asterisks*) are seen. Numerous adhesive interactions between SSRBCs (*arrows*) and an adherent WBC may also be observed. Bar, 15μm. This video sequence and others that demonstrate these interactions may be downloaded from http://www.mssm.edu/labs/frenette/microcirc.shtml. (*From* Frenette PS. Sickle cell vasoocclusion: heterotypic, multicellular aggregations driven by leukocyte adhesion. Microcirculation 2004;11:169; with permission.)

interactions occurred with adherent WBCs (Fig. 1). Interestingly, SSRBC-WBC interactions did not occur during the early phase of inflammation, despite the abundance of adherent WBCs during this period. Instead, SSRBC–WBC interactions were found to increase significantly with time and the progression of vascular inflammation in this model, suggesting that additional activation signals may be required for WBCs or SSRBCs to participate in this interaction.

This unexpected observation generated yet another paradigm in the pathogenesis of sickle cell vaso-occlusion, in which activation of the venular endothelium in the microcirculation promotes leukocyte recruitment and activation and subsequent participation in direct adhesive interactions with circulating erythrocytes. SSRBCs then become secondarily trapped, leading to complete vaso-occlusion [61,62]. From this perspective, inhibition of leukocyte recruitment would be expected to prevent vaso-occlusion and improve blood flow. Because leukocyte recruitment is severely impaired in mice lacking endothelial P- and E-selectins [63,64], sickle cell mice deficient in endothelial P- and E-selectin were generated by bone marrow transplantation and observed likewise under intravital microscopy. These mice demonstrated a dramatic decrease in leukocyte recruitment, protection from vaso-occlusion, and markedly improved survival during the experimental procedure [59]. Given these findings, it is likely that the mechanisms that mediate leukocyte adhesion to the endothelium will provide exciting targets for potential new therapies in sickle cell vaso-occlusion.

While investigating the role of specific adhesion molecules using inhibitory antibodies, the authors found that nonspecific control IgG interfered with the interactions between adherent WBCs and SSRBCs. Commercial preparations of intravenous immunoglobulin (IVIgG) could, in this model, also inhibit SSRBC–WBC interactions in a dose-dependent manner. The administration of IVIgG at doses of 200 mg/kg and 400 mg/kg resulted in a significant decrease in the number of adherent WBCs, a dramatic reduction in SSRBC–WBC interactions, and markedly improved microcirculatory blood flow and survival of the sickle transgenic mice, even after further inflammatory challenge with TNF-α (Fig. 2)

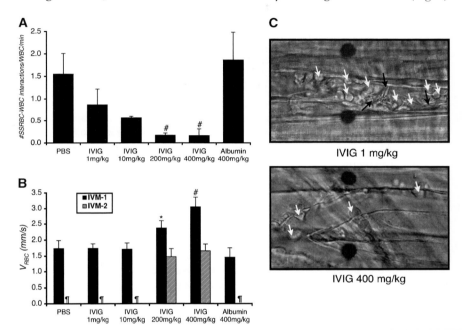

Fig. 2. IVIgG administration decreased SSRBC–WBC interactions, increased blood flow, and protected sickle cell mice from vaso-occlusion. (*A*) IVIgG reduced SSRBC–WBC interactions in vivo in a dose-dependent manner; differences were significant for the groups treated with IVIG at 200 mg/kg or more. # denotes $P \leq .01$ compared with phosphate-buffered saline (PBS)-treated control group; $P < .05$ compared with albumin-treated control group. (*B*) During the first 75 minutes after surgical preparation of the cremaster (intravital microscopy [IVM] 1), IVIgG 400 mg/kg improved centerline RBC velocities (V_{RBC}) in venules as measured by an optical Doppler velocimeter in real time. The effect was sustained after TNF-α administration (IVM 2). * denotes $P < .05$ compared with the albumin group; # denotes $P < .05$ compared with both the PBS and albumin groups; ¶ denotes groups in which the numbers of live mice and venules were too small for reliable determination. (*C*) Representative still frames of venules from sickle mice treated with 1 mg/kg or 400 mg/kg IVIgG, after TNF-α administration. In venules of sickle mice treated with 1 mg/kg IVIG, there persisted numerous interactions between SSRBCs (*black arrows*) and adherent WBCs (*white arrows*). Fewer SSRBC–WBC interactions and adherent WBCs were observed in sickle mice treated with 400 mg/kg IVIgG. Bar, 10 μm. The videos corresponding to these still frames may be downloaded from http://www.mssm.edu/labs/frenette/sickle_ivig.shtml. (*From* Turhan A, Jenab P, Bruhns P, et al. Intravenous immune globulin prevents venular vaso-occlusion in sickle cell mice by inhibiting leukocyte adhesion and the interactions between sickle erythrocytes and adherent leukocytes. Blood 2004;103:2399; with permission.)

[65]. Although the mechanism underlying the beneficial effect of IVIgG on vaso-occlusion is still unknown, it is appealing to speculate that IVIgG may be clinically useful to prevent or treat acute pain crises or other vaso-occlusive processes. However, this issue needs to be studied in the setting of a well-designed, prospective clinical trial, because IVIgG therapy has been associated with thrombotic complications in patients without sickle cell disease [66,67].

These studies offer an intriguing new view into the pathogenesis of vaso-occlusion; it is certainly plausible, given these findings, that recruited leukocytes could initiate vascular obstruction through their adhesive interactions with circulating erythrocytes. Observations of SSRBC–WBC interactions in this model have suggested that these interactions may be restricted to certain leukocyte subclasses. It follows that the identification of the particular leukocyte subclasses recruited to the endothelium, and of the subclasses that are capable of supporting interactions with erythrocytes, may prove particularly valuable as an entry into potential new therapeutic targets. The authors have initiated intravital microscopic observations in sickle cell mice using simultaneously multiple fluorescence-conjugated, lineage-specific leukocyte markers. Preliminary data suggest that neutrophils not only compose the leukocyte subclass most abundantly recruited to the endothelium but also participate in the vast majority of interactions with circulating erythrocytes. It will be interesting to test whether the disruption of neutrophil recruitment in this disease model will thereby prohibit SSRBC–WBC interactions and, presumably, prevent vaso-occlusion. Because leukocyte recruitment is itself a sequential, multistep process, there are multiple potential therapeutic targets in each step of leukocyte rolling, activation, and firm adhesion, all of which are valuable avenues of investigation.

PLATELETS AND PLASMA COAGULATIVE FACTORS: POTENTIAL ROLE OF THROMBOGENESIS

Activation of factors involved in hemostasis is unmistakable in sickle cell disease, given the observations of ongoing platelet activation, thrombin generation, and fibrinolytic activity. However, the role these processes play in vaso-occlusion is still unclear. Significantly, circulating platelets in sickle cell disease exhibit an abnormally activated phenotype both during steady state and during vaso-occlusive crises [68]. Increased release of platelet contents, including β-thromboglobulin, platelet factor–4, TSP, and IL-1, points to this markedly activated phenotype, as does increased expression of platelet P-selectin and activated GPIIb/IIIa [24,69]. During steady-state or noncrisis periods, platelet survival appears to be normal, yet decreased platelet counts have been found during acute pain episodes, indicating increased platelet consumption during vaso-occlusion [70,71]. Platelet aggregation, along with the generation of platelet-derived microparticles, may be abnormally increased [68,69]. Circulating tissue factor–bearing microparticles, shed from activated monocytes and, to a lesser extent, from endothelial cells, have also been described [72]. Activated platelets, like membrane-injured SSRBCs, expose phosphatidylserine on the outer layer of their cell membranes, so that both cell types provide a platform for the association of coagulation factors and promote circulating procoagulant activity [73,74].

However, antiplatelet therapy in sickle cell disease has yielded inconclusive results to date. Two uncontrolled trials, evaluating the effect of aspirin with or without dipyridamole, reported a modest clinical benefit of aspirin in decreasing pain crisis frequency and increasing hemoglobin levels [75,76]. By contrast, a randomized placebo-controlled trial assessing low-dose aspirin did not show any decrease in the frequency of pain crises [77]. Ticlopidine, a platelet ADP receptor antagonist, reduced platelet release products β-thromboglobulin and platelet factor–4 yet demonstrated no improvement in platelet survival or in pain crisis frequency [78,79]. Unfortunately, these trials were not designed to exclude the possibility of benefit, and it is still controversial whether antiplatelet therapy at appropriate doses may have beneficial effects in sickle cell vaso-occlusion. Anticoagulants may also yield therapeutic benefit in vaso-occlusion. Heparin has been shown to inhibit SSRBC adhesion to endothelial cells [25,80,81]; its additional anti-inflammatory effect may be of particular benefit in sickle cell disease. Oral anticoagulants, though associated with major bleeding complications during chronic use, show promise with lower dosing. In two small studies of patients who had sickle cell disease and took oral anticoagulation, the elevated plasma levels of biochemical markers of thrombin generation were normalized, and elevated plasma levels of D-dimer during pain crisis were significantly lowered [82,83]. However, various markers of endothelial cell activation were not shown to be significantly different in patients taking low-dose oral anticoagulation, and clinical benefit, such as in pain crisis frequency, has not yet been shown from this therapy [84,85].

It may be that platelets participate in a more complex, multicellular process during vaso-occlusion, in which platelet activation leads to the release of cytoadhesive proteins and exposure of phospholipid surfaces or promotes the adhesion of circulating erythrocytes, leukocytes, and the endothelium as a bridging mechanism. Interestingly, SSRBC adhesion to cultured human umbilical vein endothelial cells in vitro was found to increase in the presence of autologous platelets [86]. In the blood of patients who have sickle cell disease, flow cytometric analyses have identified the presence of circulating platelet-RBC and platelet-WBC complexes [87]. The increased number of platelet-erythrocyte aggregates in children who have sickle cell disease compared with nonsickle controls was found to be associated with reduced nocturnal oxygen saturation as measured by overnight pulse oximetry [88]. Nocturnal hypoxemia is of particular interest, because it has been shown to be associated with anemia and inversely correlated with erythrocyte adhesivity and markers of leukocyte, endothelial, and platelet activation [89]. These findings suggest a role for nocturnal hypoxemia in vaso-occlusive episodes and cerebrovascular complications of sickle cell disease. It is thus conceivable that platelets may also be involved in the adhesion of circulating SSRBCs to adherent leukocytes or to the endothelium. Future studies in which microcirculatory platelet behavior is directly visualized in vivo are needed to address this compelling question.

THE VASO-OCCLUSION MODEL: NEW EXPANSIONS, FUTURE DIRECTIONS

The vaso-occlusion model has evolved impressively over the past several decades from polymerization-based concepts to a complex, wide-ranging schema that involves multistep, heterogeneous, and interdependent interactions among the SSRBCs, adherent leukocytes, endothelial cells, plasma proteins, and other factors (Fig. 3) [62]. Endothelial activation, induced directly or indirectly by the proinflammatory behavior of SSRBCs, is the most likely initiating step toward vaso-occlusion. The resultant activation of endothelial NF-κB and upregulation of endothelial adhesion molecules promote the recruitment of leukocytes and help propagate the syndrome of chronic vascular inflammation so prominent in this disease. Adherent leukocytes and circulating erythrocytes, with or without additional activation signals, then form adhesive bonds that lead to multicellular aggregates within the microvasculature. It is possible that platelets and hemostatically active microparticles, with or without plasma coagulative elements, participate in these aggregates, although such interactions have not yet been fully investigated. In addition, the molecular mediators of these intercellular interactions have not yet been characterized. Much work has been performed with purified blood cells in vitro to characterize multiple adhesion pathways between erythrocytes and endothelial cells, and in vitro flow systems are increasingly used to approximate more closely cellular interactions in vivo. However, given the complexity and dynamic relationships of the potential mechanisms leading to vaso-occlusion, further in vivo studies in relevant sickle

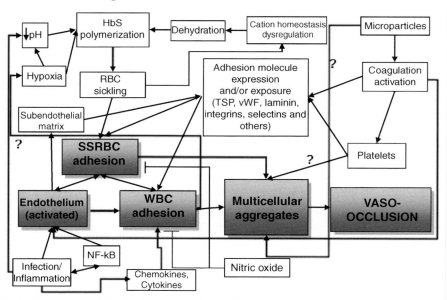

Fig. 3. Dynamic relationships among cellular elements, plasma proteins, and systemic conditions that may contribute to the multistep, multicellular process of sickle cell vaso-occlusion.

cell animal models will most likely yield the greatest advances and promote the development of novel, more effective therapeutic strategies.

References

[1] Herrick JB. Peculiar elongated and sickle-shaped red blood corpuscles in a case of severe anemia. Arch Intern Med 1910;6:517–21.

[2] Hahn E, Gillespie E. Sickle cell anemia. Arch Intern Med 1927;39:233–4.

[3] Hansen-Pruss O. Experimental studies of the sickling of red blood cells. J Lab Clin Med 1936;22:311–5.

[4] Scriver J, Waugh T. Studies on a case of sickle cell anemia. Can Med Assoc J 1930; 23:375–80.

[5] Pauling L, Itano HA, et al. Sickle cell anemia a molecular disease. Science 1949;110:543–8.

[6] Ingram VM. Gene mutations in human haemoglobin: the chemical difference between normal and sickle cell haemoglobin. Nature 1957;180:326–8.

[7] Hebbel RP, Boogaerts MA, Koresawa S, et al. Erythrocyte adherence to endothelium as a determinant of vasocclusive severity in sickle cell disease. Trans Assoc Am Physicians 1980;93:94–9.

[8] Hoover R, Rubin R, Wise G, et al. Adhesion of normal and sickle erythrocytes to endothelial monolayer cultures. Blood 1979;54:872–6.

[9] Hebbel RP, Boogaerts MA, Eaton JW, et al. Erythrocyte adherence to endothelium in sickle-cell anemia. A possible determinant of disease severity. N Engl J Med 1980;302:992–5.

[10] Kaul DK, Fabry ME. In vivo studies of sickle red blood cells. Microcirculation 2004; 11:153–65.

[11] Parise LV, Telen MJ. Erythrocyte adhesion in sickle cell disease. Curr Hematol Rep 2003; 2:102–8.

[12] Barabino GA, McIntire LV, Eskin SG, et al. Rheological studies of erythrocyte–endothelial cell interactions in sickle cell disease. Prog Clin Biol Res 1987;240:113–27.

[13] Kaul DK, Fabry ME, Nagel RL. Microvascular sites and characteristics of sickle cell adhesion to vascular endothelium in shear flow conditions: pathophysiological implications. Proc Natl Acad Sci U S A 1989;86:3356–60.

[14] Mohandas N, Evans E. Sickle erythrocyte adherence to vascular endothelium. Morphologic correlates and the requirement for divalent cations and collagen-binding plasma proteins. J Clin Invest 1985;76:1605–12.

[15] Stone PC, Stuart J, Nash GB. Effects of density and of dehydration of sickle cells on their adhesion to cultured endothelial cells. Am J Hematol 1996;52:135–43.

[16] Lew VL, Bookchin RM. Ion transport pathology in the mechanism of sickle cell dehydration. Physiol Rev 2005;85:179–200.

[17] Mueller BU, Brugnara C. Prevention of red cell dehydration: a possible new treatment for sickle cell disease. Pediatr Pathol Mol Med 2001;20:15–25.

[18] Steinberg MH, Brugnara C. Pathophysiological-based approaches to treatment of sickle cell disease. Annu Rev Med 2003;54:89–112.

[19] Parsons SF, Lee G, Spring FA, et al. Lutheran blood group glycoprotein and its newly characterized mouse homologue specifically bind alpha5 chain–containing human laminin with high affinity. Blood 2001;97:312–20.

[20] Udani M, Zen Q, Cottman M, et al. Basal cell adhesion molecule/lutheran protein. The receptor critical for sickle cell adhesion to laminin. J Clin Invest 1998;101:2550–8.

[21] Murphy MM, Zayed MA, Evans A, et al. Role of Rap1 in promoting sickle red blood cell adhesion to laminin via BCAM/LU. Blood 2005;105:3322–9.

[22] Hines PC, Zen Q, Burney SN, et al. Novel epinephrine and cyclic AMP-mediated activation of BCAM/Lu-dependent sickle (SS) RBC adhesion. Blood 2003;101:3281–7.

[23] Zennadi R, Hines PC, De Castro LM, et al. Epinephrine acts through erythroid signaling pathways to activate sickle cell adhesion to endothelium via LW-alphavbeta3 interactions. Blood 2004;104:3774–81.

[24] Browne PV, Mosher DF, Steinberg MH, et al. Disturbance of plasma and platelet thrombospondin levels in sickle cell disease. Am J Hematol 1996;51:296–301.

[25] Gupta K, Gupta P, Solovey A, et al. Mechanism of interaction of thrombospondin with human endothelium and inhibition of sickle erythrocyte adhesion to human endothelial cells by heparin. Biochim Biophys Acta 1999;1453:63–73.

[26] Brittain JE, Han J, Ataga KI, et al. Mechanism of CD47-induced alpha4beta1 integrin activation and adhesion in sickle reticulocytes. J Biol Chem 2004;279:42393–402.

[27] Kaul DK, Tsai HM, Liu XD, et al. Monoclonal antibodies to alphaVbeta3 (7E3 and LM609) inhibit sickle red blood cell–endothelium interactions induced by platelet-activating factor. Blood 2000;95:368–74.

[28] Wick TM, Moake JL, Udden MM, et al. Unusually large von Willebrand factor multimers increase adhesion of sickle erythrocytes to human endothelial cells under controlled flow. J Clin Invest 1987;80:905–10.

[29] Wick TM, Moake JL, Udden MM, et al. Unusually large von Willebrand factor multimers preferentially promote young sickle and nonsickle erythrocyte adhesion to endothelial cells. Am J Hematol 1993;42:284–92.

[30] Manodori AB, Barabino GA, Lubin BH, et al. Adherence of phosphatidylserine-exposing erythrocytes to endothelial matrix thrombospondin. Blood 2000;95:1293–300.

[31] Setty BN, Kulkarni S, Stuart MJ. Role of erythrocyte phosphatidylserine in sickle red cell–endothelial adhesion. Blood 2002;99:1564–71.

[32] Embury SH, Matsui NM, Ramanujam S, et al. The contribution of endothelial cell P-selectin to the microvascular flow of mouse sickle erythrocytes in vivo. Blood 2004;104:3378–85.

[33] Wood KC, Hebbel RP, Granger DN. Endothelial cell P-selectin mediates a proinflammatory and prothrombogenic phenotype in cerebral venules of sickle cell transgenic mice. Am J Physiol Heart Circ Physiol 2004;286:H1608–14.

[34] Belcher JD, Bryant CJ, Nguyen J, et al. Transgenic sickle mice have vascular inflammation. Blood 2003;101:3953–9.

[35] Solovey A, Lin Y, Browne P, et al. Circulating activated endothelial cells in sickle cell anemia. N Engl J Med 1997;337:1584–90.

[36] Kaul DK, Liu XD, Choong S, et al. Anti-inflammatory therapy ameliorates leukocyte adhesion and microvascular flow abnormalities in transgenic sickle mice. Am J Physiol Heart Circ Physiol 2004;287:H293–301.

[37] Solovey AA, Solovey AN, Harkness J, et al. Modulation of endothelial cell activation in sickle cell disease: a pilot study. Blood 2001;97:1937–41.

[38] Belcher JD, Mahaseth H, Welch TE, et al. Critical role of endothelial cell activation in hypoxia-induced vaso-occlusion in transgenic sickle mice. Am J Physiol Heart Circ Physiol 2005;288(6):H2715–25 [Epub 2005 Jan 21].

[39] Reiter CD, Gladwin MT. An emerging role for nitric oxide in sickle cell disease vascular homeostasis and therapy. Curr Opin Hematol 2003;10:99–107.

[40] Manodori AB, Matsui NM, Chen JY, et al. Enhanced adherence of sickle erythrocytes to thrombin-treated endothelial cells involves interendothelial cell gap formation. Blood 1998;92:3445–54.

[41] Croizat H. Circulating cytokines in sickle cell patients during steady state. Br J Haematol 1994;87:592–7.

[42] Francis Jr RB, Haywood LJ. Elevated immunoreactive tumor necrosis factor and interleukin-1 in sickle cell disease. J Natl Med Assoc 1992;84:611–5.

[43] Selvaraj SK, Giri RK, Perelman N, et al. Mechanism of monocyte activation and expression of proinflammatory cytochemokines by placenta growth factor. Blood 2003;102:1515–24.

[44] Perelman N, Selvaraj SK, Batra S, et al. Placenta growth factor activates monocytes and correlates with sickle cell disease severity. Blood 2003;102:1506–14.

[45] Belcher JD, Marker PH, Weber JP, et al. Activated monocytes in sickle cell disease: potential role in the activation of vascular endothelium and vaso-occlusion. Blood 2000;96:2451–9.

[46] Okpala I. The intriguing contribution of white blood cells to sickle cell disease—a red cell disorder. Blood Rev 2004;18:65–73.

[47] Platt OS, Brambilla DJ, Rosse WF, et al. Mortality in sickle cell disease. Life expectancy and risk factors for early death. N Engl J Med 1994;330:1639–44.

[48] Kinney TR, Sleeper LA, Wang WC, et al. Silent cerebral infarcts in sickle cell anemia: a risk factor analysis. The Cooperative Study of Sickle Cell Disease. Pediatrics 1999; 103:640–5.

[49] Vichinsky EP, Styles LA, Colangelo LH, et al. Acute chest syndrome in sickle cell disease: clinical presentation and course. Cooperative Study of Sickle Cell Disease. Blood 1997; 89:1787–92.

[50] Charache S, Terrin ML, Moore RD, et al. Effect of hydroxyurea on the frequency of painful crises in sickle cell anemia. Investigators of the Multicenter Study of Hydroxyurea in Sickle Cell Anemia. N Engl J Med 1995;332:1317–22.

[51] Abboud M, Laver J, Blau CA. Granulocytosis causing sickle-cell crisis. Lancet 1998; 351:959.

[52] Adler BK, Salzman DE, Carabasi MH, et al. Fatal sickle cell crisis after granulocyte colony-stimulating factor administration. Blood 2001;97:3313–4.

[53] Grigg AP. Granulocyte colony-stimulating factor–induced sickle cell crisis and multiorgan dysfunction in a patient with compound heterozygous sickle cell/beta+ thalassemia. Blood 2001;97:3998–9.

[54] Hofstra TC, Kalra VK, Meiselman HJ, et al. Sickle erythrocytes adhere to polymorphonuclear neutrophils and activate the neutrophil respiratory burst. Blood 1996;87:4440–7.

[55] Lum AF, Wun T, Staunton D, et al. Inflammatory potential of neutrophils detected in sickle cell disease. Am J Hematol 2004;76:126–33.

[56] Fadlon E, Vordermeier S, Pearson TC, et al. Blood polymorphonuclear leukocytes from the majority of sickle cell patients in the crisis phase of the disease show enhanced adhesion to vascular endothelium and increased expression of CD64. Blood 1998;91:266–74.

[57] Lard LR, Mul FP, de Haas M, et al. Neutrophil activation in sickle cell disease. J Leukoc Biol 1999;66:411–5.

[58] Kaul DK, Hebbel RP. Hypoxia/reoxygenation causes inflammatory response in transgenic sickle mice but not in normal mice. J Clin Invest 2000;106:411–20.

[59] Turhan A, Weiss LA, Mohandas N, et al. Primary role for adherent leukocytes in sickle cell vascular occlusion: a new paradigm. Proc Natl Acad Sci U S A 2002;99:3047–51.

[60] Lipowsky HH, Chien S. Role of leukocyte–endothelium adhesion in affecting recovery from ischemic episodes. Ann N Y Acad Sci 1989;565:308–15.

[61] Frenette PS. Sickle cell vaso-occlusion: multistep and multicellular paradigm. Curr Opin Hematol 2002;9:101–6.

[62] Frenette PS. Sickle cell vasoocclusion: heterotypic, multicellular aggregations driven by leukocyte adhesion. Microcirculation 2004;11:167–77.

[63] Bullard DC, Kunkel EJ, Kubo H, et al. Infectious susceptibility and severe deficiency of leukocyte rolling and recruitment in E-selectin and P-selectin double mutant mice. J Exp Med 1996;183:2329–36.

[64] Frenette PS, Mayadas TN, Rayburn H, et al. Susceptibility to infection and altered hematopoiesis in mice deficient in both P- and E-selectins. Cell 1996;84:563–74.

[65] Turhan A, Jenab P, Bruhns P, et al. Intravenous immune globulin prevents venular vasoocclusion in sickle cell mice by inhibiting leukocyte adhesion and the interactions between sickle erythrocytes and adherent leukocytes. Blood 2004;103:2397–400.

[66] Hefer D, Jaloudi M. Thromboembolic events as an emerging adverse effect during high-dose intravenous immunoglobulin therapy in elderly patients: a case report and discussion of the relevant literature. Ann Hematol 2004;83:661–5.

[67] Vucic S, Chong PS, Dawson KT, et al. Thromboembolic complications of intravenous immunoglobulin treatment. Eur Neurol 2004;52:141–4.

[68] Mehta P, Mehta J. Circulating platelet aggregates in sickle cell disease patients with and without vaso-occlusion. Stroke 1979;10:464–6.

[69] Tomer A, Harker LA, Kasey S, et al. Thrombogenesis in sickle cell disease. J Lab Clin Med 2001;137:398–407.

[70] Haut MJ, Cowan DH, Harris JW. Platelet function and survival in sickle cell disease. J Lab Clin Med 1973;82:44–53.

[71] Stuart MJ, Setty BN. Hemostatic alterations in sickle cell disease: relationships to disease pathophysiology. Pediatr Pathol Mol Med 2001;20:27–46.

[72] Shet AS, Aras O, Gupta K, et al. Sickle blood contains tissue factor–positive microparticles derived from endothelial cells and monocytes. Blood 2003;102:2678–83.

[73] de Jong K, Larkin SK, Styles LA, et al. Characterization of the phosphatidylserine-exposing subpopulation of sickle cells. Blood 2001;98:860–7.

[74] Tait JF, Gibson D. Measurement of membrane phospholipid asymmetry in normal and sickle-cell erythrocytes by means of annexin V binding. J Lab Clin Med 1994;123:741–8.

[75] Chaplin Jr H, Alkjaersig N, Fletcher AP, et al. Aspirin-dipyridamole prophylaxis of sickle cell disease pain crises. Thromb Haemost 1980;43:218–21.

[76] Osamo NO, Photiades DP, Famodu AA. Therapeutic effect of aspirin in sickle cell anaemia. Acta Haematol 1981;66:102–7.

[77] Greenberg J, Ohene-Frempong K, Halus J, et al. Trial of low doses of aspirin as prophylaxis in sickle cell disease. J Pediatr 1983;102:781–4.

[78] Cabannes R, Lonsdorfer J, Castaigne JP, et al. Clinical and biological double-blind-study of ticlopidine in preventive treatment of sickle-cell disease crises. Agents Actions Suppl 1984; 15:199–212.

[79] Semple MJ, Al-Hasani SF, Kioy P, et al. A double-blind trial of ticlopidine in sickle cell disease. Thromb Haemost 1984;51:303–6.

[80] Barabino GA, Liu XD, Ewenstein BM, et al. Anionic polysaccharides inhibit adhesion of sickle erythrocytes to the vascular endothelium and result in improved hemodynamic behavior. Blood 1999;93:1422–9.

[81] Matsui NM, Varki A, Embury SH. Heparin inhibits the flow adhesion of sickle red blood cells to P-selectin. Blood 2002;100:3790–6.

[82] Ahmed S, Siddiqui AK, Iqbal U, et al. Effect of low-dose warfarin on D-dimer levels during sickle cell vaso-occlusive crisis: a brief report. Eur J Haematol 2004;72:213–6.

[83] Wolters HJ, ten Cate H, Thomas LL, et al. Low-intensity oral anticoagulation in sickle-cell disease reverses the prethrombotic state: promises for treatment? Br J Haematol 1995;90:715–7.

[84] Schnog JB, Kater AP, Mac Gillavry MR, et al. Low adjusted-dose acenocoumarol therapy in sickle cell disease: a pilot study. Am J Hematol 2001;68:179–83.

[85] Schnog JB, Mac Gillavry MR, Rojer RA, et al. No effect of acenocoumarol therapy on levels of endothelial activation markers in sickle cell disease. Am J Hematol 2002;71: 53–5.

[86] Antonucci R, Walker R, Herion J, et al. Enhancement of sickle erythrocyte adherence to endothelium by autologous platelets. Am J Hematol 1990;34:44–8.

[87] Wun T, Cordoba M, Rangaswami A, et al. Activated monocytes and platelet-monocyte aggregates in patients with sickle cell disease. Clin Lab Haematol 2002;24:81–8.

[88] Inwald DP, Kirkham FJ, Peters MJ, et al. Platelet and leucocyte activation in childhood sickle cell disease: association with nocturnal hypoxaemia. Br J Haematol 2000;111:474–81.

[89] Setty BN, Stuart MJ, Dampier C, et al. Hypoxaemia in sickle cell disease: biomarker modulation and relevance to pathophysiology. Lancet 2003;362:1450–5.

Hematol Oncol Clin N Am 19 (2005) 785–802

HEMATOLOGY/ONCOLOGY CLINICS
OF NORTH AMERICA

Pain Management of Sickle Cell Disease

Samir K. Ballas, MD[a,b],*

[a]Cardeza Foundation for Hematologic Research, 1015 Walnut Street, Philadelphia, PA 19107, USA
[b]Department of Medicine, Jefferson Medical College, Thomas Jefferson University, Philadelphia, PA, USA

Sickle cell disease (SCD) is an inherited disorder of hemoglobin structure that has no established cure in adult patients. Cure has been achieved in selected children with sickle cell anemia using allogeneic bone marrow transplantation [1] or cord blood transplantation [2]. SCD is a quadrumvirate of (1) pain syndromes, (2) anemia and its sequelae, (3) organ failure, including infection, and (4) comorbid conditions. Pain, however, is the insignia of SCD and dominates its clinical picture throughout the life of the patients (Fig. 1). Pain may precipitate or be itself precipitated by the other three components of the quadrumvirate. Moreover, management of sickle cell pain must be within the framework of the disease as a whole and not in isolation. SCD is unlike other pain syndromes where the provider can make decisions on treatment based solely on the pain and its associated behavior. A primary care physician, for example, taking care of a middle-aged patient with job-related low back pain may decide to expel the patient from his or her care if the patient in question demonstrates suspicious drug-seeking behavior. Doing the same with patients who have SCD could be counterproductive. There are anecdotes of patients with SCD who were dismissed from certain programs only to be found dead at home within 24 hours after dismissal or to be admitted to other hospitals with serious complications [3]. Sickle pain could be the prodrome of a serious and potentially fatal complication of SCD in some patients. This article focuses on the pathogenesis and management of acute and chronic sickle cell pain.

CLASSIFICATION OF PAINFUL EPISODES IN SICKLE CELL SYNDROMES

Box 1 lists the major types of pain syndromes in patients with SCD. These are divided into those secondary to the disease itself, those associated with therapy, and those that are due to comorbid conditions. The acute sickle cell painful episode is the insignia of the disease; it is unpredictable in nature and may be

Supported in part by the Sickle Cell Program of the Department of Health of the Commonwealth of Pennsylvania.
* Cardeza Foundation for Hematologic Research, 1015 Walnut Street, Philadelphia, PA 19107. E-mail address: samir.ballas@jefferson.edu

0889-8588/05/$ – see front matter
doi:10.1016/j.hoc.2005.07.008

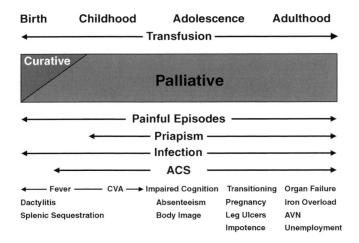

Fig. 1. Sequence of complications of sickle cell anemia from birth through adult life. Cure is possible in selected children. The mainstay of management in most patients is palliative, with pain management being most important. ACS, acute chest syndrome; AVN, avascular necrosis; CVA, cerebrovascular accident. (*Modified from* Ballas SK. Sickle cell disease: current clinical management. Semin Hematol 2001;38(4):308; with permission.)

precipitated by known or unknown factors. Sickle pain may involve any part of the body, and the severity, location, and duration of the pain vary latitudinally among patients and longitudinally in the same individual. The serum concentration of some acute phase reactants may increase in acute painful episodes and interfere with the efficacy of treatment with opioid analgesics [4]. Objective signs are often absent in the patient with a sickle cell crisis, especially within 1 to 2 days of its onset, an absence that engenders problematic attitudes in some care providers treating patients who have sickle pain [5].

ACUTE SICKLE CELL PAIN
Acute Sickle Cell Painful Episodes (Crises)
Pathogenesis

The most important pathophysiologic event in sickle cell anemia, which explains most of its clinical manifestations, is vascular occlusion; this may involve both the micro- and macrovasculature [6,7]. The primary process that leads to vascular occlusion is the polymerization of sickle hemoglobin (Hb) on deoxygenation, which in turn results in distortion of the shape of red blood cells (RBC), cellular dehydration, and decreased deformability and stickiness of RBC, which promotes their adhesion to and activation of the vascular endothelium.

Adherence of sickle RBC to vascular endothelium results in intimal hyperplasia in larger vessels, which may lead to vascular occlusion and tissue

---

Box 1: Classification of painful episodes in sickle cell disease

Pain Secondary to the Disease Itself

    Acute pain syndromes

        Recurrent acute painful episodes (crises)

        Acute chest syndrome

        Hepatic crisis

        Priapism

        Calculus cholecystitis

        Hand-foot syndrome[a]

        Splenic sequestration[a]

    Chronic pain syndromes

        • With objective signs

            Aseptic (avascular) necrosis

            Arthropathies

            Leg ulcers

            Chronic osteomyelitis

        • Without objective signs

            Intractable chronic pain

    Neuropathic pain

Pain Secondary to Therapy

    Withdrawal

    Loose prosthesis (hip or shoulder)

    Postoperative pain

Pain Due to Comorbid Conditions

    Trauma

    Arthritis (septic, degenerative, rheumatoid, collagen disease)

    Peptic ulcer disease

    Other conditions

   [a] Occurs in infants and children.

---

infarction [8,9]. Moreover, recent in vivo studies in transgenic mice suggest that vascular occlusion results in the creation of an inflammatory state [10,11], which in turn contributes to the sensation of pain.

The sequence of pathophysiologic events that lead to the perception of pain in SCD is not well known. It is agreed that tissue ischemia due to vascular occlusion resulting from in situ sickling causes infarctive tissue damage, which in turn initiates a secondary inflammatory response. The secondary response may enhance sympathetic activity by means of interactions with neuroendocrine pathways and trigger release of norepinephrine. In the setting of tissue injury, this release causes more tissue ischemia, creating a vicious cycle. It is the combination of ischemic tissue damage and secondary inflammatory response that makes the pain of SCD unique in its acuteness and severity. Tissue injury generates several major pain mediators [12–15], including but not limited to interleukin-1, bradykinin, K^+, H^+, histamine, substance P, and calcitonin gene-related peptide (CGRP). Interleukin-1 is an endogenous pyrogen and also upregulates the cyclo-oxygenase gene, leading to synthesis of prostaglandins E_2 and I_2. Bradykinin, K^+, H^+, and histamine activate nociceptive afferent nerve fibers and evoke a pain response. Prostaglandins sensitize peripheral nerve endings and facilitate the transmission of painful stimuli along A-δ and C fibers that reach the cerebral cortex via the spinal cord and the thalamus. Moreover, activated nociceptors release stored substance P, which itself facilitates the transmission of painful stimuli. Bradykinin, substance P, and CGRP also cause vasodilation and extravasation of fluids that can lead to local swelling and tenderness. The pathway for painful stimuli is subject not only to activators, sensitizers, and facilitators but also to inhibitors. Serotonin, enkephalin, β-endorphin, and dynorphin are endogenous central pain inhibitors. Thus, in a given patient, the net outcome of tissue ischemia may be severe or mild pain, depending on the extent of tissue damage and the net balance of pain stimulators versus pain inhibitors. This situation may explain, in part, the considerable variation in the frequency and severity of painful crisis among patients and longitudinally in the same patient.

Clinical picture

The clinical picture of sickle cell pain is protean. Sickle cell pain has unique features. Pathophysiologically, it is nociceptive (ie, secondary to tissue damage). It may be acute or chronic, somatic or visceral, unilateral or bilateral, localized or diffuse and mild, moderate or severe [16]. Typically, acute painful episodes affect long bones and joints, with the low back being the most frequently reported site of pain [17]. Other regions of the body, including the scalp, face, jaw, abdomen, and pelvis, may be involved. A severe acute sickle cell painful episode has been defined as one that requires treatment in a medical facility with parenteral opioids for 4 or more hours [18,19]. The occurrence of three or more such crises indicates that the affected patient has severe SCD. The words most often used to describe sickle pain include "throbbing," "sharp," "dull," "stabbing," and "shooting," in decreasing order of frequency [17].

Phases and objective signs

Objective signs of a painful crisis, such as fever, leukocytosis, joint effusions, and tenderness, occur in about 50% of patients at initial presentation [5]. During the evolution of the painful crisis, however, objective laboratory signs become evident in most patients, provided that these parameters are determined serially [20]. The acute sickle cell painful episode that requires hospitalization appears to evolve along four distinct phases: prodromal, initial, established, and resolving [21]. Each phase may be associated with certain clinical and laboratory findings. As the pain of a crisis intensifies, the percentage of dense RBC increases with a concomitant decease in RBC deformability. Some patients develop hyper-hemolysis during the evolution of the acute painful episode, with decrease in Hb level and increase in the reticulocyte count [21]. As pain resolves, the pattern is reversed, with a decrease in the number of dense red cells and an increase in RBC deformability [20].

Pain management

Pain is the hallmark of SCD, and the acute sickle cell painful episode (painful crisis) is the most common cause of more than 90% of hospital admissions among adult patients who have SCD [16]. Effective management of sickle cell pain is complex and entails thorough understanding of the issues that are associated with the treatment of pain of an incurable disease on a chronic basis [16,22]. Major prerequisites for an effective and rational management of sickle cell pain pertain to the patient, the pathophysiology of the disease, the pharmacology of analgesics, and the attitude of the health care provider.

A patient is a unique human entity. The more a provider knows the patient, the more effective pain management becomes. Knowledge of the patient should not be limited to age, sex, precise diagnosis, complications, and previous pain management methods. It should also take into consideration the biopsychosocial fabric of the patients' lives, including their level of education, employment status, occupation, family structure, source of income, ethnicity, housing conditions, fears, religion, beliefs, habits, hobbies, and perception of the severity and prognosis of their disease. This approach allows the physician to individualize pain management and avoid unfounded generalizations about patients and their consumption of opioid analgesics. Such generalizations, for instance, may result in oversedation of a patient naïve to opioids or in undertreatment of a patient too tolerant of them.

Sickle cell pain is unique and, like other types of pain, is a complex human experience that is strongly affected not only by pathophysiologic factors but also by psychologic, social, cultural, and spiritual ones. It is, however, consequent to tissue damage generated by the sickling process and occlusion of the microvasculature, as described in the preceding discussion.

An important aspect of effective management of sickle cell pain is the intent of the care provider. Do the providers in question endeavor to treat patients in an empathetic manner by listening to, respecting, and believing them? Or do they stigmatize them as drug addicts demonstrating drug-seeking behavior and thereby justify the expulsion of some patients from their system? Do the providers actively seek management of sickle cell pain, or are they passively forced by the system to which they belong to treat patients in a cursory manner? These are difficult questions to answer and research. The outcome of management of sickle cell pain relies heavily on the ethical principles to which the providers in question subscribe.

Effective management of acute sickle cell pain in the emergency room and hospital may be achieved by following four major sequential stages: (1) assessment, (2) treatment, including choice of the analgesic, the dose, and the route and method of administration, (3) reassessment to evaluate the effectiveness of the treatment stage and implement changes as needed, and (4) adjustment, including titration of the dose of opioid to achieve adequate pain relief, rescue, tapering, and switching to oral medications, driven by the feedback loops of reassessment.

Assessment. Assessment is the cornerstone of effective pain management. It should be conducted before and periodically after the administration of analgesics [16,22–24]. Because pain is subjective in nature, the patient's self-report is the most important factor in the hierarchy of pain management. Assessment relies heavily on the patient's self-report. Other factors in the process of assessment should include the presence or absence of other complications of the disease, such as infection, family members' report, and vital signs, including temperature, blood pressure, pulse, respiratory rate, and pulse oximetry. The patient's self-report should include multidimensional scales describing intensity, quality, location, distribution, onset, duration, mood, sedation, pain relief, and factors that aggravate or relieve pain [22–24].

Initial pain assessment establishes a baseline against which the effectiveness of analgesics in achieving pain relief will be compared. Assessment allows the patient and the treatment team to discuss management strategies and treatment objectives. Periodic assessment with rating and categorizing of pain will delineate multiple pain syndromes, which may occur as the pain progresses over time. Thorough assessment will thus result in intervention and modification of the treatment plan when necessary. Any change in therapy that does not take the patient's self-report into consideration by means of periodic assessment, especially a change in the dose and frequency of administration of analgesics, may be doomed to fail and to create misunderstanding between the patient and provider.

The intensity of pain can be assessed using any of several available scales, such as the visual analogue scale, verbal scale, numerical scale, or Wong-Baker faces scale for children. It is important, however, to stick to one scale and use it routinely, so that both the patient and provider become familiar with it and with its significance to a particular patient. Nociceptive sickle cell pain typically is sharp or throbbing in nature. Pain that is burning, shooting, lancinating, or tingling suggests the presence of a neuropathic component that entails the use of certain adjuvants, to be discussed later [5,22].

Initial pain assessment establishes a baseline against which the effectiveness of analgesics in achieving pain relief is compared. Subsequent assessment may lead to increasing the dose of analgesics to achieve desirable pain relief, tapering the dose of analgesics as the painful episode resolves, and identifying adverse effects of therapy or the emergence of complications of the disease that allow intervention and modification of the treatment plan as needed.

Nonpharmacologic management of pain. Nonpharmacologic management of pain includes cutaneous stimulation (transcutaneous electrical nerve stimulation), heat, cold and vibration, distraction, relaxation, massage, music, guided imagery, self-hypnosis, self-motivation, acupuncture, and biofeedback. Although there are no well-controlled clinical trials of the efficacy of these methods in the management of sickle cell pain, there are many anecdotal reports of their efficacy in pain management.

Pharmacologic management of pain. Pharmacologic management of pain includes three major classes of compounds: nonopioids, opioids, and adjuvants [5,22,23]. A major difference between nonopioids and opioids is that the former have a "ceiling effect," a term that refers to a dose above which there is no additive analgesic effect [25]. Nonopioids include acetaminophen, nonsteroidal anti-inflammatories (NSAIDs), topical agents, tramadol, and corticosteroids.

Acetaminophen has analgesic and antipyretic effects but no anti-inflammatory component [26]. The daily total adult dose must not exceed 4 g in four to six divided doses [27]. High dosages damage the liver and could be fatal. The daily dose should be decreased in the presence of liver disease. The daily dose of combination medications (medications that contain acetaminophen plus an opioid) must be controlled so that the 4-g limit of acetaminophen is met.

NSAIDs (Table 1) include nonselective cyclo-oxygenase (COX) inhibitors and selective and partially selective COX-2 inhibitors [28–30]. NSAIDs have an anti-inflammatory effect in addition to their analgesic and antipyretic potential. They act primarily at the level of nociceptors where pain impulses originate and hence are often referred to as peripherally acting analgesics. They exert their analgesic effect by inhibiting COX enzymes and decreasing the synthesis of prostaglandins [28], thus decreasing or abolishing the sensitization of nociceptors by prostanoids. The traditional nonselective NSAIDs inhibit both the house-keeping COX-1 and the inducible COX-2 enzymes. Selective NSAIDs inhibit only the COX-2 enzyme and spare COX-1, which is needed to produce physiologic levels of prostaglandins.

NSAIDs have potentially serious, systemic adverse effects. They include gastropathy, nephropathy, and hemostatic defects. NSAIDs should not be administered to patients with renal disease or history of peptic ulcer disease. It is advisable not to administer them continuously for more than 5 days to patients with SCD. Moreover, certain NSAIDs are associated with idiosyncratic (non–prostaglandin-mediated) reactions [28]. Most recently reported among these is immune thrombocytopenia resulting from sensitivity to metabolites of naproxen and acetaminophen [31]. The antibodies described were mostly specific to Glyco Protein (GP) IIb/IIIa and less often specific to GP Ib/IX/V. COX-2 inhibitors are associated with significantly fewer gastrointestinal and hemostatic adverse effects [29,30] than the nonselective NSAIDs, but their effect on renal function appears to be the same [32,33]. The concomitant administration of ketorolac with opioids is reported to exert an additional analgesic effect and decrease the quantity of opioids consumed for the treatment of acute painful episodes [34].

Table 1
Nonopioid pharmacologic agents commonly used in the management of pain

Drug (Brand name)	Maximum daily dose (mg)	Half-life (T 1/2, h)
Acetaminophen[a]	4000	1–3
Non-steroidal anti-inflammatory drugs		
Nonselective COX inhibitors		
Salicylates		
Acetylsalicylic acid (aspirin)[a]	4000	4–15
Nonacetylated salicylates		
Salicyl salicylate	3000	4–15
Diflunisal	1500	7–15
Choline magnesium trisalicylate	3000	4–15
Propionic acid derivatives[a]		
Ibuprofen[a]	3200	2
Naproxen[a,b]	1500	13
Fenoprofen	3200	2
Ketoprofen[a,b]	300	2
Flurbiprofen	300	3–4
Acetic acid derivatives		
Indomethacin[b]	200	3–11
Ketorolac orally	40	3–11
Ketorolac intramuscular/intravenous	120	3–8
Sulindac	400	16
Tolmetin	1800	1–2
Diclofenac[b]	150	2
Etodolac[b]	1000	7.3
Nabumetone	2000	22.5–30
Anthranilic acid derivatives		
Mefenamic acid	1000	2–4
Meclofenamate	400	2–3
Oxicams		
Piroxicam	20	30–86
Selective COX-2 inhibitors		
Celecoxib	400	11–12
Partially selective COX-2 inhibitors		
Meloxicam	15	15–20

Abbreviation: COX, cyclo-oxygenase.
  [a] Available over the counter.
  [b] Available in delayed/extended release forms.

On September 30, 2004, Merck voluntarily withdrew Rofecoxib from world-wide use. This decision was based on a study that was designed to detect benefits of Rofecoxib (25 mg) in preventing recurrence of cancerous polyps over 3 years. Two thousand six hundred patients enrolled (62% males, 40 to 60 years old, 16% on aspirin). After 18 months, the patients taking Rofecoxib had significantly higher incidence of cardiovascular disease compared with those taking a placebo. This finding made all other coxib inhibitors suspect of causing cardiac problems. It is therefore recommended to monitor patients taking COX-2 inhibitors care-fully, with special attention to cardiac and renal functions.

Tramadol [35] is a synthetic, centrally acting analgesic that is not chemically related to opioids. It acts as a weak agonist with preferential affinity to the μ-receptors. Moreover, it inhibits neuronal reuptake of both serotonin and norepinephrine and stimulates the release of serotonin. Thus, it has functional properties of an opioid and an antidepressant. This drug received an initial enthusiastic reception based on the perception that it was not associated with clinically significant respiratory depression or addiction potential; this enthusiasm waned after reports indicated that seizures may be an adverse effect and that abuse potential is increasing. Currently, tramadol is not a scheduled drug. It appears to be as effective as acetaminophen with codeine, with the added advantage of a tricyclic antidepressant–like effect. Tramadol may be administered by the oral or parenteral route, and it is available in slow-release form. Only the oral form is currently approved for marketing in the United States. Anecdotally, tramadol appears to be effective in the management of mild or moderately severe pain in some patients with sickle cell anemia.

Opioid analgesics [36] have fewer systemic adverse effects than NSAIDs, but their use in SCD is associated with many myths about drug-seeking behavior and addiction. Four major classes of opioids exist: agonists, partial agonists, mixed agonists-antagonists, and antagonists (Box 2).

Traditionally, opioid antagonists have been regarded as having no analgesic effect, and their use is primarily limited to counteracting the depressive effects of opioid agonists. Recently, however [37], there have been reports showing that small doses of antagonists in combination with agonists appear to enhance the analgesic effect and to prevent or delay tolerance to opioid agonists. Should this approach be proved by controlled trials, it would be a novel tool in the management of pain.

Opioid agonists are most often used in the management of sickle cell pain, especially in adults. They decrease or modify the perception of pain at the level of the central nervous system. They exert their effect by binding to μ-, κ-, and, to a lesser extent, δ-receptors [36]. Opioid agonists can be administered by several routes (eg, orally, subcutaneously, intramuscularly, intravenously, transdermally) and methods, including continuous intravenous drip, patient-controlled analgesia pump, and intermittent injection. Meperidine, morphine, and hydromorphone are the major opioid analgesics used in the treatment of severe pain in the emergency department and hospital. Controlled-released opioids, such as controlled-release (CR) oxycodone and morphine CR, are useful in the management of chronic pain and in combination with short-acting opioids for breakthrough pain. Fentanyl is available in parenteral, transdermal, and transmucosal formulations. Methadone is a true long-acting opioid that can be used in combination with short-acting opioids in selected patients.

Adverse effects of opioid analgesics include itching, nausea, vomiting, sedation, and respiratory depression. Seizures may be associated with opioids, especially with the prolonged use of meperidine and the consequent accumulation of its major metabolite, normeperidine, in some patients. The effects of meperidine and normeperidine on seizure induction are more pronounced in the

Box 2: Classification of opioids

Opioid Agonists

- Codeine
- Hydrocodone and dihydrocodeine
- Oxycodone
- Morphine
- Meperidine
- Hydromorphone
- Levorphanol
- Oxymorphone
- Methadone
- Fentanyl
    Parenteral formulation
    Transdermal patch
    Transmucosal lozenge

Partial Agonists

- Buprenorphine

Mixed Agonists-Antagonists

- Pentazocine
- Nalbuphine
- Butorphanol

Antagonists

- Naloxone
- Nalmefene
- Naltrexone

presence of renal disease. Tolerance and physical dependence occur in some patients, but addiction is rare [5]. Methadone may be associated with prolongation of the QTc interval [38].

As a group, opioid analgesics have no ceiling effect (with the possible exception of codeine); hence the only limiting factor on their dose is adverse effects. Severe sedation and respiratory depression are the most important adverse effects. Hospitalized patients receiving opioid analgesics on a regular basis should be monitored for their respiratory rate and sedation level. A respiratory rate of less than ten per minute or severe sedation justifies skipping, decreasing, or delaying the dose or discontinuing the opioid in question until the depressive effects disappear. Opioid analgesics should be used carefully in patients with impaired ventilation, asthma, increased intracranial pressure, and liver failure. The dosage of meperidine and morphine should be adjusted in the presence of renal failure. Moreover, morphine is the most histaminergic of all opioids [39], and histamine release may trigger bronchospasm or initiate allergic reactions. The presence of acetaminophen in combination with codeine or oxycodone limits the daily dose that may be safely used so that the maximum allowable dose of acetaminophen is not exceeded. The use of meperidine in conjunction with monoamine oxidase inhibitors may cause a severe adverse reaction characterized by excitation, hyperpyrexia, convulsions, and death [40]. The coadministration of antipsychotics with meperidine may cause neuromuscular disorders, including akathisia, dystonia, tardive dyskinesia, and neuroleptic malignant syndrome [41].

Adjuvants include antihistamines, antidepressants, benzodiazpines, and anticonvulsants. These are heterogeneous compounds that potentiate the analgesic effect of opioids, ameliorate their side effects, and have their own mild analgesic effect. The most commonly used adjuvants in the management of sickle cell pain are listed in Box 3. The role of selective serotonin reuptake inhibitors in sickle cell anemia is not clear at present. Adjuvants must be used with care, and patients should be monitored carefully when receiving them. Adjuvants also have adverse effects, some of which precipitate or worsen manifestations of sickle cell anemia [5].

Acute painful episodes of mild or moderate severity are usually treated at home using a combination of nonpharmacologic and pharmacologic modalities. Home treatment of pain usually follows the three-step analgesic ladder proposed by the World Health Organization [42]. Mild pain is treated with nonpharmacologic agents alone or in combination with a nonopioid. More severe pain entails the addition of an opioid with or without an adjuvant. Data from the Multi-center Study of Hydroxyurea (MSH) [18,19] in sickle cell anemia showed that oxycodone/acetaminophen formulation was the opioid most often used for the home treatment of pain [43]. However, this report preceded the advent of the new formulations of opioids, such as oxycodone CR. Whether oxycodone/acetaminophen continues to be the first choice in this scenario of pain management remains to be seen.

Severe acute sickle cell painful episodes are usually treated in a medical facility using parenteral analgesics. A mark of progress in this area is the advent of day hospitals where patients are promptly evaluated by a team of experts in the management of sickle cell pain, without the delay that is common in hospital emergency rooms [44]. Available data in the literature show that management of patients with severe acute painful episodes in such facilities, especially those that operate on a 24-hour basis, reduces the frequency of hospital admissions. These findings should encourage other metropolitan hospitals in cities with large populations of African Americans to follow suit by establishing acute care facilities specifically designed for patients who have sickle cell disease. The establishment of such facilities nationwide may, in turn, verify the cost-saving potential of this approach to health care.

Box 3: Adjuvants commonly used in the management of sickle cell pain

Antihistamines

- Hydroxyzine
- Diphenhydramine

Benzodiazepines

- Diazepam
- Alprazolam

Tricyclic Antidepressants

- Amitriptyline
- Nortriptyline
- Doxepin

Anticonvulsants

- Phenytoin
- Carbamazepine
- Gabapentin
- Topiramate
- Clonazepam

Phenothiazines

- Prochlorperazine
- Promethazine

Data from the MSH showed that the parenteral opioid most often used in the management of acute sickle cell painful episodes in the emergency department or hospital was meperidine [43]. Since this report from 1996, there have been anecdotal reports from many hospitals of switching to opioids other than meperidine, but detailed studies to confirm this transition are not yet available.

Patients with chronic sickle cell pain and those with frequent acute painful episodes are best managed with a combination of long-acting opioids and a short-acting opioid for breakthrough pain. Again, anecdotal reports suggest that this approach decreases the frequency of admissions to the emergency department or hospital, but data to confirm this finding are not available to date. Oxycodone CR appears to be unique in that it has both an immediate analgesic effect and a delayed long-acting one. These properties have made oxycodone CR popular among drug abusers who have learned to remove the mesh and release a high dose of pure oxycodone that has an immediate "euphoric" effect [45].

Care providers should exert caution in prescribing oxycodone CR and other opioids and should keep records of assessment and plans of management for their patients.

Measures to reduce the morbidity and mortality of sickle cell anemia include prophylactic penicillin therapy (or a macrolide when there is sensitivity to penicillin) in infants and children [46] and hydroxyurea in adults [18,19]. Patients who responded to hydroxyurea experienced significant reduction in the incidence of acute painful episodes, acute chest syndrome, transfusion requirement, and mortality [18,19,47]. The beneficial effects of hydroxyurea are thought to be due to its induction of Hb F production. Any increase in Hb F level appears to have a salutary effect on the clinical picture of sickle cell anemia.

CHRONIC SICKLE CELL PAIN

Chronic pain, in simple terms, is pain that does not go away. Some investigators define it as pain that persists for 3 or more months. The major feature of chronic pain is that it has no useful biologic function. Acute pain, or eudynia, has biologic usefulness in that it alerts the patient to noxious events and elicits flight and fight mechanisms that activate the sympathetic nervous system. Chronic pain, or maldynia, has no biologic usefulness. It becomes a disease in its own right with no activation of the sympathetic system. Having chronic pain is a daunting experience. Emotional distress and behavioral dysfunction are major components of chronic pain syndromes. Such pain disrupts the mind-over-body interaction so that the body, rather than the mind, becomes the operator. Chronic pain induces changes in the brain that culminate in physical deconditioning, pain behaviors, altered mood, irritability, depression, anxiety, sleep disturbance, loss of interest in sex, family stress, financial concerns, decreased self-esteem, frequent visits to health care providers, heavy use of analgesic medications, and fear.

There are two types of chronic sickle cell pain (see Box 1): chronic pain due to obvious pathology (avascular necrosis and leg ulcers) and intractable pain with no obvious signs.

Chronic Pain with Obvious Pathology
Leg ulcers
Leg ulceration [48,49] is a painful and sometimes disabling complication of sickle cell anemia that occurs in 5% to 10% of adult patients. Severe pain may necessitate the use of opioid analgesics. Leg ulcers are more common in men and older patients and less common in patients with α-gene deletion, high total Hb level, or high levels of Hb F. Treatment of leg ulcers includes wound care using wet to dry dressings soaked in saline or Burrow's solution. With good localized treatment, many ulcers heal within a few months. Leg ulcers that persist beyond 6 months may require blood transfusion or skin grafting, although results of the latter treatment have been disappointing. Because leg ulcers may recur after minimal trauma, wearing pressure stockings may appear to be an

effective preventive measure. Principles of management of leg ulcers include education, protection, infection control, debridement, and compression bandages. The efficacy of blood transfusion or exchange transfusion, hyperbaric oxygen, and skin grafting is anecdotal. Recent advances in management include the use of platelet-derived growth factor, prepared either autologously (Procuren) or by recombinant technology (Regranex). The use of newly described semipermeable polymenic membrane dressing may promote healing.

Avascular necrosis

Avascular necrosis [50–53] (also called ischemic necrosis or osteonecrosis) is the most commonly observed complication of SCD in adults. Although it tends to be most severe and disabling in the hip area, it is a generalized bone disorder in that the femoral and humeral heads and the vertebral bodies may be equally affected. The limited terminal arterial blood supply and the paucity of collateral circulation make these three areas especially vulnerable to sickling and subsequent bone damage. Patients with sickle cell anemia and α-gene deletion have a higher incidence of avascular necrosis, because their high hematocrit increases blood viscosity and thus enhances microvasculopathy in the aforementioned anatomic sites. Treatment of avascular necrosis is symptomatic and includes providing nonopioid or opioid analgesics in the early stages of the illness; advanced forms of the disease require total joint replacement. Core decompression appears to be effective in the management of avascular necrosis if performed during its early stages.

Intractable Chronic Pain Without Obvious Pathology

This is the worst scenario of chronic sickle cell pain. It is not associated with obvious signs. The only complaint is the patient's self-report of pain that does not go away. Often it is difficult to distinguish a persistent acute painful episode from a chronic pain syndrome. The distinction, however, may not be relevant, because the outcome and treatment are eventually the same or show considerable overlap. Worse still is a patient who is chronic pain, is maintained on high-dose oral opioids, and develops an acute painful episode over and above the chronic pain syndrome: a situation where the dose of opioids must increase to phenomenal levels to achieve pain relief. The pathophysiology of intractable chronic pain is unknown. It appears to result from "central sensitization": a situation where repeated and frequent pain stimuli lower the pain threshold to the degree that ambient innocuous events cause severe pain. It is unknown at which point this occurs or which are the factors that may transform an acute painful episode into a chronic pain syndrome. Surgery, a severe acute painful episode, and severe emotional stresses are some of the proposed causes [15].

Management of chronic sickle cell pain must be multidisciplinary. Leg ulcers necessitate the input of wound care centers, whereas avascular necrosis entails the involvement of orthopedics, physical therapy, rehabilitation, and rheumatology. Intractable pain (central sensitization) dictates the use of nonpharmacologic approaches, of adjuvants, and inevitably, in sickle cell chronic pain, of long-acting or CR opioids with short-acting opioids for breakthrough pain.

NEUROPATHIC PAIN

Neuropathic pain is characterized by sensations of burning, tingling, shooting, lacinating, and numbness. These symptoms may occur in the presence or absence of obvious central or peripheral nerve injury. The mechanism of neuropathic pain presumably involves aberrant somatosensory processing in the central or peripheral nervous system. Sickle cell pain could have a neuropathic component [54,55]. A thorough history and physical examination are essential to determining whether sickle cell pain is associated with a neuropathic component. Mental nerve necropathy [56,57], trigeminal neuralgia [58], acute proximal median mononeuropathy [59], entrapment neuropathy [54], and acute demyelinating polyneuropathy have [54] been described in SCD.

Management of neuropathic pain involves anticonvulsants (see Box 3). Gabapentin appears to be the anticonvulsant that is generally used for this complication.

SPECIFIC RECOMMENDATIONS FOR THE READER

- Recognize that sickle cell pain is protean in nature. Although the acute sickle cell painful episode is the hallmark of the disease, other types of pain are often present. Thus sickle cell pain may be acute, subacute, chronic with objective signs, or chronic without obvious signs. Moreover, the pain could be somatic or visual, nociceptive or neuropathic, localized or diffuse, unilateral or bilateral, and moderate or severe.
- The first step in the management of sickle cell pain is assessment to identify the factors, if any, that precipitated the painful episode. Thorough assessment will also identify the type of pain a patient has and thus make it possible to implement the appropriate plan of management.
- A key component of the process of assessment is believing the patient. Patients who have SCD are the authorities on their pain, and their self-reports must be taken seriously.
- In managing sickle cell pain, consider both the nonpharmacologic and pharmacologic approaches to pain control. Details of these approaches were discussed earlier.
- Recognize that the goal of pain management is to achieve adequate pain relief. The use of nonopioids, opioids, and adjuvants together is more effective in achieving adequate pain relief.
- Be aware that some patients who have SCD suffer from intractable chronic pain without obvious pathologic conditions. Management of these patients requires patience, compassion, regular follow-up, and the use of a multidisciplinary approach.

SUMMARY

The clinical manifestations of SCD fall into four major categories: (1) pain, (2) anemia and its sequelae, (3) organ failure, including infection, and (4) comorbid conditions.

Advances in the pathogenesis of SCD focused on the sequence of events that occur between polymerization of deoxyhemoglobin S and vaso-occlusion. Cellular dehydration, inflammatory response, and reperfusion injury appear to be important pathophysiologic mechanisms.

Management of SCD continues to be primarily palliative in nature, including supportive, symptomatic, and preventive approaches to therapy. There are three major types of sickle cell pain: acute, chronic, and neuropathic pain. The acute painful episode is the insignia of the disease and the most common cause of hospitalization. Its management entails the use of nonpharmacologic and pharmacologic modalities. Pain management should follow certain principles that include an assessment stage, treatment stage, reassessment stage, and adjustment stage. Chronic sickle cell pain may be due to certain complications of the disease, such as leg ulcers and avascular necrosis; intractable chronic pain may be due to central sensitization. Management of chronic pain should take a multidisciplinary approach.

The ultimate goals of management of sickle cell pain should be pain relief, improved physical functioning, reduced psychosocial distress, and improved quality of life.

References

[1] Walters MC, Patience M, Leisenring W, et al. Bone marrow transplantation for sickle cell disease. N Engl J Med 1996;335:369–76.

[2] Gore L, Lane PA, Quinones RR, et al. Successful cord blood transplantation for sickle cell anemia from a sibling who is human leukocyte antigen–identical: implications for comprehensive care. J Pediatr Hematol Oncol 2000;22:437–40.

[3] Ballas SK, Branden Z. Misinterpretation of pain escalation in an adult patient with sickle cell anemia defers accurate diagnosis. Pain Digest 1997;7:208–10.

[4] Williams WD, Chung H. Protein binding diminishes the efficiency of meperidine. Blood 1985;66(Suppl 1):67a.

[5] Ballas SK, Larner J, Smith ED, et al. Rheologic predictors of the severity of the painful sickle cell crisis. Blood 1988;72:1216–23.

[6] Serjeant GR. Sickle cell disease. 3rd edition. New York: Oxford University Press; 2001.

[7] Embury SH, Hebbel RP, Mohandas N, editors. Sickle cell disease. Basic principles and clinical picture. New York: Raven Press; 1994.

[8] Stockman JA, Nigro MA, Mishkin MM, et al. Occlusion of large cerebral vessels in sickle cell anemia. N Engl J Med 1972;287:846–50.

[9] Rothman SM, Fulling KH, Nelson JS. Sickle cell anemia and central nervous system infarction: a neuropathological study. Ann Neurol 1986;20:684–90.

[10] Kaul DK, Hebel RP. Hypoxia/reoxygenation causes inflammatory response in transgenic sickle mice but not in normal mice. J Clin Invest 2000;106:411–20.

[11] Platt OS. Sickle cell anemia as an inflammatory disease. J Clin Invest 2000;106:337–8.

[12] Fields HL. Pain. New York: McGraw-Hill; 1987.

[13] Cousins MJ. Acute post operative pain. In: Wall PD, Melzack R, editors. Textbook of pain. 3rd edition. New York: Churchill Livingstone; 1994. p. 357–85.

[14] Katz N, Ferrante FM. Nociception. In: Ferrante FM, VadeBoncoeur TR, editors. Post operative pain management. New York: Churchill Livingstone; 1993. p. 17–67.

[15] Wall PD, Melzack R, editors. Textbook of pain. 4th edition. New York: Churchill Livingstone; 1999.

[16] Ballas SK. Sickle cell pain. Progress in pain research and management, Vol. II. Seattle (WA): IASP Press; 1998.

[17] Ballas SK, Delengowski A. Pain measurement in hospitalized adults with sickle cell painful episodes. Ann Clin Lab Sci 1993;23:358–61.

[18] Charache S, Terrin ML, Moore RD, et al. Effect of hydroxyurea on the frequency of painful crises in sickle cell anemia. N Engl J Med 1995;332:1317–22.

[19] Charache S, Barton FB, Moore RD, et al. Hydroxyurea and sickle cell anemia: clinical utility of a myelosuppressive "switching" agent: the Multi-Center Study of Hydroxyurea in Sickle Cell Anemia. Medicine 1996;75:300–26.

[20] Ballas SK, Smith ED. Red cell changes during the evolution of the sickle cell painful crisis. Blood 1992;79:2154–63.

[21] Ballas SK. The sickle cell painful crisis in adults: phases and objective signs. Hemoglobin 1995;19:323–33.

[22] Benjamin LJ, Dampier CD, Jacox A, et al. Guideline for the management of acute and chronic pain in sickle cell disease. Glenview (IL): American Pain Society; 1999.

[23] Benjamin LJ. Nature and treatment of the acute painful episode in sickle cell disease. In: Steinberg MH, Forget BG, Higgs DR, et al, editors. Disorders of hemoglobin: genetics, pathophysiology, and clinical management. Cambridge: Cambridge University Press; 2001. p. 671–710.

[24] Cleeland CS. Strategies for improving cancer pain management. J Pain Symptom Manage 1993;8:361–4.

[25] Beaver WT. Impact of non-narcotic oral analgesics on pain management. Am J Med 1988;84:3–15.

[26] Lipton RB, Stewart WF, Ryan RE, et al. Efficacy and safety of acetaminophen, aspirin and caffeine in alleviating migraine headache pain. Arch Neurol 1998;55:210–7.

[27] Sunshine A, Olson NZ. Non-narcotic analgesics. In: Wall PD, Melzack R, editors. Textbook of pain. 3rd edition. New York: Churchill Livingstone; 1994. p. 923–42.

[28] Ferrante MF. Non-steroidal anti-inflammatory drugs. In: Ferrante FM, VedeBoncouer TR, editors. Postoperative pain management. New York: Churchill Livingstone; 1993. p. 133–43.

[29] Hawkey CJ. COX-2 inhibitors. Lancet 1999;353:307.

[30] Day R, Morrison B, Luza A, et al. A randomized trial of the efficacy and tolerability of the COX-2 inhibitor rofecoxib vs ibuprofen in patients with osteoarthritis. Arch Intern Med 2000;160:1781–7.

[31] Bougie D, Aster R. Immune thrombocytopenia resulting from sensitivity to metabolites of naproxen and acetaminophen. Blood 2001;97:3846–50.

[32] Perazella MA, Eras J. Are selective COX-2 inhibitors nephrotoxic? Am J Kidney Dis 2000;35:937.

[33] Whelton A, Schulman G, Wallemark C, et al. Effects of celecoxib and naproxen on renal function in the elderly. Arch Intern Med 2000;160:1465–70.

[34] Perlin E, Finke H, Castro O, et al. Enhancement of pain control with kerorolac tromethamine in patients with sickle cell vaso-occlusion crisis. Am J Hematol 1994;46:43–7.

[35] Abel SR. Tramadol: an alternative analgesic to traditional opioids and NSAIDS. Journal of Pharmaceutical Care in Pain & Symptom Control 1995;3:5–29.

[36] Ferrante MF. Opioids. In: Ferrante FM, VedeBoncouer TR, editors. Postoperative pain management. New York: Churchill Livingstone; 1993. p. 145–209.

[37] Crain SM, Shen KF. Antagonists of excitatory opioid receptor functions enhance morphine's analgesic potency and attenuate tolerance/dependence liability. Pain 2000; 84:121–31.

[38] Krantz MJ, Kutinsky IB, Robertson AD, et al. Dose-related effects of methadone on CPT-prolongation in a series of patients with Torsade de Pointes. Pharmacotherapy 2003; 23:802–5.

[39] Beneditti C, Butler SH. Systemic analgesics. In: Bonica JJ, editor. The management of pain. 2nd edition. Philadelphia: Lea & Febiger; 1990. p. 1640–75.

[40] Inturrisi CE, Umans JG. Meperidine biotransformation and central nervous system toxicity in animals and humans. In: Foley KM, Inturrisi CE, editors. Opioid analgesics in the management of clinical pain. Advances in pain research and therapy, Vol. 8. New York: Raven Press; 1986. p. 143–54.

[41] Mercandante S. Opioids and akathisia. J Pain Symptom Manage 1986;10:415.

[42] World Health Organization. Cancer pain relief and palliative care. World Health Organization technical report series 804. Geneva (Switzerland): World Health Organization; 1990.

[43] Ballas SK, Barton F, Castro O, et al. Narcotic analgesic use among adult patients with sickle cell anemia [abstract 2554]. Blood 1995;86(Suppl 1):642.

[44] Benjamin LJ, Swinson GI, Nagel RL. Sickle cell anemia day hospital: an approach for the management of uncomplicated painful crises. Blood 2000;95:1130–7.

[45] Kalb C. Playing with pain killers. Newsweek April 9, 2001:45–51.

[46] Gaston MH, Verter JI, Woods G, et al. Prophylaxis with oral penicillin in children with sickle cell anemia. N Engl J Med 1986;314:1593–9.

[47] Steinberg MH, Barton F, Castro O, et al. Effect of hydroxyurea on mortality and morbidity in adult sickle cell anemia: risks and benefits up to 9 years of treatment. JAMA 2003;289:1645–51.

[48] Koshy M, Entsuah R, Koranda A, et al. Leg ulcers in patients with sickle cell disease. Blood 1989;75:1403–8.

[49] Blackman JD, Senseng D, Quinn L, et al. Clinical evaluation of a semi-permeable polymeric membrane dressing for the treatment of chronic diabetic foot ulcers. Diabetes Care 1994;17:322–5.

[50] Ballas SK, Talacki CA, Rao VM, et al. The prevalence of avascular necrosis in sickle cell anemia: correlation with α-thalassemia. Hemoglobin 1989;13:649–55.

[51] Milner PF, Kraus AP, Sebes JL, et al. Sickle cell disease as a cause of osteonecrosis of the femoral head. N Engl J Med 1991;325:1476–81.

[52] Saito S, Saito MT, Nishina T, et al. Long term results of total hip arthroplasty for osteonecrosis of the femoral head: a comparison with osteoarthritis. Clin Orthop 1989; 244:198–207.

[53] Styles K, Vichinsky E. Core decompression in avascular necrosis of the hip in sickle cell disease. Am J Hematol 1996;52:103–7.

[54] Ballas SK, Reyes PE. Peripheral neuropathy in adults with sickle cell disease. Am J Pain Med 1997;71:53–8.

[55] Adams RJ. Neurological complications. In: Embury SH, Hebbel RP, Mohandas N, editors. Sickle cell disease: basic principles and clinical practice. New York: Raven Press; 1994. p. 599–621.

[56] Konotey-Ahulu FID. Mental nerve neuropathy: a complication of sickle cell crisis. Lancet 1972;2:388.

[57] Kirson LE, Tomaro AJ. Mental nerve paresthesis secondary to sickle cell crisis. Oral Surg 1979;48:509–12.

[58] Asher SW. Multiple cranial neuropathies, trigeminal neuralgia, and vascular headaches in sickle cell disease: a possible common mechanism. Neurology 1980;30:210–1.

[59] Shields Jr RW, Harris JW, Clark M. Mononeuropathy I sickle cell anemia: anatomical and pathophysiological basis for its rarity. Muscle Nerve 1991;14:370–4.

HEMATOLOGY/ONCOLOGY CLINICS OF NORTH AMERICA

Transfusion Management in Sickle Cell Disease

Sam O. Wanko, MD[a], Marilyn J. Telen, MD[b],*

[a]*Duke University Medical Center, DUMC Box 3841, Durham, NC 27710, USA*
[b]*Duke University Medical Center, DUMC Box 2615, Durham, NC 27710, USA*

S ickle cell disease (SCD) [1] is most commonly seen in individuals whose genetic origins are in sub-Saharan Africa, southern India, and the Mediterranean. Approximately 1 in 350 African Americans are born with HbSS, whereas 1 in 835 have HbSC and 1 in 1700 have HbSβ-thalassemia, making SCD the most common inherited disease in the United States [2]. In England, an estimated 140 to 175 infants are born annually with SCD [3], with a total in 1997 of about 9000 cases [4].

Pathophysiologically, SCD is a hemoglobin structure disorder in which glutamic acid at the sixth residue of the β chain of hemoglobin is substituted by valine, resulting in the formation of a poorly soluble hemoglobin tetramer (α_2/β_2^S) [5]. There are a variety of sickle cell syndromes, including homozygosity for HbS (the most common) and a number of symptomatic heterozygous states, including HbSC, HbSβ-thalassemia, and HbSO$_{Arab}$. In all of these disorders, the abnormal hemoglobin molecules associate with each other, forming paracrystals within the red blood cells, fundamentally altering the cell membrane structure, and resulting in the typical crescent or sickle-shaped appearance owing to deformation by hemoglobin polymers formed while hemoglobin is in the deoxygenated state [6]. The hallmarks of SCD are anemia and vasculopathy, which has protean clinical manifestations. The vasculopathy is characterized by increased whole blood viscosity, adherence of red blood cells to the endothelial surface with consequent vaso-occlusion, and activation of the coagulation cascade and additional adhesion molecules [7]. The anemia is a result of multiple factors, most prominent of which are chronic hemolysis and a shortened red blood cell half-life. Whether the aforementioned crystal formation is reversible in the presence of oxygen, leading to regain of red blood cell function, or whether the crystals become irreversible ultimately contributes to the severity

Dr. Telen was supported in part by National Institutes of Health grant U54 HL70769 from the National Heart, Lung, and Blood Institute. Dr. Wanko received support from the US Department of the Navy.
* Corresponding author. *E-mail address:* marilyn.telen@duke.edu (M.J. Telen).

of the clinical manifestation [5]. The major sources of morbidity and mortality in SCD are acute painful syndromes, severe anemia, infections, acute chest syndrome, and organ failure. An autopsy investigation in 306 patients revealed that the most common causes of death for all sickle cell variants and for all age groups were infection (33% to 48%), stroke (9.8%), splenic sequestration (6.6%), pulmonary thromboemboli (4.9%), renal failure (4.1%), pulmonary hypertension (2.9%), hepatic failure (0.8%), massive hemolysis/red cell aplasia (0.4%), and left ventricular failure (0.4%) [8]. The same study demonstrated that death was sudden and unexpected in 40.8% of patients and usually occurred in the context of an acute event.

In the current context of limited therapeutic approaches to affect the basic pathophysiology of SCD, blood transfusion can be life saving and can ameliorate some of the complications of SCD. Nevertheless, blood transfusions, even when correctly used, are not without immunologic and nonimmunologic complications [9]. Therefore, there is a continued need to set appropriate transfusion policy at centers caring for these patients and to continue refining the indications for transfusion through clinical research. This article reviews the commonly used transfusion methods, the generally accepted indications and controversial indications for blood transfusion, and the clinical situations in which transfusion is generally not considered. In addition, blood product selection, the complications of blood transfusion, and strategies to prevent them are discussed.

TRANSFUSION METHODS
Simple Transfusion
This modality is the oldest and most widely used form of transfusion. Its undisputable advantage lies in its ease of administration, wide availability outside of major medical centers, and lower donor exposure at any single point in time. In contrast to physical removal of HbS in exchange transfusion, simple transfusion reduces the concentration of HbS by hemodilution. Simple transfusion is most useful when restoration of circulating volume or improvement in oxygen-carrying capacity is needed [9,10]. It is readily available on an emergent basis, although exchange transfusion has been used emergently as well. The disadvantages of this method include the risks of volume and iron overload as well as exposure to whole blood viscosity. As long as at least 20% to 30% of circulating red blood cells contain predominantly HbS, patients should generally not be transfused to Hb levels above 11 g/dL, because whole blood viscosity in such a setting is markedly increased.

Exchange Transfusion
Exchange transfusion can be performed manually or by automated erythrocytapheresis. It is indicated in acute stroke and acute chest syndrome, as well as in some circumstances when iron overload is expected or limits desired chronic transfusion [6,9]. When used acutely, exchange transfusion has the advantage of reducing the concentration of HbS while limiting the volume administered and minimizing hyperviscosity [10]. Chronic exchange transfusion

reduces iron overload and has proved useful as a primary and secondary preventive strategy for stroke as well as to ameliorate other types of end-organ damage. A comparative analysis of exchange and simple transfusion in 10 children over 16 months found that exchange transfusion was well tolerated, even in children younger than 5 years. Children receiving exchange transfusion had equivalent alloimmunization rates and lower ferritin levels when compared with children receiving simple transfusion [11]. The cost of exchange transfusion was higher, as was blood use, which increased by as much as 50% [12]. Nonetheless, some investigators speculate that the increased cost may be offset by the cost of chelation therapy associated with chronic simple transfusion.

The appropriate goals for emergent and long-term exchange programs remain somewhat controversial. Although some clinicians advocate maintaining the HbS level around 30%, others argue that HbS concentrations below 50% are adequate to prevent stroke.

INDICATIONS FOR BLOOD TRANSFUSIONS

The indications for transfusion can be divided broadly into acute and chronic, with the common goals of increasing oxygen-carrying capacity lowered by anemia and improving end-organ perfusion by decreasing the proportion of circulating HbS cells (Table 1). The most common indications for acute transfusion include severe symptomatic anemia, acute splenic sequestration, acute

Table 1		
Indications for transfusion therapy in sickle cell disease		
Generally accepted	Possibly effective	Not indicated
Acute cerebrovascular accident	Preoperative/preprocedural, in which relative ischemia might be induced, such as operations involving general anesthesia and cerebral angiography	Compensated anemia
Primary and secondary stroke prevention	Recurrent or persistent priapism	Infections other than aplastic anemia
Retinal artery occlusion	Advanced pulmonary or cardiac disease, such as pulmonary hypertension and heart failure	Uncomplicated acute painful crisis
Acute and recurrent splenic sequestration	Progressive renal failure	Minor surgeries without anesthesia
Intrahepatic cholestasis	Unusually frequent or severe painful crisis	Nonsurgically managed aseptic necrosis
Acute chest syndrome	Pregnancy with exacerbation of anemia, especially if symptomatic	Uncomplicated pregnancy
Aplastic crisis	—	—
Acute blood loss (eg, traumatic splenic rupture)	—	—

chest syndrome, and acute organ damage such as stroke. Preparation for major surgery requiring general anesthesia is also a common indication for transfusion. Primary and secondary stroke prevention and, increasingly, pulmonary hypertension are common reasons for chronic transfusion.

INDICATIONS FOR ACUTE TRANSFUSION

Transient red cell aplasia and acute end-organ damage constitute the major reasons for acute transfusion. Acute end-organ damage includes acute splenic or hepatic sequestration, acute chest syndrome, acute neurologic syndromes such as stroke and retinal artery occlusion, and acute multiorgan failure. Transfusion is also often indicated in preparation for major surgery requiring general anesthesia.

Transient Red Cell Aplasia

Transient red cell aplasia is caused by human parvovirus B19, which invades proliferating erythroid progenitor cells, resulting in erythropoietic arrest and reticulocytopenia with consequent exacerbation of anemia [13,14]. The estimated prevalence in patients with SCD is 30% to 32% [15,16]. The anemia can be particularly life threatening in SCD due to the underlying chronic hemolysis and high demand for erythrocyte production. When compared with normal cohorts with human parvovirus B19 infections, SCD patients in the peri-infection period have 58 times higher risk for further complications, including pain crisis, acute chest syndrome, congestive heart failure, splenic sequestration, and cerebrovascular accidents [14,16].

Blood transfusion is required to correct the severe anemia caused by aplastic crisis and to prevent other organ complications. Simple transfusion is sufficient and should be continued until erythroid progenitors recover and the reticulocyte count rises, which usually occurs within 4 to 14 days [17]. With transfusion support, outcomes are generally good [13]. In addition, patients usually gain long lasting protective immunity after parvovirus B19–induced transient aplasia, making such infection a one-time event for most patients [16].

Acute Splenic and Hepatic Sequestration

Acute visceral organ sequestration typically involves the spleen and less often the liver. Both conditions are believed to share the same pathophysiologic basis, which is the trapping of red blood cells in small end-organ vessels and sinusoids, resulting in massive organ enlargement and dysfunction [18]. Clinically, both types of organ sequestration present with variable degrees of anemia, fever, and acute anatomically localized abdominal pain. A transient twofold to threefold elevation in transaminases and bilirubin along with painful hepatomegaly can be seen with hepatic sequestration [19]. Splenic sequestration is considered a medical emergency and presents with rapid, often painful, splenic enlargement associated with sudden and severe anemia, thrombocytopenia, and reticulocytosis. Fatality can occur from circulatory collapse owing to the rapid decrease in circulating red cell volume. Although the factors that trigger acute organ sequestration are unclear, some episodes have been associated with infection. In a study of 308 children with SCD followed up from birth, 29.9% experienced 132 clinically significant splenic sequestration episodes, with a 10% fatality rate over a 10-year period [20]. The first event occurred between the age of 3 months to 6 years, and 40% of patients had associated respiratory symptoms, although none had bacteria isolated from the blood.

Early blood transfusion can be life saving, especially in the presence of hypotension and severe anemia. Because the infusion of normal red blood cells can lead to the release of sequestered cells, overtransfusion should be avoided. The combination of transfusion and reversal of sequestration may lead to polycythemia, increased whole blood hyperviscosity with consequent sludging, and further end-organ damage [21]. An initial small simple transfusion volume (5–10 mL/kg in children) should be administered during the first hour. This volume is often sufficient to treat splenic sequestration. When indicated, further transfusion should be administered slowly over the course of hours [5,21]. The therapeutic goal is the re-establishment of an adequate circulatory volume. For hepatic sequestration of moderate severity, simple or exchange transfusion has been used successfully [22–24]. As is true in transfusion for splenic sequestration, hyperviscosity induced by overly aggressive transfusion can result in additional organ damage and sometimes fatality [22–25]. Given these potential pitfalls, exchange transfusion is probably preferable in hepatic sequestration, especially in the absence of significant circulatory collapse. Although splenectomy has been suggested and sometimes undertaken to manage splenic sequestration, no large randomized clinical trials have compared splenectomy with blood transfusion. A recent large literature review found that full splenectomy prevented splenic sequestration [26], whereas partial splenectomy was shown in at least one study to decrease recurrence [27]. Partial or full splenectomy may be considered for patients with frequent recurrences requiring blood transfusion.

Acute Chest Syndrome

Acute chest syndrome is a descriptive term given to a heterogeneous group of acute pulmonary illnesses that may occur in isolation or as complications of other sickle cell–related events [28]. Clinically, acute chest syndrome is characterized by chest pain, fever, and an infiltrate on chest radiography and is the leading cause of death in SCD [29–31]. Potential triggers, which are sometimes difficult to prove, include local infection, vaso-occlusion by HbS cells, thromboembolism, and fat embolism resulting from bone marrow ischemia or necrosis [29]. In a multicenter study of 538 patients in which 671 episodes of acute chest syndrome occurred, Vichinsky and coworkers found specific causes in only 38% of the patients. Most encouragingly, treatment with partially phenotypically matched transfusions improved oxygenation with only a 1% alloimmunization rate.

Early transfusion is thought to be a necessary component of therapy for acute chest syndrome [30]. Although simple transfusion can be used, exchange transfusion in this setting has the distinct advantage of dramatically lowering the concentration of HbS without raising the hematocrit too high and seems to result in improved outcomes [30,32,33]. The target HbS should be less than 30% and 30% to 50% in children and adults, respectively. Efforts to predict acute chest syndrome and potentially forestall its onset with transfusion are ongoing. Styles and colleagues [34] reported that serum concentrations of secreted phospholipase A_2, an enzyme that cleaves fatty acid, directly correlated with the onset, peak, and resolution of acute chest syndrome. Similarly, levels of soluble vascular cell adhesion molecule-1 (sVCAM-1) have been suggested as a biomarker for acute chest syndrome and have been shown to correlate with its onset and resolution. sVCAM-1 was also lower in transfused patients [35]. Validation of these potential biomarkers of acute chest syndrome could transform the treatment of this deadly complication by allowing early treatment with transfusion.

Acute Neurologic Syndromes

Acute stroke is the most common acute neurologic disorder seen in SCD, occurring in 10% or more of patients [1]. A less frequent but sight-threatening neurologic event is acute retinal artery occlusion. Acute stroke and retinal artery occlusion are believed to be caused by intracranial arteriopathy resulting from damaged vascular endothelium. An initial event is followed by intimal proliferation and cell adhesion, which causes occlusion of the terminal internal carotid, proximal middle cerebral, or distal arteries [36,37]. This vasculopathy may become fixed as suggested by the finding that, even after transfusion, cerebral oxygenation remains significantly lower in SCD patients when compared with non-SCD patients with anemia from other causes [38].

In the large Cooperative Study of Sickle Cell Disease, which observed 4082 patients from 1978 to 1988, the prevalence rate of stroke in HbSS disease was 4.01%, with an incidence of 0.61 cases per 100 patient-years [39]. Infarctive stroke was more likely to occur in children, but no deaths were reported among this group. In contrast, hemorrhagic strokes were more frequent in young adults (20–29 years), with an associated mortality rate of 26% in the first 2 weeks following the event. Identified risk factors for infarctive stroke included a prior transient ischemic attack, a low steady-state hemoglobin concentration, high blood pressure, and the frequency of acute chest syndrome. Hemorrhagic stroke was associated with a low steady-state hemoglobin and high leukocyte count. Higher stroke rates of 11% to 15% have been reported in smaller studies. Infarctive strokes represented 75% of the cases and occurred primarily in children (starting about age 7 years), whereas intracranial hemorrhages occurred in 25% and mostly in adults [12,37,40].

Exchange transfusion should be accomplished as soon as possible after an acute stroke, although the indication for transfusion is more established in infarctive than hemorrhagic stroke. In infarctive stroke, exchange transfusion is the treatment of choice [21], especially for patients presenting with a hemoglobin level greater 10g/dL. Simple transfusion to restore cerebral oxygenation may be warranted after an infarctive stroke in patients who present with significantly lower hemoglobin levels, but that treatment should be followed as soon as possible by exchange transfusion to decrease the concentration of HbS to less than 30% [41]. In infarctive stroke, exchange transfusion started 6 to 12 hours after the onset of neurologic symptoms may completely reverse the presenting neurologic deficits [21]. This response may also be seen in acute retinal artery occlusion.

Secondary prevention is vital following the resolution of an acute stroke in order to decrease recurrences with their associated morbidity and mortality. In the large Cooperative Study, the rate of stroke recurrence among all types of stroke was about 14% [39]. Life-long transfusion is efficacious in this setting and should be an integral part of a secondary prevention strategy.

Multiple Organ Failure

Although acute single organ damage is most often encountered, life-threatening multiorgan damage is not infrequent in patients with SCD. In their small series of 14 patients, Hassell and coworkers [42] reported 17 episodes (suggesting recurrence in some patients) of acute multiorgan failure, a syndrome that occurred mostly during severe painful crisis. Onset was heralded by fever, a rapid fall in the hemoglobin level and platelet count, nonfocal encephalopathy, and rhabdomyolysis. A low baseline hemoglobin level was a predisposing factor, and all of the patients except one recovered with blood transfusion. A retrospective review from four European SCD centers over a 10-year period reported a 25% mortality rate from this syndrome [43]. Widespread vaso-occlusion was believed to be the major underlying etiology, and aggressive exchange transfusion therapy was associated with improved survival and rapid recovery of organ function [42,44].

Preparation for Major Surgery Requiring General Anesthesia

Orthopedic procedures, cholecystectomies, and splenectomies are the most common operations performed in SCD patients, with serious complications reported in as many as 67%, especially after hip replacement [45]. For reasons not yet completely defined, major surgeries requiring general anesthesia may induce postoperative vaso-occlusive complications and sometimes fatality. Of the 3765 patients observed in the Cooperative Study of Sickle Cell Disease, 12 deaths occurred among 717 patients who underwent over 1000 surgical procedures, including cholecystectomy, splenectomy, dilation and curettage, cesarean section or hysterectomy, tonsillectomy or adenoidectomy, hip replacement, removal, or revision, and myringotomies [46]. Of the 12 patients who died, 11 had been transfused before surgery, 10 were homozygous for HbS, and all had intra-abdominal surgeries. Nine patients were believed to have died of comorbid medical complications and SCD-related multiorgan failure, whereas three patients died of surgery-related complications, including severe anemia from delayed transfusion reactions and massive intra-abdominal hemorrhage. Surprisingly, regional anesthesia was associated with more complications than general anesthesia, with painful episodes being the most common postoperative event.

Routine perioperative transfusions have been standard practice for SCD patients undergoing major surgery, but the data supporting this practice have been mixed. While Janik and Seeler [47] did not observe any major complications in 35 children who underwent a total of 46 surgical procedures over an 11-year period and who received preoperative transfusion to achieve a target hematocrit of at least 36%, other investigators have reported major complications with a similar preoperative transfusion strategy. In a study of 16 SCD patients who underwent 32 hip arthroplasties, Ould amar and coworkers [48] found that perioperative transfusions were frequently associated with episodes of hemolysis, vaso-occlusive crisis, and chest syndrome, whereas many patients were able to undergo the procedure without transfusion. They recommended against prophylactic preoperative transfusion. Different conclusions were reached in the National Preoperative Transfusion in Sickle Cell Disease Group study [49], which had randomized and nonrandomized arms and evaluated 364 SCD patients who underwent cholecystectomy. In the randomized arm, 110 patients received aggressive (exchange) transfusion designed to decrease the hemoglobin S level to less than 30%, whereas 120 patients were treated with conservative (simple) transfusions designed to increase the hemoglobin level to 10 g/dL. In the nonrandomized arm, 37 patients were transfused, whereas 97 patients did not receive transfusions. The overall perioperative complication rate in the study was 39% and included sickle cell events (19%), intraoperative or recovery room events (11%), transfusion complications (10%), postoperative surgical events (4%), and death (1%). There was no improvement in the complication rate in patients randomized to the aggressive transfusion arm when compared with the conservative transfusion regimen, whereas complications were more frequent in the nonrandomized, nontransfused subjects (32%). These observations led the investigators to recommend the use of simple preoperative transfusion over exchange transfusion; however, the study was limited by the fact that only about 25% of the patients who were randomized were over the age of 20 years, and relatively few had baseline hypoxemia or abnormal chest radiographs. Even for this single type of surgery, no data are available to help manage sicker and older patients.

The study of cholecystectomy was part of an even larger Preoperative Transfusion Study Group of 604 operations [50] in which two groups of SCD patients were prospectively assigned to the aggressive or conservative regimen described previously. In this larger study, there was also no statistically significant difference in the number of serious complications occurring in the two groups (31% in the aggressive group and 35% in the conservative group). The investigators concluded that a conservative preoperative transfusion regimen was as effective as aggressive transfusion but had the advantage of reduced transfusion-related complications. Even for patients undergoing orthopedic surgery, which carried the highest rate of perioperative complications, conservative transfusion seemed to be as helpful as a more aggressive transfusion strategy

[45]. A retrospective review of surgeries (mostly cholecystectomy and splenectomy) performed on 92 SCD patients who received aggressive transfusion support to reduce HbS to 30% or less performed at Duke University from 1986 to 1995 demonstrated a major complication rate of 12%. That rate was appreciably lower than the nearly 33% rate reported in the Preoperative Transfusion Study Group, leading some clinicians to continue advocating for the use of preoperative exchange transfusion therapy in children with SCD who are scheduled for major surgical procedures. Relatively few patients in these studies were aged more than 21 years or had baseline cardiopulmonary dysfunction; therefore, the optimal management of older patients undergoing major surgeries is undefined. Preparation for major surgery in sickle cell patients should generally involve a consultation with physicians highly familiar with the care of these patients. A likely predictor of the need for transfusion in older patients may be the patient's prior history of complications associated with anesthesia.

INDICATIONS FOR CHRONIC TRANSFUSION

The prevention of stroke and the amelioration of other chronic organ damage are the most common reasons for chronic transfusion. Cerebral infarction often occurs during childhood, whereas failure of other organs such as the kidneys (glomerulosclerosis), pulmonary hypertension, and heart failure occur during young adulthood and adulthood [51]. Efforts to predict the risk and rate of progression of end-organ damage are ongoing. It is hoped these findings will become useful in stratifying risks of progression and the need and timing of chronic transfusion. Currently, the ability to predict the risk for complications of SCD preventable by transfusion is limited. Powars and colleagues [52] have shown that the β-globin haplotype correlates with hematologic laboratory findings, clinical severity, and the risk of major organ failure. In their study, Central African Republic haplotype carriers had the highest risk of irreversible end-organ failure, whereas morbidity was consistently lower in Senegalese haplotype carriers, who also had higher hemoglobin F levels. In all haplotype combinations, the presence of α-thalassemia-2 was associated with a decreased risk of organ failure. In contrast, low hemoglobin and elevated platelet counts, leukocyte counts, and plasma fibrinogen portended worse clinical morbidity. Unfortunately, these findings have not been well validated in larger studies; therefore, the use of chronic blood transfusion remains a clinical event-driven decision.

Chronic blood transfusion is intended to stabilize rather than reverse fixed lesions and to prevent further tissue damage. Following a first event, stroke recurs in as many as 70% of patient within 3 years [53], splenic sequestration in as many as 50% of children [21], and acute chest syndrome in as many as 20% to 80% of patients [54], making secondary prevention of further end-organ damage such as recurrent stroke the most common reason for chronic blood transfusion. There is now unequivocal evidence that chronic blood transfusion can reduce or prevent a first infarctive stroke in children at high risk, as identified by transcranial Doppler examination. Other conditions for which chronic transfusions have been advocated, despite a lack of large carefully designed studies, include renal damage, congestive heart failure, pulmonary hypertension, and chronic pain. Exchange transfusion and simple transfusion targeted to maintain HbS levels around 30% are often used for chronic transfusion [9].

Primary Stroke Prevention

Stroke occurs in 7% to 10% of children with SCD [1,55]. Efforts to identify patients at risk and to determine the efficacy of treatment have been active areas of research. The Stroke Prevention in Sickle Cell Anemia (STOP I) trial was a pivotal study in which 5613 transcranial Doppler studies on 2324 children aged 2 to 16 years were used to identify 130 high-risk children (transcranial Doppler velocity >200 m/s in the internal carotid and middle cerebral arteries). These children were then randomized to receive standard care (n=67) or transfusions (n=63) to reduce the HbS concentration to less than 30% to prevent a first stroke. At baseline, the transfusion group had a slightly lower mean hemoglobin concentration (7.2 versus 7.6 g/dL, $P=.001$) and hematocrit (20.4% versus 21.7%, $P=.002$). Ten patients dropped out of the transfusion group, and two patients crossed over from the standard care group to the transfusion group. The trial was terminated early after detecting a 90% reduction in the rate of first stroke in favor of the transfusion arm. Ten cerebral infarctions and one intracerebral hemorrhage occurred in the standard care arm compared with one infarctive stroke in the transfusion arm ($P<.001$) [55–57]. For children identified to be at high risk by transcranial Doppler examination, the number needed to treat to prevent one stroke per year was 10 [28]. It is now standard in most centers treating large numbers of SCD patients to identify children at risk for stroke with transcranial Doppler imaging. In recent studies, silent ischemia identified on brain MRI is emerging as another independent predictor of the risk for clinical overt stroke [58].

Secondary Prevention of Vaso-Occlusive Stroke

Chronic transfusions have been reported to reduce the rate of recurrent cerebral infarction from 46% to 90% to less than 10% [55]. Initial studies of transfusions for secondary stroke prevention set the target HbS to less than 30%, but the associated transfusion cost and complications with this strategy prompted some investigators to recommend a higher HbS target of 50%, which may be equally effective. Using this approach, Cohen and colleagues [59] reported a high rate of protection against recurrent cerebral infarction using simple transfusion or exchange transfusion. Wang and colleagues [60] addressed the question of how long transfusion should be continued following an initial stroke by prospectively discontinuing transfusions in 10 patients with SCD after a median transfusion duration of 9.5 years (range, 5 to 12 years). There was a 50% recurrence of ischemic events within 12 months after discontinuing transfusion, with 20% resulting in massive intracranial hemorrhage and 10% in fatality. Cerebral angiography, cranial MRI, neuropsychologic testing, electroencephalography, and neurologic examination performed before cessation of transfusions were not predictive of recurrent stroke. These findings led to the recommendation of indefinite blood transfusion or a suitable therapeutic alternative in sickle cell patients with a history of stroke. Regrettably, the high rates of stroke recurrence in this small study have made it difficult to design further clinical studies addressing this issue. A 2004 Cochrane review did not find any randomized controlled trial investigating the use of transfusion for preventing recurrence of stroke or the length of time after an event at which transfusion could safely be stopped [61].

The National Heart, Lung and Blood Institute [1] sponsored the STOP II study, which was designed to test whether chronic transfusions for primary stroke prevention could be discontinued safely in children who had not had an overt stroke and who reverted to low-risk transcranial Doppler velocity with chronic transfusion therapy. The study was discontinued prematurely in 2004 when an interim analysis showed a highly significant difference in the composite endpoints of transcranial Doppler reversion to high risk and overt stroke between the transfusion and nontransfusion arms. Among the 41 patients randomized to come off transfusion, 16 endpoints had occurred. Fourteen reversions from low- to high-risk transcranial Doppler (without stroke) were noted, and two ischemic strokes occurred immediately after reversion to high-risk transcranial Doppler findings. Six other subjects (crossovers) were returned to periodic transfusion therapy primarily owing to recurrent acute chest syndrome and other sickle cell–related painful episodes [1].

Recurrent Acute Chest Syndrome and Pulmonary Hypertension

Recurrent acute chest syndrome, chronic hemolytic anemia, recurrent infection, regional pulmonary hypoxia, and resistance to hydroxyurea have been proposed as risk factors for the development of pulmonary hypertension [51,62,63], which, in turn, is associated with premature mortality. A recent study in which 195 consecutive patients with SCD were screened by echocardiography demonstrated a substantial risk of death in the 63 patients with tricuspid regurgitant jet velocity greater than 2.5 m/s [64]. Among these patients, 17 had severe pulmonary hypertension (tricuspid regurgitant jet velocity of ≥3.0 m/s). Of these subjects, 10 of 11 patients who began an aggressive transfusion program or inhaled nitric oxide therapy were still alive. The prevalence rate of pulmonary hypertension was 32%, although some retrospective studies have shown prevalence rates as high as 60% [63].

Although several pilot studies suggest that blood transfusion can reverse early pulmonary hypertension, only about 10% of patients outside comprehensive centers are currently screened for this deadly entity [63]. In the pivotal STOP I trial, compliance with aggressive chronic transfusion was associated with a reduction in the frequency of acute chest syndrome and pain episodes [65]. Successful prevention and treatment of pulmonary hypertension may depend on adopting the same strategy of early detection performed in primary stroke prevention to identify risk groups.

Identifying predictors that might lead to early treatment for SCD-related pulmonary disease, such as acute chest syndrome, may go a long way toward ameliorating its morbidity. In a series reported on by Sakhalkar and colleagues [35], 15 patients who had acute chest syndrome and who were chronically transfused demonstrated a statistically significant lower level of sVCAM-1 in a comparison with asymptomatic SCD patients ($P = .003$). Nevertheless, there is no routine and accepted method for predicting acute chest syndrome or for identifying patients at risk other than establishing a prior history of acute chest syndrome.

Until further studies addressing the timing of screening and the best therapy for pulmonary hypertension are available, it seems reasonable to screen SCD patients starting by 20 years of age. More frequent identification of patients with pulmonary hypertension and the identification of associated risk factors should lead to future randomized clinical trials in which patients with tricuspid regurgitant jet velocity greater than 2.5 m/s can be enrolled to investigate the utility of various proposed therapies, including blood transfusion.

CONTROVERSIAL INDICATIONS

Priapism

Priapism is a common and often dramatic complication seen in 30% to 80% of male patients [66–68]. It can occur in an acute, recurrent, acute on chronic, or stuttering fashion [69]. In the prepubertal age group, only the cavernosa is involved, the duration tends to be shorter, and symptoms are usually more amenable to nonsurgical therapy than in the postpubertal age group, in whom the inverse is more often true [70]. Priapism, especially when recurrent and severe, is a predictor of other end-organ damage and mortality. In a review of 25 years' experience with 461 SCD patients, Sharpsteen and colleagues identified 38 patients with priapism. Of these patients, 9 (25%) died within 5 years of their first episode of priapism, and other vaso-occlusive complications occurred with higher frequency in patients with priapism. Although exchange transfusion has been used successfully in some cases of priapism [71–73], other investigators have reported a lack of detumescence or acute pain control using the same modality [74]. In addition, the ASPEN syndrome (Association of SCD, Priapism, Exchange transfusion, and Neurologic events) has been described, in which headache, seizures, mental status changes, focal neurologic defects, and strokes occur after transfusion for priapism [73]. Several reports have suggested that medical therapy may be effective in preventing recurrent priapism, obviating the need for transfusion. Currently, the issue of whether to transfuse and what modality to use remains largely unanswered, with most treatment choices made based on available resources and institutional preferences at the time of presentation.

Pregnancy

Pregnancy outcomes have improved in the last two decades with advances in obstetric technology. Nevertheless, significant SCD-related complications of pregnancy can affect the fetus, the mother, or both. There are conflicting data regarding the benefit of regular transfusion during pregnancy. A United Kingdom multicenter study compared pregnancy complications in 81 sickle cell patients with those in 100 other pregnant women of black African descent without hemoglobinopathies [75]. Pregnancy complications, including anemia, preterm delivery, proteinuric hypertension, and low birth weight, were higher in the sickle cell cohort when compared with the controls and were more likely to occur in the third trimester. These findings prompted the investigators to recommend the use of prophylactic transfusion starting at 28 weeks' gestation to reduce these complications. A reduction in the complications of pregnancy with transfusion has been reported by other investigators [76–78].

Other investigators have not observed a reduction in pregnancy complications with prophylactic transfusion and have recommended selective transfusion targeted to treat clearly identifiable medical and obstetric complications, such as increasing hypoxemia, progressive symptomatic anemia, acute chest syndrome, twin pregnancy, splenic sequestration syndrome, pre-eclampsia, septicemia, or in preparation for general anesthesia and surgery [79]. The well-known complications of transfusion, such as infections, allergic reactions, and alloimmunization, can have compounding effects in pregnancy, and such risks must be weighed carefully against potential benefits. A Cochrane Pregnancy and Childbirth Group review of controlled trials that addressed the question of routine versus selective blood transfusion in pregnant women with SCD identified only one such trial that enrolled 72 women. Of the 72 patients, 36 received blood transfusions if their hemoglobin level fell below 6 g/dL (selective transfusion), whereas the other half received 2 units of blood every week for 3 weeks, or until the hemoglobin level was 10 to 11 g/dL. Pregnancy outcomes were similar in both groups, although the selective transfusion group had more frequent pain crises. It was concluded that there was not enough evidence to draw conclusions about the prophylactic use of blood transfusion for sickle cell anemia during pregnancy [80]. Currently, most centers that provide care for large populations of patients with SCD follow a policy of selective transfusion targeted to address specific problems that arise during pregnancy. Nevertheless, in the United States, limited data have been obtained during the last 15 to 20 years regarding the effectiveness of this strategy on pregnancy outcomes.

Leg Ulcers

Leg ulcers are common in sickle cell disease. In the Cooperative Study of Sickle Cell Disease, 2.5% of patients aged 10 years and older were affected [81]. The pathologic mechanism of ulceration is not well defined but may involve compromised venous microcirculation and decreased skin perfusion [82]. Anatomically, ulcers often occur at the medial or lateral malleolus, either spontaneously or incited by minor trauma. Superinfection is common and often complicates healing. Identified risk factors include male gender, low steady-state hemoglobin, a genotype other than sickle β^+-thalassemia and HbSC, and low fetal hemoglobin [81,83]. Hydroxyurea, which increases the expression of fetal hemoglobin, has been used for leg ulcers with good results [84], although there are rare and controversial reports that hydroxyurea may predispose to ulceration or at least poor wound healing [85,86].

The basis for contemplating blood transfusion as an adjunctive therapy for leg ulcers stems from the notion that improving microcirculation might improve healing. A paucity of clinical data support transfusion for leg ulcers, although some investigators have reported accelerated ulcer healing in transfused patients [87].

Precontrast Media Infusion

Complications such as multiple cerebral infarction and the induction of vaso-occlusive crisis have been reported after using hyperosmolar contrast solution in patients with SCD [88,89]. It is thought that red blood cell dehydration may occur after intravenous hyperosmolar contrast injection, rendering the cells even less deformable than at baseline and leading to microcirculatory impairment [90,91]. Thankfully, this problem has been recognized and circumvented by using isotonic contrast medium. In rare instances when hyperosmolar contrast must be given, the clinician may want to consider simple transfusion to increase the number of normal red blood cells that are less prone to dehydration.

CLINICAL SITUATIONS NOT REQUIRING TRANSFUSION

In general, stable compensated anemia, infections without aplastic crisis, non-surgically managed aseptic necrosis, minor surgeries without general anesthesia, and uncomplicated acute painful crisis do not required blood transfusion and can be managed with other appropriate medical and supportive measures.

COMPLICATIONS OF BLOOD TRANSFUSION AND CONSIDERATIONS IN BLOOD PRODUCT SELECTION

Immunologic Complications

Immunologic consequences of blood transfusions include two related events— alloimmunizations and hemolytic reactions. Alloimmunization occurs in 5% to 50% of SCD patients after multiple transfusions [92–94], and the rate may be even higher given that some antibodies are only transiently detected [21]. The principal reason for the high rate of alloimmunization is the antigenic discrepancy between the donor population, which is mostly Caucasian, and the recipient, who is mostly of African descent [21,95]. Antigenic frequency mismatch between Caucasians and African Americans has been described in the Rh, Kell, Kidd, MNS, and Duffy blood groups, among others (Tables 2 and 3). The consequences of alloimmunization are difficulty in locating compatible donor blood, which may limit needed therapy, as well as severe hemolytic transfusion reactions, which can occur acutely or as delayed hemolytic transfusion reactions (DHTR) days to weeks after transfusion.

Hemolytic reactions are seen in as many as 4% to 11% of transfused SCD patients [94,96]. The most common causes are clerical errors (leading to transfusion of incompatible blood) and previous undetected alloimmunization [96,97]. Signs and symptoms of hemolytic transfusion reactions may include fever, chills,

Table 2
Frequency of Rh gene complexes in Caucasians and African Americans

		Gene frequency in the US population	
RH gene complex	Antigens expressed	Caucasians	African Americans
R_0	cDe	0.04	0.44
r	ce	0.37	0.26
R_1	Cde	0.42	0.17
R_2	cDE	0.14	0.11
r'	Ce	0.02	0.02
r''	cE	0.01	<0.01
R_z	CDE	<0.01	<0.01
r_y	CE	<0.01	<0.01

tachycardia, and even circulatory collapse resulting in death [98–100]. Other severe complications, including acute chest syndrome, congestive heart failure, pancreatitis, and acute renal failure, have been reported in some series [96]. Furthermore, hemolytic reactions can present with symptoms typical of vaso-occlusive crises, making recognition a challenge; therefore, DHTR should always be included in the differential diagnosis of a recently transfused patient who has SCD and vaso-occlusive crisis. On laboratory evaluation, one frequently finds a positive antiglobulin test (DAT), elevated lactate dehydrogenase, and bilirubin above the patient's baseline.

Acute hemolytic transfusion reactions usually occur as a result of major ABO mismatch and are usually clinically apparent within minutes to hours. DHTRs are the result of anamnestic immune responses in previously alloimmunized

Table 3
Frequency of other commonly encountered antigens in Caucasians and African Africans

		Antigen frequency (%)	
Blood group	Antigens expressed	Caucasians	African Americans
Kell	K	9.0	2.0
	k	99.8	>99.9
	Kp^a	2.0	<0.1
	Js^a	<0.1	20.0
	Js^b	>99.9	99.0
Kidd	Jk^a	77.0	92.0
	Jk^b	74.0	49.0
MNS	M	78.0	70.0
	N	72.0	74.0
	S	55.0	31.0
	S	89.0	97.0
	S-S-U-[1]	0	1.0
Duffy	Fy^a	66.0	10.0
	Fy^b	83.0	23.0
	Fy(a-b-)[1]	<0.01	68.0

[1] Null phenotypes in the MNS and Duffy blood group systems.

patients and occur 2 to 14 days after red blood cell transfusion. In SCD, there is often hemolysis of transfused cells as well as autologous red blood cells, leading to anemia that can be profound. For reasons not well understood, DHTRs are also often accompanied by reticulocytopenia. Further transfusion, even of blood compatible in a crossmatching test, often leads to further hemolysis and a decrease in the Hb level. When possible, additional transfusions should be avoided, because they may exacerbate the degree of anemia. In some cases, the DAT remains negative despite an apparent accelerated destruction of transfused cells, which can be demonstrated by serial hemoglobin electrophoresis [94,101,102].

Corticosteroids and intravenous gamma globulin have been used successfully in the management of DHTRs in patients with SCD, and erythropoietin has been used for cases accompanied by reticulocytopenia [94,103–105]. Because DHTRs can mimic sickle cell crisis, treating physicians must remain vigilant to this possibility in patients with recent transfusion who present with sickle crisis. Maintenance of accurate records and a request and review of outside hospital records for previously identified antibodies are policy measures that can reduce the rate of DHTRs.

Nonimmunologic Complications

Infections

Viral infection, including hepatitis, HIV, HTLV types I and II, and parvovirus B19, are among the most common infections transmitted by blood transfusions. There is a correlation between the rate of infection and the frequency and number of units transfused [106,107]. The risks of parvovirus B19 and hepatitis C are 1 in 10,000 and 1 in 200,000 per unit transfused, respectively. Hepatitis C is currently seen in as many as 10% of SCD patients in the United States and in as many as 70% in developing countries [107,108]. The risk of HIV is less than 1 in 2 million per unit of transfused blood, but the prevalence of actual transmission is unknown. Bacteria can sometimes be transmitted as well and can manifest with fever and hemodynamic changes during or after transfusion. Patients developing these symptoms should receive prompt attention, starting with discontinuation of transfusion, laboratory evaluation of the blood product, including Gram stain and culture, and supportive care, including antibiotics if indicated. All patients with SCD should receive hepatitis B vaccine. Those with hepatitis C should be monitored closely by an appropriate medical specialist knowledgeable about the complexities of treating such patients with interferon, peginterferon alfa-2a, or the combination of one of these agents with ribavirin. Although ribavirin is associated in some patients with hemolysis, this drug has been used successfully in patients with SCD, and one reports suggests that pretreatment with hydroxyurea can ameliorate this hemolytic side effect [109].

Iron overload

Multiple simple blood transfusions on an episodic basis over decades can lead to iron overload with consequent morbidity and mortality. The prevalence of iron overload is as high as 33% among patients with SCD [110]. Norol and colleagues reported an inverse correlation between low versus high iron values and painful crisis (38% versus 64%), organ failure (19% versus 71%), and mortality (64% versus 5%). Because ferritin levels do not always correlate with tissue iron stores, experts have recommended monitoring the cumulative quantity of blood transfused in conjunction with ferritin at steady state for determining the status of iron stores. Ferritin may be increased during vaso-occlusive crises and should therefore be viewed as an approximation of iron storage in SCD patients. The gold standard for quantifying iron overload remains hepatic tissue biopsy. Noninvasive measurement of hepatic magnetic susceptibility by super-conducting quantum interference device (SQUID) susceptometry or MR sus-ceptometry may replace liver biopsy as the gold standard in the near future [111]. Current studies are also focusing on the use of T2* MRI of the heart to assess cardiac iron stores, because these are believed to be poorly predicted from measurement of hepatic iron.

Exchange transfusion and the use of iron chelation therapy may prevent or delay the onset of iron overload. Deferoxamine is the standard chelation therapy; however, the need for long hours of parenteral administration limits patients' compliance and has led to the development of deferiprone, an orally bioavailable alternative that is currently only licensed in Europe. ICL670, a newer oral chelator, is being tested in large clinical trials. In the future, improved chelation may be achievable through a combination of parenteral and oral agents [112].

Patients with iron overload and particularly those on chelator therapy are predisposed to infection with *Yersinia enterocolitica*. Unlike most bacteria, *Yersinia* is unable to produce iron chelators known as siderophores; therefore, in the presence of iron overload and especially in patients treated with deferox-amine, *Yersinia enterocolitica* becomes more virulent. Treatment includes an-tibiotics such as cefotaxime or an aminoglycoside, as well as temporary discontinuation of deferoxamine [92,113,114].

Blood Product Selection

Because of the increased risk of alloantibodies in patients with SCD, as well as the lifelong probability of the need for future transfusions, special steps are recommended to reduce the rate of alloimmunization and other transfusion-related complications. It has become standard in centers with large numbers of patients with SCD to use blood products that are phenotypically typed for ABO, Rh (Cc, D, Ee), and Kell. This strategy was shown in the multicenter Stroke Prevention Trial to reduce the alloimmunization rate from 3% to 0.5% per unit of blood and to reduce hemolytic transfusion reactions by 90% [93,115,116]. Similarly, Castro and coworkers reported a 53.3% reduction in alloantibodies achieved by matching phenotypes for the same antigens, with a reduction in alloimmunization of more than 70% if a more extensive matching involving S, Fy, and Jk antigens was undertaken. Unfortunately, such extensive phenotypic matching for all SCD patients requiring transfusion is probably impractical on a national scale because of the costs involved [93]. A recent proficiency testing survey by the College of American Pathologists concluded that most North American hospital transfusion service laboratories do not determine the red blood cell antigen phenotype of nonalloimmunized SCD patients beyond ABO and D, and that when such testing is performed, it is usually in preparation for needed blood transfusion [117]. In this survey of 1182 laboratories, only 37.1% (439) routinely performed phenotype testing of SCD patients for antigens other than ABO and D. When phenotype-matched donor red blood cells were used in the latter laboratories, 85% of the matching was for C, E, and K. At the authors' center, all patients are prospectively typed for all major antigens before first transfusion or at their first clinic visit. They are also provided blood matched for D, Ce, Ee, and K, irrespective of previous alloimmunization. These practices are currently recommended by the National Heart, Lung and Blood Institute. In chronically transfused patients in whom serologic typing may eventually become difficult, DNA typing of blood groups by PCR-RFLP of peripheral blood white cells has been found to select donor units accurately, although such typing is currently available at only a few centers [118]. Cytometric typing of reticulocytes is being explored as another nonserologic method of donor blood selection in difficult-to-type patients, because reticulocytes are often easily isolated from the blood of even transfused SCD patients. Traditional capillary agglutination typing of reticulocytes can also routinely be achieved by most blood bank reference laboratories. Although all patients are routinely screened for alloantibodies before blood transfusion, clinicians caring for SCD patients need to maintain accurate records and obtain outside hospital records of previously identified antibodies.

No good data suggest that patients with SCD need specially prepared blood products. Although leukoreduction has theoretical advantages and leads to lower instances of febrile transfusion reactions and viral transmission overall, no data prove a particular benefit for the leukoreduction of blood products to be transfused to patients with SCD. In fact, when red blood cells are extensively antigen matched, the likelihood of selecting an African American donor with sickle cell trait is increased. Blood from patients with the sickle cell trait usually passes through leukoreduction filters adequately when filtration is performed soon after the blood is drawn ("prestorage leukoreduction"), whereas such blood often clogs filters if the "bedside" filtration method is used after storage of blood in the routine manner. Likewise, there are no special indications for washed red blood cells outside of the usual indication of repeated allergic reactions to transfusion. Irradiated blood products should be reserved for bone marrow transplant candidates or after transplant. Because HbSS red blood cells do not store or freeze well, autologous transfusion, although it has been attempted, is rarely successful.

Some clinicians caring for SCD patients recommend transfusing only blood that is not positive in Sickledex testing, which identifies blood carrying one copy of HbS; however, sickle cell trait red blood cells do not normally sickle in physiologic conditions and are not generally responsible for SCD-type clinical syndromes. The advantage of transfusing Sickledex-negative blood products may be primarily the ease with which the results of transfusion and the survival of transfused cells can be followed by hemoglobin electrophoresis when only HbS-negative cells are transfused.

SUMMARY

Blood transfusion is a critical and, in many circumstances, life-saving part of evolving strategies for the treatment of patients with SCD. Because of the complications associated with transfusions, and to a lesser extent the cost, many areas of controversy remain regarding some indications for transfusions. Clinicians caring for patients who have SCD should be knowledgeable of national and institutional guidelines regarding the indications, contraindications, and surveillance and treatment of complications of transfusions. Therapy for SCD has increasingly become a multidisciplinary endeavor. Consultations with physicians specializing in the management of these patients should be sought liberally.

References

[1] National Heart, Lung, and Blood Institute. Clinical alert from the National Heart, Lung, and Blood Institute (December 5, 2004). Available at: http://www.nhlbi.nih.gov/health/prof/blood/sickle/clinical-alert-scd.htm. Accessed March 15, 2005.

[2] Bonds DR. Three decades of innovation in the management of sickle cell disease: the road to understanding the sickle cell disease clinical phenotype. Blood Rev 2005;19(2): 99–110.

[3] Hickman M, Modell B, Greengross P, et al. Mapping the prevalence of sickle cell and beta thalassaemia in England: estimating and validating ethnic-specific rates. Br J Haematol 1999;104(4):860–7.

[4] Okpala I, Thomas V, Westerdale N, et al. The comprehensiveness care of sickle cell disease. Eur J Haematol 2002;68(3):157–62.

[5] Rosse WF, Telen MJ, Ware RE. Transfusion support for patients with sickle cell disease. Bethesda (MD): AABB Press; 1998.

[6] Ballas SK. Sickle cell anaemia: progress in pathogenesis and treatment. Drugs 2002; 62(8):1143–72.

[7] Kaul DK, Fabry ME, Costantini F, et al. In vivo demonstration of red cell–endothelial interaction, sickling and altered microvascular response to oxygen in the sickle transgenic mouse. J Clin Invest 1995;96(6):2845–53.

[8] Manci EA, Culberson DE, Yang YM, et al. Causes of death in sickle cell disease: an autopsy study. Br J Haematol 2003;123(2):359–65.

[9] Germain S, Brahimi L, Rohrlich P, et al. [Transfusion in sickle cell anemia]. Pathol Biol (Paris) 1999;47(1):65–72 [in French].

[10] Eckman JR. Techniques for blood administration in sickle cell patients. Semin Hematol 2001;38(Suppl 1):23–9.

[11] Adams DM, Schultz WH, Ware RE, et al. Erythrocytopheresis can reduce iron overload and prevent the need for chelation therapy in chronically transfused pediatric patients. J Pediatr Hematol Oncol 1996;18(1):46–50.

[12] Hilliard LM, Williams BF, Lounsbury AE, et al. Erythrocytopheresis limits iron accumulation in chronically transfused sickle cell patients. Am J Hematol 1998;59(1):28–35.

[13] Wierenga KJ, Serjeant BE, Serjeant GR. Cerebrovascular complications and parvovirus infection in homozygous sickle cell disease. J Pediatr 2001;139(3):438–42.

[14] Rao SP, Miller ST, Cohen BJ. Transient aplastic crisis in patients with sickle cell disease: B19 parvovirus studies during a 7-year period. Am J Dis Child 1992;146(11):1328–30.

[15] Sant'Anna AL, Garcia Rde C, Marzoche M, et al. Study of chronic hemolytic anaemia patients in Rio de Janeiro: prevalence of anti-human parvovirus B19 IgG antibodies and the development of aplastic crises. Rev Inst Med Trop Sao Paulo 2002; 44(4):187–90.

[16] Smith-Whitley K, Zhao H, Hodinka RL, et al. Epidemiology of human parvovirus B19 in children with sickle cell disease. Blood 2004;103(2):422–7.

[17] Saarinen UM, Chorba TL, Tattersall P, et al. Human parvovirus B19-induced epidemic acute red cell aplasia in patients with hereditary hemolytic anemia. Blood 1986;67(5): 1411–7.

[18] Roshkow JE, Sanders LM. Acute splenic sequestration crisis in two adults with sickle cell disease: US, CT, and MR imaging findings. Radiology 1990;177(3):723–5.

[19] Ojuawo A, Adedoyin MA, Fagbule D. Hepatic function tests in children with sickle cell anaemia during vaso-occlusive crisis. Cent Afr J Med 1994;40(12):342–5.

[20] Emond AM, Collis R, Darvill D, et al. Acute splenic sequestration in homozygous sickle cell disease: natural history and management. J Pediatr 1985;107(2):201–6.

[21] Telen MJ. Principles and problems of transfusion in sickle cell disease. Semin Hematol 2001;38(4):315–23.

[22] Morrow JD, McKenzie SW. Survival after intrahepatic cholestasis associated with sickle cell disease. J Tenn Med Assoc 1986;79(4):199–200.

[23] Shao SH, Orringer EP. Sickle cell intrahepatic cholestasis: approach to a difficult problem. Am J Gastroenterol 1995;90(11):2048–50.

[24] Sheehy TW, Law DE, Wade BH. Exchange transfusion for sickle cell intrahepatic cholestasis. Arch Intern Med 1980;140(10):1364–6.

[25] Lee ES, Chu PC. Reverse sequestration in a case of sickle crisis. Postgrad Med J 1996;72(850):487–8.

[26] Owusu-Ofori S, Riddington C. Splenectomy versus conservative management for acute sequestration crises in people with sickle cell disease. Cochrane Database Syst Rev 2002;4:CD003425.

[27] Svarch E, Vilorio P, Nordet I, et al. Partial splenectomy in children with sickle cell disease and repeated episodes of splenic sequestration. Hemoglobin 1996;20(4):393–400.

[28] Buchanan GR, Debaun MR, Quinn CT, et al. Sickle cell disease. Hematology (Am Soc Hematol Educ Program) 2004;35–47.

[29] Vichinsky EP, Neumayr LD, Earles AN, et al. Causes and outcomes of the acute chest syndrome in sickle cell disease: National Acute Chest Syndrome Study Group. N Engl J Med 2000;342(25):1855–65.

[30] Emre U, Miller ST, Gutierez M, et al. Effect of transfusion in acute chest syndrome of sickle cell disease. J Pediatr 1995;127(6):901–4.

[31] Platt OS, Brambilla DJ, Rosse WF, et al. Mortality in sickle cell disease: life expectancy and risk factors for early death. N Engl J Med 1994;330(23):1639–44.

[32] Lombardo T, Rosso R, La Ferla A, et al. Acute chest syndrome: the role of erythro-exchange in patients with sickle cell disease in Sicily. Transfus Apheresis Sci 2003;29(1):39–44.

[33] Davies SC, Luce PJ, Win AA, et al. Acute chest syndrome in sickle-cell disease. Lancet 1984;1(8367):36–8.

[34] Styles LA, Aarsman AJ, Vichinsky EP, et al. Secretory phospholipase A(2) predicts impending acute chest syndrome in sickle cell disease. Blood 2000;96(9):3276–8.

[35] Sakhalkar VS, Rao SP, Weedon J, et al. Elevated plasma sVCAM-1 levels in children with sickle cell disease: impact of chronic transfusion therapy. Am J Hematol 2004;76(1): 57–60.

[36] Kirkham FJ, DeBaun MR. Stroke in children with sickle cell disease. Curr Treat Options Neurol 2004;6(5):357–75.

[37] Dickerhoff R, Pongratz E, Scheel-Walter HG. [Cerebral infarct and hemorrhage in patients with sickle cell disease]. Klin Padiatr 1994;206(5):381–4 [in German].

[38] Nahavandi M, Tavakkoli F, Hasan SP, et al. Cerebral oximetry in patients with sickle cell disease. Eur J Clin Invest 2004;34(2):143–8.

[39] Ohene-Frempong K, Weiner SJ, Sleeper LA, et al. Cerebrovascular accidents in sickle cell disease: rates and risk factors. Blood 1998;91(1):288–94.

[40] Jones A, Granger S, Brambilla D, et al. Can peak systolic velocities be used for prediction of stroke in sickle cell anemia? Pediatr Radiol 2005;35(1):66–72.

[41] Dabrow MB, Wilkins JC. Hematologic emergencies: management of transfusion reactions and crises in sickle cell disease. Postgrad Med 1993;93(5):183–90.

[42] Hassell KL, Eckman JR, Lane PA. Acute multiorgan failure syndrome: a potentially catastrophic complication of severe sickle cell pain episodes. Am J Med 1994;96(2): 155–62.

[43] Perronne V, Roberts-Harewood M, Bachir D, et al. Patterns of mortality in sickle cell disease in adults in France and England. Hematol J 2002;3(1):56–60.

[44] Green M, Hall RJ, Huntsman RG, et al. Sickle cell crisis treated by exchange transfusion: treatment of two patients with heterozygous sickle cell syndrome. JAMA 1975;231(9): 948–50.

[45] Vichinsky EP, Neumayr LD, Haberkern C, et al. The perioperative complication rate of orthopedic surgery in sickle cell disease: report of the National Sickle Cell Surgery Study Group. Am J Hematol 1999;62(3):129–38.

[46] Koshy M, Weiner SJ, Miller ST, et al. Surgery and anesthesia in sickle cell disease: Cooperative Study of Sickle Cell Diseases. Blood 1995;86(10):3676–84.

[47] Janik J, Seeler RA. Perioperative management of children with sickle hemoglobinopathy. J Pediatr Surg 1980;15(2):117–20.

[48] Ould Amar AK, Delattre O, Godbille C, et al. [Assessment of the use of transfusion therapy and complications in orthopedic surgery in patients with sickle-cell anemia: retrospective study]. Transfus Clin Biol 2003;10(2):61–6 [in French].

[49] Haberkern CM, Neumayr LD, Orringer EP, et al. Cholecystectomy in sickle cell anemia patients: perioperative outcome of 364 cases from the National Preoperative Transfusion Study. Preoperative Transfusion in Sickle Cell Disease Study Group. Blood 1997;89(5): 1533–42.

[50] Vichinsky EP, Haberkern CM, Neumayr L, et al. A comparison of conservative and aggressive transfusion regimens in the perioperative management of sickle cell disease: The Preoperative Transfusion in Sickle Cell Disease Study Group. N Engl J Med 1995; 333(4):206–13.

[51] Powars DR. Sickle cell anemia and major organ failure. Hemoglobin 1990;14(6): 573–98.

[52] Powars DR, Meiselman HJ, Fisher TC, et al. Beta-S gene cluster haplotypes modulate hematologic and hemorheologic expression in sickle cell anemia: use in predicting clinical severity. Am J Pediatr Hematol Oncol 1994;16(1):55–61.

[53] Powars D, Wilson B, Imbus C, et al. The natural history of stroke in sickle cell disease. Am J Med 1978;65(3):461–71.

[54] Dreyer ZE. Chest infections and syndromes in sickle cell disease of childhood. Semin Respir Infect 1996;11(3):163–72.

[55] Adams RJ, McKie VC, Brambilla D, et al. Stroke prevention trial in sickle cell anemia. Control Clin Trials 1998;19(1):110–29.

[56] Adams RJ, McKie VC, Hsu L, et al. Prevention of a first stroke by transfusions in children with sickle cell anemia and abnormal results on transcranial Doppler ultrasonography. N Engl J Med 1998;339(1):5–11.

[57] Adams RJ, Brambilla DJ, Granger S, et al. Stroke and conversion to high risk in children screened with transcranial Doppler ultrasound during the STOP study. Blood 2004; 103(10):3689–94.

[58] Miller ST, Macklin EA, Pegelow CH, et al. Silent infarction as a risk factor for overt stroke in children with sickle cell anemia: a report from the Cooperative Study of Sickle Cell Disease. J Pediatr 2001;139(3):385–90.

[59] Cohen AR, Martin MB, Silber JH, et al. A modified transfusion program for prevention of stroke in sickle cell disease. Blood 1992;79(7):1657–61.

[60] Wang WC, Kovnar EH, Tonkin IL, et al. High risk of recurrent stroke after discontinuance of five to twelve years of transfusion therapy in patients with sickle cell disease. J Pediatr 1991;118(3):377–82.

[61] Riddington C, Wang W. Blood transfusion for preventing stroke in people with sickle cell disease. Cochrane Database Syst Rev 2002;1:CD003146.

[62] Fauroux B, Muller MH, Quinet B, et al. [The sickle cell anemia lung from childhood to adulthood]. Rev Mal Respir 1998;15(2):159–68 [in French].

[63] Vichinsky EP. Pulmonary hypertension in sickle cell disease. N Engl J Med 2004; 350(9):857–9.

[64] Gladwin MT, Sachdev V, Jison ML, et al. Pulmonary hypertension as a risk factor for death in patients with sickle cell disease. N Engl J Med 2004;350(9):886–95.

[65] Miller ST, Wright E, Abboud M, et al. Impact of chronic transfusion on incidence of pain and acute chest syndrome during the Stroke Prevention Trial (STOP) in sickle-cell anemia. J Pediatr 2001;139(6):785–9.

[66] Emond AM, Holman R, Hayes RJ, et al. Priapism and impotence in homozygous sickle cell disease. Arch Intern Med 1980;140(11):1434–7.

[67] Fowler Jr JE, Koshy M, Strub M, et al. Priapism associated with the sickle cell hemoglobinopathies: prevalence, natural history and sequelae. J Urol 1991;145(1):65–8.

[68] Mantadakis E, Cavender JD, Rogers ZR, et al. Prevalence of priapism in children and adolescents with sickle cell anemia. J Pediatr Hematol Oncol 1999;21(6):518–22.

[69] Okpala I, Westerdale N, Jegede T, et al. Etilefrine for the prevention of priapism in adult sickle cell disease. Br J Haematol 2002;118(3):918–21.

[70] Sharpsteen Jr JR, Powars D, Johnson C, et al. Multisystem damage associated with tricorporal priapism in sickle cell disease. Am J Med 1993;94(3):289–95.

[71] Walker Jr EM, Mitchum EN, Rous SN, et al. Automated erythrocytapheresis for relief of priapism in sickle cell hemoglobinopathies. J Urol 1983;130(5):912–6.

[72] Campbell LC, Von Burton G, Holcombe RF. Transfusion therapy in sickle cell disease patients: methods and acute indications. J La State Med Soc 1993;145(12):515–21.

[73] Danielson CF. The role of red blood cell exchange transfusion in the treatment and prevention of complications of sickle cell disease. Ther Apher 2002;6(1):24–31.

[74] McCarthy LJ, Vattuone J, Weidner J, et al. Do automated red cell exchanges relieve priapism in patients with sickle cell anemia? Ther Apher 2000;4(3):256–8.

[75] Howard RJ, Tuck SM, Pearson TC. Pregnancy in sickle cell disease in the UK: results of a multicentre survey of the effect of prophylactic blood transfusion on maternal and fetal outcome. Br J Obstet Gynaecol 1995;102(12):947–51.

[76] Moussaoui DR, Chouhou L, Guelzim K, et al. [Severe sickle cell disease and pregnancy: systematic prophylactic transfusions in 16 cases]. Med Trop (Mars) 2002;62(6):603–6 [in French].

[77] Cunningham FG, Pritchard JA, Mason R. Pregnancy and sickle cell hemoglobinopathies: results with and without prophylactic transfusions. Obstet Gynecol 1983;62(4): 419–24.

[78] Morrison JC, Schneider JM, Whybrew WD, et al. Prophylactic transfusions in pregnant patients with sickle hemoglobinopathies: benefit versus risk. Obstet Gynecol 1980; 56(3):274–80.

[79] Koshy M, Chisum D, Burd L, et al. Management of sickle cell anemia and pregnancy. J Clin Apheresis 1991;6(4):230–3.

[80] Mahomed K. Prophylactic versus selective blood transfusion for sickle cell anaemia during pregnancy. Cochrane Database Syst Rev 2000;2:CD000040.

[81] Koshy M, Entsuah R, Koranda A, et al. Leg ulcers in patients with sickle cell disease. Blood 1989;74(4):1403–8.

[82] Mohan JS, Marshall JM, Reid HL, et al. Postural vasoconstriction and leg ulceration in homozygous sickle cell disease. Clin Sci (Lond) 1997;92(2):153–8.

[83] Adedeji MO, Ukoli FA. Haematological factors associated with leg ulcer in sickle cell disease. Trop Geogr Med 1987;39(4):354–6.

[84] Bachir D, Galacteros F. [Potential alternatives to erythrocyte transfusion in hemoglobinopathies: hydroxyurea (HU), erythropoietin (EPO), butyrate derivatives, blood substitutes]. Transfus Clin Biol 1994;1(1):35–9 [in French].

[85] Chaine B, Neonato MG, Girot R, et al. Cutaneous adverse reactions to hydroxyurea in patients with sickle cell disease. Arch Dermatol 2001;137(4):467–70.

[86] de Montalembert M, Begue P, Bernaudin F, et al. Preliminary report of a toxicity study of hydroxyurea in sickle cell disease: French Study Group on Sickle Cell Disease. Arch Dis Child 1999;81(5):437–9.

[87] De Montalembert M, Girot R, Boiteux F, et al. [Long-term blood transfusion in sickle-cell anemia]. Arch Fr Pediatr 1987;44(5):349–54 [in French].

[88] Rao AK, Thompson R, Durlacher L, et al. Angiographic contrast agent-induced acute hemolysis in a patient with hemoglobin SC disease. Arch Intern Med 1985;145(4): 759–60.

[89] Banna M. Post-angiographic blindness in a patient with sickle cell disease. Invest Radiol 1992;27(2):179–81.

[90] Gulley ML, Ross DW, Feo C, et al. The effect of cell hydration on the deformability of normal and sickle erythrocytes. Am J Hematol 1982;13(4):283–91.

[91] Losco P, Nash G, Stone P, et al. Comparison of the effects of radiographic contrast media on dehydration and filterability of red blood cells from donors homozygous for hemoglobin A or hemoglobin S. Am J Hematol 2001;68(3):149–58.

[92] Vichinsky EP. Current issues with blood transfusions in sickle cell disease. Semin Hematol 2001;38(Suppl 1):14–22.

[93] Castro O, Sandler SG, Houston-Yu P, et al. Predicting the effect of transfusing only phenotype-matched RBCs to patients with sickle cell disease: theoretical and practical implications. Transfusion 2002;42(6):684–90.

[94] Talano JA, Hillery CA, Gottschall JL, et al. Delayed hemolytic transfusion reaction/ hyperhemolysis syndrome in children with sickle cell disease. Pediatrics 2003;111(6 Pt 1): e661–5.

[95] Sosler SD, Jilly BJ, Saporito C, et al. A simple, practical model for reducing alloimmunization in patients with sickle cell disease. Am J Hematol 1993;43(2):103–6.

[96] Cox JV, Steane E, Cunningham G, et al. Risk of alloimmunization and delayed hemolytic transfusion reactions in patients with sickle cell disease. Arch Intern Med 1988; 148(11):2485–9.

[97] Honig CL, Bove JR. Transfusion-associated fatalities: review of Bureau of Biologics reports 1976–1978. Transfusion 1980;20(6):653–61.

[98] Kalyanaraman M, Heidemann SM, Sarnaik AP, et al. Anti-s antibody-associated delayed hemolytic transfusion reaction in patients with sickle cell anemia. J Pediatr Hematol Oncol 1999;21(1):70–3.

[99] Mintz PD, Williams ME. Cerebrovascular accident during a delayed hemolytic transfusion reaction in a patient with sickle cell anemia. Ann Clin Lab Sci 1986;16(3):214–8.

[100] Rao KR, Patel AR. Delayed hemolytic transfusion reactions in sickle cell anemia. South Med J 1989;82(8):1034–6.

[101] Diamond WJ, Brown Jr FL, Bitterman P, Klein HG, et al. Delayed hemolytic transfusion reaction presenting as sickle-cell crisis. Ann Intern Med 1980;93(2):231–4.

[102] Fabron Jr A, Moreira Jr G, Bordin JO. Delayed hemolytic transfusion reaction presenting as a painful crisis in a patient with sickle cell anemia. Sao Paulo Med J 1999; 117(1):38–9.

[103] Cullis JO, Win N, Dudley JM, et al. Post-transfusion hyperhaemolysis in a patient with sickle cell disease: use of steroids and intravenous immunoglobulin to prevent further red cell destruction. Vox Sang 1995;69(4):355–7.

[104] Telen MJ, Combs M. Management of massive delayed hemolytic transfusion reaction in patients with sickle cell disease. Transfusion 1999;39(Suppl):97.

[105] Win N, Doughty H, Telfer P, et al. Hyperhemolytic transfusion reaction in sickle cell disease. Transfusion 2001;41(3):323–8.

[106] al-Fawaz I, Ramia S. Decline in hepatitis B infection in sickle cell anaemia and beta thalassaemia major. Arch Dis Child 1993;69(5):594–6.

[107] Hasan MF, Marsh F, Posner G, et al. Chronic hepatitis C in patients with sickle cell disease. Am J Gastroenterol 1996;91(6):1204–6.

[108] Norol F, Bachir D, Bernaudin F, et al. Frozen blood and transfusion-transmitted hepatitis C virus. Vox Sang 1993;64(3):150–3.

[109] Hassan M, Hasan S, Castro O, et al. HCV in sickle cell disease. J Natl Med Assoc 2003;95(9):864–7, 872–4.

[110] Ballas SK. Iron overload is a determinant of morbidity and mortality in adult patients with sickle cell disease. Semin Hematol 2001;38(Suppl 1):30–6.

[111] Brittenham GM, Sheth S, Allen CJ, et al. Noninvasive methods for quantitative assessment of transfusional iron overload in sickle cell disease. Semin Hematol 2001;38(Suppl 1): 37–56.

[112] Kwiatkowski JL, Cohen AR. Iron chelation therapy in sickle-cell disease and other transfusion-dependent anemias. Hematol Oncol Clin North Am 2004;18(6):1355–77.

[113] Wong WY. Prevention and management of infection in children with sickle cell anaemia. Paediatr Drugs 2001;3(11):793–801.

[114] Pierron H, Gillet R, Perrimond H, et al. [Yersinia infection and hemoglobin disorder: apropos of 4 cases]. Pediatrie 1990;45(6):379–82 [in French].

[115] Vichinsky EP, Luban NL, Wright E, et al. Prospective RBC phenotype matching in a stroke-prevention trial in sickle cell anemia: a multicenter transfusion trial. Transfusion 2001; 41(9):1086–92.

[116] Tahhan HR, Holbrook CT, Braddy LR, et al. Antigen-matched donor blood in the transfusion management of patients with sickle cell disease. Transfusion 1994;34(7): 562–9.

[117] Osby M, Shulman IA. Phenotype matching of donor red blood cell units for non-alloimmunized sickle cell disease patients: a survey of 1182 North American laboratories. Arch Pathol Lab Med 2005;129(2):190–3.

[118] Castilho L, Rios M, Bianco C, et al. DNA-based typing of blood groups for the management of multiply-transfused sickle cell disease patients. Transfusion 2002;42(2): 232–8.

Hematol Oncol Clin N Am 19 (2005) 827–837

HEMATOLOGY/ONCOLOGY CLINICS
OF NORTH AMERICA

Arterial Blood Pressure and Hyperviscosity in Sickle Cell Disease

Cage S. Johnson, MD

Comprehensive Sickle Cell Center, Keck School of Medicine, University of Southern California, RMR 304, 2025 Zonal Avenue, Los Angeles, CA 90033, USA

Abnormal rheologic behavior of sickle cells is the result of increased viscosity of the blood caused by the polymerization of hemoglobin S (HbS) and the resultant production of dense, dehydrated sickle erythrocytes. As the viscosity of sickle cells increases, there is a negative impact on blood flow, which contributes to the vascular occlusion process, the hallmark of the sickling disorders. Blood flow is directly proportional to the blood pressure and inversely proportional to the blood viscosity. Blood flow has important implications for the diagnosis and management of hypertension in sickle cell patients and for transfusion therapy for the acute and chronic complications of this disease.

ARTERIAL BLOOD PRESSURE REGULATION

Control of arterial blood pressure involves a series of complex interactions between the heart, kidneys, vascular endothelium, and the central and peripheral nervous systems. In brief, the arterial blood pressure is continuously monitored and regulated by sensors throughout the body to maintain blood flow to critical organs (central nervous system, heart, lungs) at the relative expense of less critical organs (skin, muscle, kidneys). Blood pressure is primarily a function of the cardiac output and total peripheral resistance. Peripheral resistance is important to blood pressure regulation because of its effect on blood flow and venous return to the heart [1]. The relationships between blood flow, blood pressure, and vascular resistance are described in the Hagen-Poiseuille equation [2]:

$$Q = \frac{\Delta P \pi R^4}{8 L \eta}$$

where blood flow (Q) is directly proportional to the pressure gradient (ΔP) between the arterial and venous pressures, but is inversely proportional to the

This work was supported by National Institutes of Health grants HL 15162, HL 48484, and HL 070595.
E-mail address: cagejohn@email.usc.edu

peripheral resistance. Resistance is determined by the length (L) and radius (R) of the blood vessels and by the viscosity (η) of the blood. Thus, flow is directly proportional to the pressure and inversely proportional to the viscosity.

Short-term control of blood pressure is maintained by baroreceptors in the heart and great vessels, which signal via central integration at the dorsal medulla oblongata through sympathetic and parasympathetic nerve pathways to the heart blood vessels (vasoconstriction and dilation). These baroreceptors sense changes in arterial pressure and in pressure and volume changes in the atria and the central venous blood volume. Acute changes in blood pressure alter the balance between sympathetic and parasympathetic activity. A decrease in blood pressure causes an increase in sympathetic activity, and a reciprocal decrease in parasympathetic tone, in an effort to return the blood pressure to normal. Stimulation of sympathetic activity increases arteriolar tone, which increases peripheral resistance by vasoconstriction. Sympathetic activity further affects the blood pressure by increasing both heart rate and stroke volume, thus increasing the cardiac output. Stroke volume is increased via increased venous tone and increased fluid resorption, which leads to increases in blood volume and blood return to the heart. An increase in blood pressure has the opposite effect [3,4].

Long-term regulation of blood pressure is primarily accomplished by changes in renal blood flow that are modulated by hormonal mechanisms through renal control of blood volume. Low blood pressure causes an increase in renal vascular resistance, which results in a decrease in renal blood flow, an increase in fluid resorption, and a decrease in urine output. Increasing fluid resorption restores the blood volume and blood pressure. When osmoreceptors in the hypothalamus are stimulated, Vasopressin, (antidiuretic hormone, ADH) is released from the anterior pituitary, which regulates water resorption from the collecting ducts. ADH is also regulated by the atrial stretch reflex. The renin-angiotensin system is further regulated by the kidney in response to alterations in blood pressure or renal blood flow. The juxta-glomerular apparatus senses changes in blood pressure or renal blood flow, and secretes renin in response to changes. Renin cleaves circulating angiotensinogen to anigiotensin I, which is further cleaved by an angiotensin-converting enzyme (ACE) in the lungs to angiotensin II. Anigiotensin II causes constriction of small arteries and arterioles to increase peripheral resistance and aldosterone secretion by the adrenal gland; aldosterone increases sodium and water retention by the kidneys, thereby increasing blood volume and ultimately blood pressure [5,6]. Other components are important in blood pressure control. Endothelin is the most potent endogenous vasoconstrictor and works in concert with angiotensin II to regulate vascular tone [7]. Nitric oxide (NO) is a potent vasodilator produced by the endothelium from the amino acid, L-arginine, via NO synthase, and plays a vital role in the maintenance of blood pressure [8].

BLOOD PRESSURE

In sickle cell disease, as in other chronic anemias, the cardiac output is increased because of an increase in stroke volume. The blood volume is increased because of an increase in plasma volume, and the total peripheral resistance is decreased. However, these changes are more profound in sickle cell disease than in other anemias [9]. A sustained increase in blood volume or cardiac output is expected to increase blood pressure unless peripheral resistance falls, as indicated in the Hagen-Poiseuille equation. Moreover, with correction of the anemia, the blood pressure rises, sometimes to hypertensive levels. The peripheral resistance rises, as does the blood viscosity, and both are likely responsible for the increase in blood pressure. In patients who have sickle cell disease, endothelin levels [10] and NO metabolites are increased, which suggests increased catabolism and possible depletion of NO in this disease [11]. Taken together, these findings predict that an elevated blood pressure might be expected in sickle cell disease.

However, studies reported from Los Angeles on the arterial blood pressure in 187 adult patients [12] showed that, when compared with age- and sex-matched African American controls taken from national databases, individuals who had a sickling disease had significantly lower blood pressures than controls. In addition, the trend of blood pressure rising with age was not seen. Moreover, the number of sickle cell patients who had hypertension (3.2%) was significantly lower than the usual 29% in the control population. These findings, although unexpected, were subsequently confirmed by studies from Jamaica and the Netherlands. In Jamaica [13], blood pressure in 64 adult subjects who had sickle cell anemia and normal serum creatinine levels were significantly lower than controls. Elevation of blood pressure occurred only in subjects with renal insufficiency and was mild. Data from the Netherlands [14] on 81 adults who had a sickling disease revealed generally lower values for blood pressure in most age groups. Further examination of this phenomenon in a large group of adolescents in Jamaica [15], showed that the blood pressure effect was present in patients younger than age 20 who had sickle cell anemia but not sickle C disease, and that the blood pressure difference could be explained by differences in weight. Similar findings have been reported from Turkey and Nigeria [16,17]. The coinheritance of α- thalassemia with sickle cell disease appears to reduce blood pressure in sickle cell disease, as well as possibly protect against proteinuria. More importantly, this study confirmed the association between elevated blood pressure and both proteinuria and renal insufficiency [18].

The Cooperative Study of Sickle Cell Disease examined this issue in 3317 subjects who had a sickling disease who ranged in age from 5 years to 45 years; measurements averaged 6.5 per subject [19]. Researchers detected a significantly lower blood pressure for sickle cell anemia in nearly all age ranges except for some older children and adolescent subgroups. In this large study, they were able to detect small but significant positive correlations with age and body mass index, and a negative correlation with estimated glomerular filtration rate. In patients over age 18, the frequency of elevated systolic or diastolic pressure was approximately 6%. More importantly, this study showed (1) a decrease in survival for those with the highest blood pressures, (2) a positive association of systolic blood pressure with stroke, and (3) data on blood pressure by age and gender (Table 1). Another study from Washington, DC, [20] compared patients

Table 1
Blood pressure ≥90th percentile for age and gender in sickle cell disease

Age (y)	Blood pressure (systolic/diastolic)	
	Females	Males
2–3	100/62	104/66
4–5	110/70	110/68
6–7	110/70	108/68
8–9	110/70	116/70
10–11	110/74	112/70
12–13	118/74	120/72
14–15	120/80	120/78
16–17	122/78	128/80
18–24	122/80	130/80
25–34	125/80	130/80
35–44	130/84	132/84

Data from Pegelow CH, Colangelo L, Steinberg M, et al. Natural history of blood pressure in sickle cell disease: risks for stroke and death associated with relative hypertension in sickle cell anemia. Am J Med 1997;102:171–7.

who had sickle cell anemia and β-thalassemia and found that the blood pressure was lower in both groups than in controls, but noted that the β-thalassemia group was lower than the sickle cell anemia group, even though the thalassemia patients had higher hemoglobin. They attributed this difference to the elevated blood viscosity for hematocrit typical of sickle cell disease.

HYPOTHESES

It has been suggested that natriuresis and hyposthenuria, which cause blunting of a maximal plasma volume increase, are the reasons for the blood pressure observations in those patients who have sickle cell disease [12]. Since about half of the people who have sickle cell trait have hyposthenuria and an increased ADH response, one might expect blood pressures in these individuals to be lower than usual. However, studies from Columbia [21] and Nigeria [22,23] have shown no difference between subjects who had sickle cell trait and controls. Intravenous sodium loading has not shown any effect on blood pressure in subjects who have sickle cell disease [24], although the absence of sodium retention did not suggest a sustained rise in plasma volume as might have been seen in an albumin or plasma infusion. Prostaglandin stimulation by the ischemic medulla has been proposed as being responsible for the blood pressure findings [14]. However, prostaglandins are rapidly cleared from systemic circulation by the lungs and unlikely to exert any systemic effect. Moreover, when administered indomethacin, the blood pressure did not change in those patients who have sickle cell disease [25].

Plasma renin activity is significantly higher in sickling diseases than in controls, but serum catecholamine levels are normal [24]. Plasma renin activity increased with sodium restriction, as expected, but did not affect blood pressure. The pressor response to graded infusions of angiotensin II for sickle cell patients was significantly less than for controls, but the pressor response to norepinephrine, although lower, was not significantly different from controls. These findings were interpreted to indicate tachyphylaxis. The insensitivity to the pressor response of angiotensin II and to norepinephrine suggests that receptors for these molecules are not readily available. Alternatively, NO could counteract the effects of pressor agents. NO is synthesized in endothelial cells from L-arginine by NO synthase and has multiple effects relevant to sickle cell disease. It inhibits platelet aggregation and vascular cell adhesion molecule-1 expression, it ameliorates ischemia-reperfusion injury, and it is a potent vasodilator. NO concentrations are increased by anemia and decreased by free intravascular hemoglobin, superoxide, and arginine deficiency [11]. There is considerable interest in the possible role of NO in pulmonary hypertension in sickle cell disease.

In chronic anemia, increased cardiac output and rapid flow—with its lowered hemoglobin level—might not pick up all available NO, although some NO would be scavenged by free hemoglobin. Consequently, there would be a relative excess of NO available to the vasculature for vasodilation. There are considerable data in support of this hypothesis from animal studies in which infusions of stroma-free hemoglobin solutions, developed as blood substitutes, led to occurrences of systemic hypertension and mortality related to scavenging of NO by free hemoglobin molecules [26,27].

ELEVATED BLOOD PRESSURE

Pain has a variable effect on blood pressure. Superficial or cutaneous pain may raise the blood pressure, whereas deep pain may cause diminished sympathetic tone and reduce blood pressure. In a study of eight patients from St. George's Hospital, heart rate and mean arterial pressure were slightly, but not significantly, higher at the start of a crisis compared with steady state values [28]. Data from New Orleans on 459 episodes of acute pain in 106 patients were compared with data from 100 African American patients without hypertension seen in the emergency department [29]. Again, the blood pressure was significantly lower in the group that had sickling diseases than in the control group, as was the frequency of hypertension (1% versus 20%). Those with unilateral pain had significantly higher systolic blood pressure than those with bilateral pain, but no explanation was offered.

Elevations of blood pressure in the 140/90 range or greater are almost always associated with renal disease, either proteinuria or renal insufficiency, and should prompt an assessment of renal function [18,30]. Elevation of blood pressure also may be associated with stroke [19,20]. Most importantly, those patients who have blood pressure at or above the 90th percentile have shortened survival [19]. Finally, abrupt elevation of blood pressure is an important sign of the hyperviscosity syndrome that follows transfusion.

TREATMENT OF HYPERTENSION

Currently there is no evidence-based data to guide clinicians in the selection of drugs or their timing in management of arterial hypertension in sickle cell patients. Based upon extrapolation from other patient populations and on data from the Cooperative Study of Sickle Cell Disease (see Table 1), therapy should be considered whenever blood pressure is >130/80, blood pressure rises 15 to 20 mm Hg from baseline, or blood pressure is >120/75 in the presence of proteinuria. Alternatively, one may treat all patients with proteinuria in excess of 300 mg/24 h [19]. Use of an ACE inhibitor has the dual benefit of blood pressure control and reduction of proteinuria, which delays the progression of renal insufficiency and prolongs the time to dialysis [18,31–33]. Potential adverse effects in these patients include hyper-kalemia, which may be spurious because of potassium release from high platelet counts. Calcium channel blockers require dose adjustments for hepatic and renal disease, which are common in these patients. Therapy with a β-blocker can be effective but may exacerbate bronchial asthma, which is also common in these patients. Diuretic therapy, increasing urine volume in patients who have hyposthenuria, has the disadvantage of dehydration and requires careful dose adjustment.

WHOLE BLOOD VISCOSITY

The whole blood viscosity is a function of both the number of erythrocytes and their deformability and of the plasma proteins. In sickle cell disease the viscosity is dominated by HbS gelation and the presence of dense sickle cells [2]. At a hematocrit of 25%, the viscosity is only slightly lower than that of normal blood which has a hematocrit of 45% [34,35]. Upon deoxygenation below 85%, the viscosity of sickle blood rises sharply, because of the polymerization of deoxy-HbS [34,35]. In sickle cell disease, anemia can be considered to be partially protective of microcirculatory flow because the blood viscosity is reduced, as indicated in the Hagen-Poiseuille equation. The anemia is supplemented by the known decrease in oxygen affinity and by the increase in cardiac output, which maintain efficient oxygen transport (see the article by Johnson elsewhere in this issue for further exploration of this topic). Elevation of the hematocrit by transfusion, which is now used in a growing number of clinical situations, can increase viscosity and upset this balance, resulting in hyperviscosity and clinical deterioration (see the article by Wanko and Telen elsewhere in this issue for further exploration of this topic). In anemia, oxygen transport increases with transfusion up to a hematocrit of 40%–45%. Above a hematocrit of 45%, the viscosity increases and oxygen transport begin to decline. Cardiac output and coronary blood flow begin to decrease at hematocrits above 45% as resistance to flow increases [36]. A 50% increase in blood viscosity increases total peripheral resistance by 75% and reduces flow unless the pressure rises to compensate [36,37].

HYPERVISCOSITY SYNDROME

The hyperviscosity syndrome in hemoglobinopathies was first described from Bangkok in eight thalassemia patients undergoing simple transfusion [38]. Patients developed significant increases in blood pressure, convulsions, and cerebral hemorrhage; three of these patients died. Blood pressure greater than 160/90 was seen in 6 of the 8 patients, whereas blood pressure had been below 122/80 before transfusion. Post-transfusion hematocrits ranged from 20% to 40%; most were greater than 33%. This complication was subsequently reported in sickle cell patients receiving simple or partial exchange transfusions. Two patients reported from Chicago developed a ≥20 mm rise in blood pressure several days after transfusion to hematocrits of 38% and 40% with symptoms of headache, altered mental status, and seizure; spinal fluid showed erythrocytes consistent with cerebral hemorrhage [39]. In Philadelphia, six patients underwent partial exchange transfusion for priapism and developed headaches, seizures, and increased intracranial pressure at post-transfusion hemoglobins of 10.5 to 13.4 g/dL, despite HbS levels of 33% or less; blood pressures were not reported [40]. Charache and colleagues [41] reported an interesting case of carbon monoxide poisoning in a sickle cell patient whose hemoglobin rose from a baseline of ~9.0 g/dL to 15.5 g/dL. When the carboxy-hemoglobin declined under treatment, the patient developed bizarre behavior and sustained a cardiac arrest. At autopsy, the organs were edematous and congested. These authors calculated the whole blood viscosity for sickle cells at a hematocrit of 40% as equivalent to normal blood at a hematocrit of 70%. Another case was reported by Lee and Chu [42] in which transfusion was given for hepatic sequestration. Four days after the last transfusion, there was an abrupt rise in hemoglobin from 5 g/dL to 12.4 g/dL associated with abrupt onset of hypertension, congestive heart failure, and cerebral hemorrhage. These authors postulated that the hyperviscosity syndrome was caused by a reversal of the sequestration process and return of erythrocytes into the circulation.

This post-transfusion hyperviscosity syndrome is characterized by the sudden onset of elevated blood pressure during or shortly after transfusion, in conjunction with signs of congestive heart failure and profound alterations in mental status, including stupor, coma, or features of intra-cerebral infarct or hemorrhage. The cerebral circulation is particularly sensitive to the pressure and flow relationships illustrated in the Hagen- Poiseuille equation. When studied by positron emission tomography, cerebral blood flow and cerebral blood volume in sickle cell disease are higher than controls by a factor of 1.5 and vary inversely with the degree of anemia [43]. The higher blood flow permits adequate oxygen extraction. However, when cerebral blood flow decreases in relation to tissue oxygen requirements, the fractional oxygen extraction can increase from 35%–45% to more than 90% [43]. Under conditions of low flow and increased oxygen extraction, polymerization of HbS is favored. It is likely that the intracerebral blood viscosity rises to levels that cause blood flow to be essentially stationary, despite dramatic blood pressure increases and the fact that near cessation of flow is the probable cause of the CNS symptoms. Treatment of acute hyperviscosity entails emergent venesection and volume replacement with saline, or immediate exchange transfusion.

Post-transfusion hyperviscosity syndrome is attributed to an increase in whole blood viscosity, caused by the increased hematocrit of mixed sickle (SS) and normal (AA) erythrocytes (red blood cells), which causes a reduction in blood flow. Early rheologic studies of sickle cell patients undergoing transfusion revealed that post-transfusion blood viscosity was higher than that of normal blood for the same hematocrit, consistent with the known effect of the residual sickle cells on viscosity [44]. Moreover, the venous pO_2, a measure of effective oxygen delivery, rose with transfusion up to hematocrits of 30%–35% and fell at higher hematocrits, consistent with the hypothesis that blood flow and oxygen delivery decreased as the viscosity increased beyond a threshold value. Consequently, transfusion to a hemoglobin/hematocrit no greater than 11/35 became the standard recommendation.

Further studies of mixtures of SS and AA erythrocytes confirmed the prior observations that the blood viscosity increases with hematocrit and with the percentage of sickle cells, especially at hematocrits greater than 30%, and that these effects are exaggerated by hypoxia [45]. In this study, the ratio of hematocrit to viscosity was used as an approximation of oxygen transport effectiveness, and this analysis shows that the viscosity rises faster then the hematocrit increase, consistent with the oxygen transport effectiveness model. Moreover, the presence of sickle cells accentuates the viscosity rise as hematocrit increases. The study by Schmalzer and colleagues [45] used erythrocytes suspended in buffer to avoid red cell agglutination in plasma at low shear as a confounding factor. Additional studies of mixtures of SS and AA red blood cells in autologous plasma have addressed the issue of low shear viscosity, which is relevant to blood flow in the microcirculation in sickle cell disease (Alexy et al, submitted for publication, 2005). For AA erythrocytes in plasma, the hematocrit-to-viscosity ratio provides additional support for optimum oxygen transport effectiveness at hematocrits of 40%–45% at high shear. However, for these normal cells, there was no optimum hematocrit at low shear because viscosity continued to increase as hematocrit increased. In this study of mixtures of SS and AA red blood cells at high shear, there was an optimal hematocrit of 30%–35% under both oxygenated and de-oxygenated (37 torr) conditions, with the fraction of SS cells as high as 50%. However, as with normal cells, there is no optimum hematocrit at low shear. Although these studies provide partial support for the standard transfusion recommendation, it is clear that the fraction of sickle cells has a disproportional effect on blood viscosity at low shear. Consequently, in clinical situations where diminished flow and stasis are present, as in vaso-occlusive episodes, the optimal hematocrit may be influenced by the fraction of sickle cells as well as the prevailing shear rates in the relevant organ or tissue. Thus, for tissues with low oxygen tension and low perfusion pressure, the native hematocrit might represent the optimal value, and simple transfusion might fail to improve or even worsen oxygen transport. This is consistent with observations that transfusion is not helpful in acute sickle pain and post-transfusion hematocrits as low as 34% can be detrimental [46].

For these reasons, exchange transfusion is often preferred over simple transfusion, so as to reduce the fraction of sickle cells and maximize flow in the microcirculation.

SUMMARY

Blood viscosity is an important determinant of blood pressure and blood flow in the microcirculation. Blood pressure in patients who have sickle cell disease is lower than that in control populations, and they should be considered hypertensive and treated at blood pressures lower than those for the general population. Hypertension, when present, indicates underlying renal insufficiency or proteinuria in most instances, but is variably seen in acute pain, and is seen more often when pain is mild. Acute hypertension following transfusion signals onset of the hyperviscosity syndrome and is a medical emergency that requires immediate reduction of blood viscosity by venesection or by exchange transfusion.

References

[1] Beevers G, Lip GY, O'Brien E. ABC of hypertension: the pathophysiology of hypertension. BMJ 2001;322:912–6.

[2] Stuart J, Johnson CS. Rheology of the sickle cell disorders. Baillere's Clin Haematol 1987; 1:747–75.

[3] Laitenen T, Hartikan J, Niskane L, et al. Sympathovagal balance is a major determinant of short-term blood pressure variability in healthy subjects. Am J Physiol 1999;276: H1245–52.

[4] Parati G, Lantelme P. Mechanical and neural components of the cardiac baroreflex: new insights into complex physiology. J Hypertens 2005;23:717–20.

[5] Timmerman TB. Angiotensin II receptor antagonists: an emerging new class of cardiovascular therapeutics. Hypertens Res 1999;22:147–53.

[6] Bakris G, Burstyn M, Gavras I, et al. Role of vasopressin in essential hypertension: racial differences. Am J Hypertens 1997;15:545–50.

[7] Gardener SM, March JE, Kemp PA, et al. Cardiovascular responses to angiotensins I and II in normotensive and hypertensive rats: effects of NO synthetase inhibition or ET receptor antagonism. Br J Pharmacol 1999;128:1795–803.

[8] Moncada S, Higgs A. Mechanisms of disease: the L-arginine-nitric oxide pathway. N Engl J Med 1993;329:2002–12.

[9] Covitz W, Espeland M, Gallagher D, et al. The heart in sickle cell disease. The cooperative study of sickle cell disease (CSSCD). Chest 1995;108:1214–9.

[10] Hammerman SI, Kourembanas S, Conca TJ, et al. Endothelin-1 production during the acute chest syndrome in sickle cell disease. Am J Respir Crit Care Med 1997;156:280–5.

[11] Reiter CD, Gladwin MT. An emerging role for nitric oxide in sickle cell disease vascular homeostasis and therapy. Curr Opin Hematol 2003;10:99–107.

[12] Johnson CS, Giorgio AJ. Arterial blood pressure in adults with sickle cell disease. Arch Intern Med 1981;141:891–3.

[13] Grell GA, Alleyne GA, Serjeant GR. Blood pressure in adults with homozygous sickle cell disease. Lancet 1981;2:1166.

[14] de Jong PE, Landman H, van Eps LW. Blood pressure in sickle cell disease. Arch Intern Med 1982;142:1239–40.

[15] Homi J, Homi-Levee L, Gentles S, et al. Adolescent blood pressure in a cohort study of sickle cell disease. Arch Intern Med 1993;153:1233–6.

[16] Karayaylali I, Onal M, Yildizer K, et al. Low blood pressure, decreased incidence of hypertension, and renal cardiac, and autonomic nervous system functions in patients with sickle cell syndromes. Nephron 2002;91:535–7.

[17] Aderibigbe A, Omotoso AB, Awobusuyi JO, et al. Arterial blood pressure in adult Nigerian sickle cell anaemia patients. West Afr J Med 1999;18:114–8.

[18] Guasch A, Zayas CF, Eckman JR, et al. Evidence that microdeletions in the alpha globin

gene protect against the development of sickle cell glomerulopathy in humans. J Am Soc Nephrol 1999;10:1014–9.

[19] Pegelow CH, Colangelo L, Steinberg M, et al. Natural history of blood pressure in sickle cell disease: risks for stroke and death associated with relative hypertension in sickle cell anemia. Am J Med 1997;102:171–7.

[20] Rodgers GP, Walker EC, Podgor MJ. Is "relative" hypertension a risk factor for vaso-occlusive complications in sickle cell disease? Am J Med Sci 1993;305:150–6.

[21] Rossi-Espagnet A, Newell KW, MacLennan R, et al. The relationship of sickle cell trait to variations in blood pressure. Am J Epidemiol 1968;88:33–44.

[22] Nwankwo MU, Bunker CH, Ukoli FA, et al. Blood pressure and other cardiovascular disease risk factors in black adults with sickle cell trait or glucose-6-phosphate dehydrogenase deficiency. Genet Epidemiol 1990;7:211–8.

[23] Adams-Campbell LL, Nwankwo MU, Ukoli FA, et al. The sickle gene: a marker for blood pressure? J Natl Med Assoc 1993;85:385–7.

[24] Hatch FE, Crowe LR, Miles DE, et al. Altered vascular reactivity in sickle hemoglobinopathy. A possible protective factor from hypertension. Am J Hypertens 1989;2:2–8.

[25] de Jong PE, De Jong-van den Berg LTW, Sewrajsingh GS, et al. The influence of indomethacin on renal hemodynamics in sickle cell anaemia. Clin Sci 1980;59:245–50.

[26] Lee R, Neya K, Svizzero TA, et al. Limitations of the efficacy of hemoglobin-based oxygen-carrying solutions. J Appl Physiol 1995;79:236–42.

[27] Ulatowski JA, Nishikawa T, Matheson-Urbaitis B, et al. Regional blood flow alterations after bovine fumaryl ββ-crosslinked hemoglobin transfusion on nitric oxide synthase inhibition. Crit Care Med 1996;24:558–65.

[28] Singer M, Boghossian S, Bevan DH, et al. Hemodynamic changes during sickle cell crisis. Am J Cardiol 1989;64:1211–3.

[29] Ernst AA, Weiss SJ, Johnson WD, et al. Blood pressure in acute vaso-occlusive crises of sickle cell disease. South Med J 2000;93:590–2.

[30] Guasch A, Cua M, Mitch WE. Early detection and the course of glomerular injury in patients with sickle cell anemia. Kidney Int 1996;49:786–91.

[31] Falk RJ, Scheinman J, Phillips G, et al. Prevalence and pathologic features of sickle cell nephropathy and response to inhibition of angiotensin-converting enzyme. N Engl J Med 1992;326:910–5.

[32] Lewis EJ, Hunsicker LG, Bain RP, et al. The effect of angiotensin-converting-enzyme inhibition on diabetic nephropathy. N Engl J Med 1993;329:1456–62.

[33] Maschio G, Alberti D, Janin G, et al. Effect of the angiotensin-converting-enzyme inhibitor benazepril on the progression of chronic renal insufficiency. N Engl J Med 1996; 334:939–45.

[34] Chien S, Usami S, Bertles JF. Abnormal rheology of oxygenated blood in sickle cell anemia. J Clin Invest 1970;49:623–34.

[35] Chien S. Rheology of sickle cells and erythrocyte content. Blood Cells 1977;8:283–303.

[36] Jan K-M, Chien S. Effect of hematocrit variation on coronary hemodynamics and oxygen utilization. Am J Physiol 1977;233:H106–13.

[37] Gordon RJ, Snyder GK, Tritel H, et al. Potential significance of plasma viscosity and hematocrit variations in myocardial ischemia. Am Heart J 1974;87:175–82.

[38] Wasi P, Pootrakul P, Piankijagum A, et al. A syndrome of hypertension, convulsion, and cerebral hemorrhage in thalassemic patients after multiple blood transfusions. Lancet 1978;2:602–4.

[39] Royal JE, Seeler RA. Hypertension, convulsions and cerebral hemorrhage in sickle-cell anaemia patients after blood-transfusions. Lancet 1978;II:1207.

[40] Rackoff WR, Ohene-Frempong K, Month S, et al. Neurologic events after partial exchange transfusion for priapism in sickle cell disease. J Pediatr 1992;120:882–5.

[41] Charache S, de la Monte S, Macdonald V. Increased blood viscosity in a patient with sickle cell anemia. Blood Cells 1982;8:103–9.

[42] Lee ESH, Chu PCM. Reverse sequestration in a case of sickle cell crisis. Postgrad Med J 1996;72:487–8.

[43] Herold S, Brozovic M, Gibbs J, et al. Measurement of regional cerebral blood flow, blood volume and oxygen metabolism in patients with sickle cell disease using positron emission tomography. Stroke 1986;17:692–8.

[44] Jan K, Usami S, Smith JA. Effects of transfusion on rheological properties of blood in sickle cell anemia. Transfusion 1982;22:17–20.

[45] Schmalzer EA, Lee JO, Brown AK, et al. Viscosity of mixtures of sickle and normal red cells at varying hematocrit levels. Implications for transfusion. Transfusion 1987;27: 228–33.

[46] Serjeant GR. Blood transfusion in sickle cell disease: a cautionary tale. Lancet 2003; 361:1659–60.

Hematol Oncol Clin N Am 19 (2005) 839–855

HEMATOLOGY/ONCOLOGY CLINICS
OF NORTH AMERICA

Overt and Incomplete (Silent) Cerebral Infarction in Sickle Cell Anemia: Diagnosis and Management

Wing-Yen Wong, MD[a], Darleen R. Powars, MD[b],*

[a]*Department of Pediatrics, Division of Hematology/Oncology, Children's Hospital Los Angeles, Keck School of Medicine at the University of Southern California, Los Angeles, CA, USA*
[b]*Department of Pediatrics, Division of Hematology/Oncology, Women's & Children's Hospital, Keck School of Medicine at the University of Southern California, 1240 North Mission Road, Room L902, Los Angeles, CA 90033, USA*

Cerebral vasculopathy in sickle cell anemia (HbSS) is manifest clinically as cerebral infarction and intracranial hemorrhage. The type of stroke, ischemic or hemorrhagic, is age specific with distinct differences in outcomes. Cerebral infarction with or without clinical stroke begins during early childhood and rarely causes death immediately [1,2]. Acute intracranial hemorrhage has been associated with high immediate mortality ranging from 24% to 50% [3–5].

The authors' overall calculated incidence of first overt infarction in HbSS patients by age 20 years is 11% and by age 45 years 24%. The highest frequency occurs in children aged 2 through 5 years followed by those aged 6 to 9 years. A second peak is observed in adults greater than 20 years of age (Fig. 1). The calculated median age of onset among the authors' subjects for clinically recognized cerebral infarctions is 13.88 years (range, 1.2 to 58.18) and for intracranial hemorrhage 31.75 years (range, 4.87 to 51.5 years).

The accumulative overall risk for cerebral infarction during the patient's lifetime, including clinical events and subclinical events, has been estimated to be as high as 30% [2,6,7]. This percentage rises even further if one uses improved MRI techniques, particularly fluid-attenuated inversion recovery (FLAIR) [8]. Steen and coworkers reported that 44% of patients demonstrated infarction, ischemia, or atrophy on MRI (FLAIR) and 49% had abnormal findings on MR angiography.

During the last decade, a changing prevalence pattern has been observed, with an increasing frequency of first identified clinical neurologic events at 20 to 25 years of age. Using definitive neuroimaging techniques based on the presence of areas of cerebral atrophy or old infarcts in the border zone regions, it is clear that these patients have "silent" stroke (incomplete infarctions) [9] before overt

* Corresponding author. *E-mail address:* powars@hsc.usc.edu (D.R. Powars).

0889-8588/05/$ – see front matter
doi:10.1016/j.hoc.2005.07.006

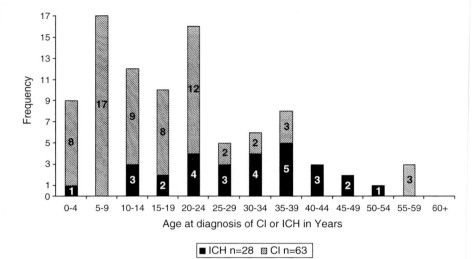

Fig. 1. Age and type of first cerebral vascular accident in hemoglobin SS subjects. The specific type of clinical stroke was identified based on neuroimaging or autopsy in 91 subjects with sickle cell anemia. Intracranial hemorrhage (ICH) was found in 28 subjects and cerebral infarction (CI) in 63. Six subjects not shown on the figure had CI followed by ICH, and 23 subjects had an unspecified CVA usually occurring before contemporary neuroimaging capability was available (N = 122).

clinical stroke becomes apparent [10]. The overall prevalence of stroke including cerebral infarction and intracranial hemorrhage is close to reaching the level observed in children between 2 and 9 years of age. The clinical demarcation line is blurring between overt stroke and incomplete infarction, particularly during the third decade of life. This phenomenon is most obvious in the patients who the authors observed during the calendar era of 1980 through 1995 as children. At that time, these patients had evidence of incomplete infarctions based on positron-emission tomography (PET) technology [11] but were not placed on transfusion therapy or hydroxyurea. They now appear with identified neurologic events during the third decade life.

RISK FACTORS

Clinical and laboratory risk factors for cerebral infarction are listed in Box 1 [3,12–16]. Seventeen percent of North American HbSS children who had three or more risk factors by age 2 years demonstrated a 38.3% frequency of subsequent clinical stroke by age 8 years [17]. In a prospective study, Glauser and coworkers [18] observed the onset of a first neurologic event between 2.4 and 6.1 years in children who had a transient ischemic attack (TIA) or effervescent neurologic symptoms. These children had incomplete infarction (silent) at a rate of 71% (12 of 17) on conventional MRI. Wang and coworkers [19] showed that 7 of 39 very young neurologically asymptomatic children had significant magnetic resonance neuroimaging abnormalities. Border zone silent infarction com-

Box 1: Cerebral infarction: factors predictive of risk

Clinical Factors

- Age 2 through 8 years (elevated cerebral flood flow)
- HbSS sibling with stroke
- Incomplete (silent) infarction
- Prior TIA
- Bacterial meningitis
- B19 infection–induced aplastic crisis
- Repeat episodes of severe acute chest syndrome with hypoxia (PaO$_2$) <60 mm Hg
- Nocturnal hypoxemia with or without sleep apnea
- Acute anemic episode (Hb 2 g/dL below normal level)
- Repeat seizure episodes
- Dactylitis before age 1 year
- Splenic dysfunction or infarction near age 1 year
- Priapism
- Systolic hypertension[a]
- Decreasing academic school performance
- Decreasing fine motor skills (Zurick fine motor examination, Perdue non-dominant hand pegboard)
- Abnormal test of variables of attention

Laboratory Risk Factors

- Hemoglobin (steady state) concentration <7.5 g/dL with high reticulo-cyte count
- Leukocyte count >15 × 10^9/L
- Platelet count >450 × 10^9/L
- Pocked (pitted) red blood cells ≥3.5% by 24 months of age
- Fetal hemoglobin ≤13% by age 24 months
- No alpha gene deletion [14]
- HLA subtypes (DPBI*0401)
- HLA-A*0102, HLA-A*2612 [13]

Observations in young children during steady state, not recently transfused, and not on chemotherapy (hydroxyurea) [3,12–16]. In a prospective natural history study. For the 17% of North American HbSS children who had three or more risk factors by age 2 years, the frequency of clinical stroke by age 8 years was 38.3% [17].

[a] Frequently associated with adult onset uremia and intracranial hemorrhage.

bined with elevated blood flow velocity on Doppler analysis increased the risk of overt clinical stroke [20]. Recently, Steen and Ogg [16] have demonstrated that HbSS children have elevated brain N-acetylaspartate, a highly specific marker for neurons. Normal glial cells express a high-affinity for N-acetylaspartate [15]. The transport into glial cells is obligatory for myelination and repair. No risk factor analysis can distinguish between the patient who will progress to clinical stroke and the patient who will sustain slowly enlarging penumbral ischemia or new incomplete infarctions. Border zone infarctions in adults that are identified during childhood seem to be a risk factor for subsequent infarction and intracranial hemorrhage. The observation that the acute chest syndrome rate and recurrence during young childhood is a risk factor for clinical stroke [21] seems to carry over as a comorbid predictor in adult patients with developing chronic pulmonary disease. Systolic hypertension, which is frequently associated with adult onset uremia, is a significant risk factor for intracranial hemorrhage.

Using the criteria in Box 1, a high-risk HbSS child should be evaluated at 3 years of age. The neuroimaging evaluation should include ultrasonography of the branches of the internal carotid arteries (ICA), distal carotid siphon (dICA), middle cerebral artery (MCA), and anterior cerebral artery (ACA) (Fig. 2). This evaluation should be followed by diffusion-weighted (DWI) or FLAIR MRI and MR angiography [22]. Abnormalities seen on this combination of studies increase the subsequent infarction risk to greater than 50% in the untreated child [1,23]. The identification of dICA and MCA stenosis, conventional MRI border zone lesions, and loss of gray matter on quantitative or FLAIR MRI is evidence of disease progression. Cognitive deficiency may be inevitable [24], although overt stroke and severe cognitive disability should be preventable with adequate treatment [25].

CLINICAL DIAGNOSIS

Clinical diagnosis of cerebral infarction with overt hemiparesis and hemisensory loss is not difficult [6,26–28]. More difficult is the diagnosis of less overt dysfunction such as the weakness of one leg or arm. TIAs are not frequently recognized during childhood and adolescence. The reason for this may be the subtleness of the findings and the transient nature of a mild hemiparesis of less than 24 hours. The problem of nonrecognition of mild stroke symptomatology or TIA has been reported in a group of children with and without sickle cell disease. Gabis and coworkers [29] identified that, in children, the time from clinical onset to first medical contact averaged 28.5 hours and the time to diagnosis 35.7 hours. Remarkably, young patients are often not taken to the physician who is aware of the risk of stroke. The patient's family becomes accustomed to pain in the child's arms and legs and often states that they thought the weakness of an extremity was secondary to a pain crisis [30].

The most important aspect of the physical examination at age 3 years during risk assessment is observing the child walking, jumping, standing on one leg, and playing. Any uneven gait or inability to use both hands and arms when

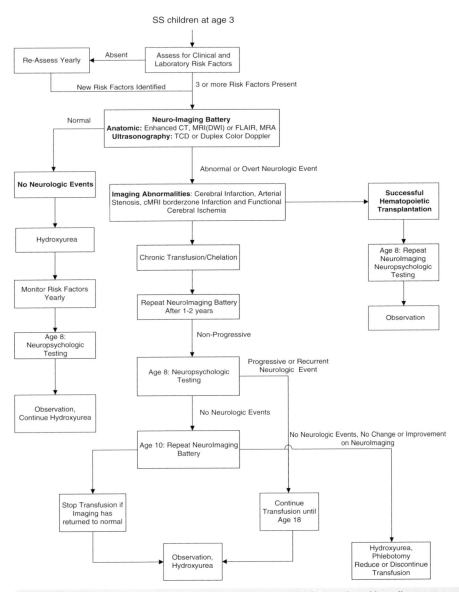

Fig. 2. Management algorithm for cerebral infarction in children with sickle cell anemia. Clinical and laboratory risk factors are listed in Box 1. cMRI, conventional MRI; CT, computed tomography; FLAIR, fluid-attenuated inversion recovery MRI; MRA, MR angiography; MRI (DWI), diffusion-weighted MRI; TCD, ultrasonography using transcranial Doppler.

placing one block upon another should heighten the sense that this child may already have had an incomplete infarction and should act as a impetus for rapid neurodiagnostic testing [18].

The association of incomplete (silent) infarction on conventional MRI with an increase in subsequent clinical stroke and cognitive dysfunction has been documented in children [20,31–35] and seems to be present in young adults. The progressive accumulation of incomplete neurovascular infarcts leads to poorer intellectual function.

The combined application of anatomic and physiologic neuroimaging modalities in high-risk young HbSS children can improve the predictive accuracy of impending stroke during the first decade of life [36,37]. Neuroimaging border zone abnormalities without a complete infarction combined with the finding of elevated velocity on ultrasonography define a "window of opportunity" that should prompt the initiation of preventative therapy before the development and diagnosis of overt stroke [1]. Fifty-two percent (52%) of children with border zone abnormalities combined with elevated transcranial Doppler ultrasonography experienced new or expanded silent (incomplete) infarctions or overt stroke. Cognitive disability is a major consequence of microvascular ischemia even without overt clinical stroke [38]. Falling off neurodevelopmental milestones is an indicator for further neuropsychologic evaluation and diagnosis.

Beyond the third decade, intracranial hemorrhage is the most common type of clinical stroke observed. After the third decade of life as end-stage renal disease and chronic lung disease with pulmonary hypertension increase in prevalence, these comorbidities enhance the risk of rupture of small fragile collateral vessels of the brain (Moyamoya like), which are often not recognized clinically to be present.

NEUROIMAGING

Essential to the diagnosis of cerebral vasculopathy in HbSS patients is the use of recently developed improvements in CT and MRI [35,39–42]. These imaging modalities confirm a clinical diagnosis of cerebral infarction in nearly 100% of HbSS subjects with hemiparetic hemisensory strokes. In addition, enhanced CT and the recently developed techniques of DWI and FLAIR MRI demonstrate exquisite detail about brain structure [43,44]. Cerebral infarction lesions appear hyperintense on T2-weighted conventional MRI images and are consistently associated with quantitative MRI (DWI) and FLAIR lesions in the contiguous penumbral cerebral lesions. Steen and coworkers [8] reported that FLAIR images demonstrated gray matter abnormalities present in 35% of HbSS subjects without known clinical stroke, similar to findings using PET technology [11,22]. Kirkham and coworkers [22] noted that perfusion abnormalities on DWI were larger than the conventional MRI infarction regions, identifying penumbral affected regions. FLAIR or DWI abnormalities are associated with soft neurologic symptoms in patients with normal conventional MRI and normal ultrasonography velocities. It is now possible to perform anatomic studies rapidly using DWI or FLAIR images and MR angiography at one time using the same equipment with additional programming. This capability allows for a rapid assessment of the state of the cerebral vasculopathy, defining complete infarctions, incomplete infarctions, early gray matter neuronal loss without overt infarction, and the extent of the affected penumbral regions (Table 1). DWI detects acute ischemia when conventional MRI with spin-echo T2-weighted images may still be normal and can be helpful in differentiating acute from chronic ischemic changes. In a small study, acute infarcts less than 6 hours old were detected correctly in only 18% of conventional MRI images, whereas all of the lesions were detected on DWI [40]. Comparison studies have shown equivalent specificity of MR angiography for the diagnosis of cerebral arterial stenosis when compared with conventional angiography or ultrasonography [37,45]. MR angiography can detect aneurysms of the circle of Willis and the narrow twisted fragile vessels characteristic of Moyamoya anomaly, which are prevalent in patients during the second, third, and fourth decades of life. Programming of T1-weighted MR angiography images can differentiate large vessel endothelial roughening with early stenosis from turbulent blood flow. Turbulence disappears after the anemia is corrected while stenosis of the major vessels remains evident. MR spectroscopy can detect significant metabolic changes in areas of recent ischemia, including the level of N-acetylaspartate. Increases in the level of lactate and glutamate and decreases in the level of N-acetylaspartate can be measured within minutes of the insult and are present for 3 to 6 hours. These acute changes are valuable in the differentiation of old infarction from new ischemic lesions in penumbral regions. In the old infarcts, readily seen on conventional MRI or enhanced CT scans, patients with stable neurologic deficits do not show specific spectral abnormalities.

Ultrasonography using transcranial Doppler or duplex color Doppler imaging provides a safe and noninvasive measure of blood flow velocity in the carotid siphon (dICA), proximal MCA, and proximal ACA [7]. The velocity of the posterior cerebral artery and basilar arteries is less well defined using transcranial Doppler imaging. The numeric velocities obtained by duplex color Doppler imaging are somewhat lower than those obtained by transcranial imaging. A velocity greater than 170 cm/s is diagnostic of significant stenosis on duplex Doppler imaging, whereas a velocity of 200 cm/s is the equivalent value on transcranial imaging [46]. Very high and very low velocities are manifestations of stenosis or incipient occlusions. Elevated blood flow velocities combined with MRI-detected incomplete infarction predict a significant risk of subsequent clinical stroke in HbSS children [1]. As HbSS patients are placed on transfusion therapy, the velocity in the MCA decreases [47].

The MRI appearance in infarction becomes more obvious in the subacute phase. The T1-weighted signal becomes more hypointense, and there are increases in the T2-weighted images making gray matter and white matter abnormalities more apparent. In HbSS patients, the most common sites of conventional MRI and CT abnormalities involve the frontal and parietal lobes. Brain atrophy is observed in approximately 20% of the patients on MRI and is better defined on enhanced CT scan.

Table 1
Brain imaging modalities

Modality	Physiologic activity	Advantages	Disadvantages
Transcranial Doppler ultrasonography (TCD)	Measures elevated blood flow velocity in dICA, MCA, ACA >200 cm/s in anemic children	Portable Best used for screening of presymptomatic cerebrovascular disease	Nonduplex (no direct visualization of vessels) Cannot demonstrate small vessel disease Requires special training Velocity decreases to normal in transfused subjects
Modifications of color duplex Doppler ultrasonography including high-resolution B-mode ultrasonography	Measures cerebral blood vessel flow Measures cerebral vessel intima/media thickness >170 cm/s in anemic children is conditionally elevated	Direct duplex visualization of cerebral vessels Good visualization of bifurcation of distal internal carotid artery, posterior cerebral artery, basilar artery Best used for screening for cerebrovascular disease Widely available in tertiary medical centers	In transfused HbSS subjects, velocities decrease to normal range Requires meticulous examination technique
Conventional MRI (cMRI)	Acute infarction visible on T1-weighted sequences as low attenuation, hyperintense T2 in completed and border zone incomplete infarction (silent infarction)	Widely available equipment allows high-resolution anatomic visualization of gray and white matter in cerebral infarction Requires modest technical experience	Confinement time in equipment is prolonged; use in unstable patients or during stroke in progression not recommended Poor identification of hemorrhage early
Diffusion- and perfusion-weighted MRI (MRI [DWI])	Identifies molecular displacement of water	Early hyperintense signal detection of acute ischemia before cMRI or CT is sensitive by 8 hours Identifies penumbral areas surrounding infarcts Can be incorporated into routine MRI procedure by adding 3 minutes to immobility time	Requires high-speed echoplanar imaging (EPI) with absolute immobility of head (single shot requires 100 ms)

(continued on next page)

Modality	Physiologic activity	Advantages	Disadvantages
Table 1 (continued)			
Fluid-attenuated inversion recovery MRI (FLAIR)	Finer definition of neuronal microanatomy Special pulse sequence	Cerebrospinal fluid appears dark White matter lesions, acute infarcts appear bright	Axial sequence is required as a part of the routine brain protocol
Quantitative MRI (qMRI)	T1 (spin-lattice relaxation time) demonstrates subtle gray matter abnormalities in subjects with normal cMRI	Very high resolution using available equipment Good correlation with regional cognitive deficiencies	Requires special software and extensive radiologic expertise
MR spectroscopy (MRS)	Spectra measures brain lactate, glutamine, N-acetyl aspartate and other metabolites	Rapid onset but short lived elevation of lactate and glutamate with ischemia in gray matter before cMRI or CT abnormalities appear	Adult norms achieved by age 2 years Difficult clinical monitoring during critical period of stroke in progression Subject immobility required
MR angiography (MRA)	High-resolution visualization of stenotic carotid and intracerebral arteries	Good correlation to conventional angiography with less adverse risk Uses available MRI equipment with slight increase in time of confinement	Endothelial roughening and irregular blood flow velocity mimics stenosis
Computed tomography (CT)	Low-attenuation regions in completed infarctions Cerebral atrophy well defined	Short acquisition time Readily available Acute hemorrhage is hyperintense and identifiable within a few hours of onset	Incomplete (silent) border zone infarctions are often not identified

Data from Refs. [8,11,22,23,39–45,48].

CT reliably demonstrates nearly 100% of cases of acute parenchymal hemorrhage and subarachnoid hemorrhage. MRI is less reliable and variable. In a small study, FLAIR MRI had a sensitivity of 100% and was comparable with CT scans in the detection of acute intracranial hemorrhage [48]. On FLAIR images, the signal of normal cerebrospinal fluid is suppressed; therefore, the signal intensity of hemorrhage is higher than that of cerebrospinal fluid and the surrounding gray matter. When possible, the physician responsible for clinical case management should request DWI or FLAIR MRI for infarction and enhanced CT for hemorrhage in the diagnostic neuroimaging of these subjects.

PREVENTION

The ideal treatment for stroke is prevention [46]. Drugs such as hydroxyurea, decitabine, and apicidin [49] that increase the proportion of fetal hemoglobin (HbF) in the sickle red blood cell show promise. Hydroxyurea demonstrates a two-pronged effect by also decreasing HbS reticulocyte adhesion to the endothelium. There is solid theoretical support but no evidenced-based clinical trials to support its use in high-risk children to prevent cerebral ischemia [50].

Ideally, the fundamental requirement of successful management is treatment of the HbSS child before neuronal loss has begun. Bone marrow or stem cell transplantation is successful if engraftment succeeds. This highly invasive therapy is only possible in the 10% to 15% of children who have HLA-compatible siblings who are not HbSS.

ACUTE MANAGEMENT

Immediate neuroprotective therapy includes control of oxygenation, blood pressure, dehydration, hypothermia, hyperglycemia, and aspiration. Cerebral ischemia and early reperfusion trigger a cascade of events that involve presynaptic release of glutamate, activation of proteases as a result of increased intracellular calcium, generation of free radicals, and subsequent inflammatory responses. Several neuroprotective agents, such as N-methyl D-aspartate receptor antagonists, glycine antagonists, calcium blockers and free radical scavengers, and anti-inflammatory agents, are under study in adult atherosclerotic patients [51,52]. Their function is to preserve the brain tissues in the penumbra areas during stroke in progression. None of these agents has been used in a research setting in patients with sickle cell anemia with infarctive stroke.

TRANSFUSION THERAPY

The early onset of cerebral vasculopathy in HbSS children is directly related to the age-specific elevated cerebral blood flow and the increased oxygen required for brain maturation [53–55]. The magnitude of the damage is compounded by anemia, abnormal red blood cell rheology, and sickle reticulocyte-induced endothelial hyperplasia. If untreated, two of three children with clinical strokes will have repeat strokes [5]. The treatment of clinical stroke during childhood has generally relied on chronic transfusion therapy, often until the patient is at least 18 years of age. If maintained on HbA red blood cell transfusion, most patients sustaining hemiparetic hemisensory strokes will demonstrate fewer recurrent clinical episodes [21,56]. The goal of transfusion therapy is to maintain the hemoglobin concentration at 12 g/dL and the HbS percentage at less than 30%. In HbSS subjects with prior stroke, transfusion is associated with a 20% reduction in mean MCA blood flow velocities as measured by ultrasound [47]. These reductions occur rapidly within the first 3 hours of transfusion and are directly correlated with a rise in the hematocrit of 29% to 34%. Blood rheology immediately improves because of the dilution of sickle cells. Transfusion therapy should be initiated as soon as the diagnosis of cerebral infarction is confirmed. The choice as to the type of transfusion includes repeated simple transfusions of leukocyte-depleted cross-matched red cells, exchange transfusion, or erythrocytapheresis. Initially, simple transfusion is given during stroke in progression because of the fragile state of the child requiring intensive care monitoring. This transfusion can be followed by exchange transfusion, erythrocytapheresis, or repeat simple transfusion. The choice is usually based on institutional preference and resources. There are no outcome data to support any specific transfusion procedure.

The cerebral vasculopathy during the first decade is not a static process. On transfusion, some patients will show an improvement in functional neuroimaging during the first year of therapy, whereas others will develop new asymptomatic penumbral lesions [55,57]. MR angiography shows occasional smoothing of previously roughened endothelium in some transfused patients but progression of large vessel disease in others [58]. Completed infarction sites do not improve, and penumbral lesion progression occurs with continued loss of neuropsychologic function [9,24,31]. Functional neurologic deficits persist and become more obvious as the child matures. In children with elevated cerebral blood flow who are less than 10 years of age, stroke frequently recurs when the transfusion program is discontinued [3]. The consensus is that transfusion should continue until approximately 18 years of age or longer. Attempts to reduce the transfusion level after a number of years because of iron overload in older adolescents and young adults have been shown to be relatively safe. The hemoglobin S percentage is allowed to rise to approximately 50% [59].

Clearly, the prevention of first stroke should be a goal of therapeutic intervention [25,46]. Adams and coworkers initiated a randomized clinical trial directed at stroke prevention. Asymptomatic young children who had elevated blood flow velocity measured by transcranial Doppler imaging of the MCA or dICA (>200 cm/s) were randomized to receive transfusion or no transfusion. Within 2.5 years, the patients who were randomly assigned to transfusion therapy had fewer overt clinical strokes than those who were maintained on standard nontransfusion therapy (11 subjects with 10 cerebral infarctions and one intracranial hemorrhage in the nontransfusion group versus one cerebral infarction in the transfusion group), a 92% difference in stroke risk. The patients with concomitant abnormal conventional MRI were at highest risk for overt clinical infarction. In a second trial (STOP II), transfused subjects with no clinical evidence of a neurologic disorder but elevated Doppler velocity were randomized to discontinuance of transfusion therapy after 30 months. Sixteen of 41 patients randomized to discontinuance of transfusion therapy reverted to high-risk transcranial Doppler findings, and two subsequently had overt clinical strokes. The combination of increased MCA and dICA velocities along with evidence of persistence of the border zone MRI abnormalities mark a high rate of progressive neuropathy of 38%; therefore, transfusion therapy cannot be safely discontinued after 30 months [57]. Currently ongoing is a multi-institutional randomized study of red blood cell transfusions versus no transfusion in children identified by conventional MRI imaging to have asymptomatic incomplete infarctions without elevated Doppler velocities.

Chronic transfusion therapy is burdensome to the patient and family and is associated with a high frequency of problems [60]. Venous access becomes a major issue. Also added to the burden is increasing adolescent resistance to nightly subcutaneous chelation therapy, which is painful and difficult to continue over many years. Iron chelation therapy requires the use of subcutaneous or intravenous deferoxamine (Desferal). Complications include skin rash, ototoxity, and, in young children, growth retardation. Compliance with home treatment in adolescents is poor, limiting its usefulness. New (non–Food and Drug Administration approved) investigational agents include deferiprone alone or in combination with deferoxamine. Deferosirox, a tridentate iron chelator, is given orally at 20 mg/kg/day dissolved in water and has shown few toxicities in phase II studies to date with some nausea and vomiting. Effectiveness is assessed using superconducting quantum interference device (SQUID) measurements of liver iron. The parents need to be informed that embarkation on a transfusion program in this clinical situation is a long-term commitment, and compliance with an iron chelation regimen is vital.

HYDROXYUREA

Hydroxyurea therapy may be useful as a replacement for transfusion [61,62]. The hematologic factors of elevated neutrophils, platelets, and reticulocyte count that predict an increased risk of cerebral vasculopathy also predict which subjects will respond best to hydroxyurea. The dose of hydroxyurea can be escalated from 15 to 35 mg/kg/day monitoring the hematologic parameters. The maximum dose for older children and adolescents is between 1000 and 1500 mg orally per day [63]. In HbSS adults without known stroke, hydroxyurea was shown to reduce the frequency of painful crisis, acute chest syndrome, and hospitalization, and the need for blood transfusion in a double-blind placebo-controlled study. Hydroxyurea decreased the risk of adult mortality in a 9-year follow-up study [64]. There are no controlled trials on the progression of cerebral vasculopathy during hydroxyurea therapy. Successful replacement of transfusion therapy with hydroxyurea in patients known to have symptomatic stroke who were unable to tolerate continued transfusion therapy has been reported [61,62,65,66]. It is thought that hydroxyurea may decrease the rate of penumbral spread to regions adjacent to already infarcted regions.

The question is whether hydroxyurea or similar agents can prevent the development of cerebral vasculopathy in the very young child. The fact that splenic germinal centers have been shown to return may be a promising model [67]. There are no data available regarding the efficacy of hydroxyurea therapy in the very young patient at 3 or 4 years in an attempt to prevent cerebral vasculopathy before clinical or radiologic evidence of central nervous system disease becomes apparent. Long-term clinical trials of hydroxyurea beginning during early childhood in a multi-institutional trial in North America are in progress [50]; however, recent neuroradiologic advances using conventional MRI or FLAIR imaging are not included in the trial. An evidenced-based randomized clinical trial monitored by neuroimaging and neuropsychologic testing is needed. To be clinically effective in the prevention of central nervous system vasculopathy, therapeutic agents must be relatively nontoxic in children, orally available, and should not impart an unpleasant odor (ie, butyrate). Long-term compliance with oral medication is a major difficulty in young children.

Published recommendations do not include data regarding seriously ill young adults with significant comorbid conditions such as renal insufficiency and chronic pulmonary disease who cannot be managed with the single focus on cerebral vasculopathy. Children who have had clinical stroke and who have been transfused for 10 to 15 years often have the complications of chronic transfusion, that is, iron overload with hemosiderosis of the liver and alloimmunization. They are frequently removed from the transfusion program, given hydroxyurea, and observed. No data are available on subjects regarding renal function or pulmonary function as their transfusion therapy is discontinued.

NEUROREHABILITATION

Rehabilitative techniques have advanced significantly during the last decade. Most large hospitals have neurorehabilitation services focusing on adult patients with stroke. These services have been underused by the pediatric population. The services go far beyond the standard physical therapy of muscle strengthening and treatment for poststroke spasticity and improvement of coordination and volitional movements [68,69]. Constraint-induced therapy has shown good success in the rehabilitation of adult patients [70]. It is possible to harness the plasticity of adaptive properties of neuronal networks in the brain through therapies that engage the patient in active voluntary use of impaired limbs [71]. Constraint-induced therapy is intended to help patients with central paresis overcome learned "nonuse" of the paretic limb and involves a physical restraint such as a mitt or sling on the functional arm or leg to encourage use of the nonfunctional extremity [70–72].

Studies are underway to determine whether the dopamine agonist ropinirole (Requip) combined with physical therapy can be associated with improved gait and motor status [73]. The hypothesis is that decreased dopamine has a role in poststroke motor deficits. If the dopamine can be increased, motor recovery is thought to be more likely. Numerous studies suggest that increasing noradrenergic activity after stroke improves motor outcome. Human trials of L-dopa and amphetamine have found significant treatment-related gains in motor status but have been marred by significant toxicities. Ropinirole or similar agents might provide the same neurobeneficial results with considerably less toxicity.

Once a patient has had an acute stroke, prevention of recurrence, close monitoring by means of imaging modalities, psychometric analyses, and ongoing rehabilitation with psychosocial support should be implemented. It is hoped that studies currently ongoing and those being planned will make significant inroads into the prevention, diagnosis, and management of HbSS individuals with cerebral infarction.

References

[1] Pegelow CH, Wang W, Granger S, et al. Silent infarcts in children with sickle cell anemia and abnormal cerebral artery velocity. Arch Neurol 2001;58:2017–21.

[2] Prengler M, Pavlakis SG, Prohovnik I, et al. Sickle cell disease: the neurological complications. Ann Neurol 2002;51:543–52.

[3] Grubb RL, Derdeyn CP, Fritsch SM, et al. Importance of hemodynamic factors in the prognosis of symptomatic carotid occlusion. JAMA 1998;280:1055–60.

[4] Ohene-Frempong K, Weiner SJ, Sleeper LA, et al, and the Cooperative Study of Sickle Cell Disease. Cerebrovascular accidents in sickle cell disease: rates and risk factors. Blood 1998;91:228–94.

[5] Powars DR, Wilson B, Imbus C, et al. The natural history of stroke in sickle cell disease. Am J Med 1978;65:461–71.

[6] Adams RJ, Ohene-Frempong K, Wang W. Sickle cell and the brain. Hematology (Am Soc Hematol Educ Program) 2001;31–46.

[7] Wang WC, Gallagher DM, Pegelow CH, et al. Multicenter comparison of magnetic resonance imaging and transcranial Doppler ultrasonography in the evaluation of the central nervous system in children with sickle cell disease. J Pediatr Hematol Oncol 2000; 22:335–9.

[8] Steen RG, Emudianughe T, Hankins GM, et al. Brain imaging findings in pediatric patients with sickle cell disease. Radiology 2003;228:216–25.

[9] Garcia JH, Lassen NJ, Weiller C, et al. Ischemic stroke and incomplete infarction. Stroke 1996;27:761–5.

[10] Koshy M, Thomas C, Goodwin J. Vascular lesions in the central nervous system in sickle cell disease (neuropathology). JAAMP 1990;1:71–8.

[11] Powars DR, Conti PS, Wong WY, et al. Cerebral vasculopathy in sickle cell anemia: diagnostic contribution of positron emission tomography. Blood 1999;93:71–9.

[12] Driscoll MC, Hurlet A, Styles L, et al. Stroke risk in siblings with sickle cell anemia. Blood 2003;101:2401–4.

[13] Hoppe C, Klitz W, Noble J, et al. Distinct HLA associations by stroke in children with sickle cell anemia. Blood 2003;101:2865–9.

[14] Hsu LL, Miller ST, Wright E, et al. Alpha thalassemia is associated with decreased risk of abnormal transcranial Doppler ultrasonography in children with sickle cell anemia. J Pediatr Hematol Oncol 2003;25:622–8.

[15] Huang W, Wang H, Kekuda R, et al. Transport of N-acetylaspartate by the Na+-dependent high-affinity dicarboxylate transporter NaDC3 and its relevance to the expression of the transporter in the brain. Pharmacology 2000;295:392–403.

[16] Steen RG, Ogg RJ. Abnormally high levels of brain N-acetylaspartate in children with sickle cell disease. AJNR Am J Neuroradiol 2005;26:463–8.

[17] Miller ST, Sleeper LA, Pegelow CH, et al. Prediction of adverse outcomes in children with sickle cell disease: a report from the Cooperative Study (CSSCD). N Engl J Med 2000; 342:83–9.

[18] Glauser TA, Siegel MJ, Lee BCP, et al. Accuracy of neurologic examination and history in detecting evidence of MRI-diagnosed cerebral infarctions in children with sickle cell hemoglobinopathy. J Child Neurol 1995;10:88–92.

[19] Wang WC, Langston JW, Steen RG, et al. Abnormalities of the central nervous system in very young children with sickle cell anemia. J Pediatr 1998;132:994–8.

[20] Miller ST, Macklin EA, Pegelow CH, et al. Silent infarction as a risk factor for overt stroke in children with sickle cell anemia: a report from the Cooperative Study of Sickle Cell Disease. J Pediatr 2001;139:385–90.

[21] Scothorn DJ, Price C, Schwartz D, et al. Risk of recurrent stroke in children with sickle cell disease receiving blood transfusion therapy for at least five years after initial stroke. J Pediatr 2002;140:348–54.

[22] Kirkham FJ, Calamante F, Bynevelt M, et al. Perfusion magnetic resonance abnormalities in patients with sickle cell disease. Ann Neurol 2001;49(4):477–85.

[23] Dobson SR, Holden KR, Nietert PJ, et al. Moyamoya syndrome in childhood sickle cell disease: a predictive factor for recurrent cerebrovascular events. Blood 2002;99:3144–50.

[24] Swift AV, Cohen MJ, Hynd GW, et al. Neuropsychologic impairment in children with sickle cell anemia. An Pediatr (Barc) 1989;84:1077–85.

[25] Adams RJ. Stroke prevention and treatment in sickle cell disease. Arch Neurol 2001;58: 565–8.

[26] Quinn CT, Rogers ZR, Buchanan GR. Survival of children with sickle cell disease. Blood 2004;103:4023–7.

[27] Powars DR. Management of cerebral vasculopathy in children with sickle cell anaemia. Br J Haematol 2000;l108:666–78.

[28] Earley CJ, Kittner SJ, Feeser BR, et al. Stroke in children and sickle-cell disease: Baltimore-Washington Cooperative Young Stroke Study. Neurology 1998;51:169–76.

[29] Gabis LV, Yangala R, Lenn NJ. Time lag to diagnosis of stroke in children. An Pediatr (Barc) 2002;110:924–8.

[30] Katz ML, Smith-Whitley K, Ruzek SB, et al. Knowledge of stroke risk, signs of stroke, and the need for stroke education among children with sickle cell disease and their caregivers. Ethn Health 2002;7:115–23.

[31] Armstrong FD, Thompson Jr RJ, Wang W, et al. Cognitive functioning and brain magnetic resonance imaging in children with sickle cell disease. An Pediatr (Barc) 1996;97: 864–70.

[32] Craft S, Schatz J, Glauser TA, et al. Neuropsychologic effects of stroke in children with sickle cell anemia. J Pediatr 1993;123:712–7.

[33] Bernaudin F, Verlhac S, Freard F, et al. Multicenter prospective study of children with sickle cell disease: radiographic and psychometric correlation. J Child Neurol 2000; 15:333–43.

[34] Schatz J, White DA, Moinuddin A, et al. Lesion burden and cognitive morbidity in children with sickle cell disease. J Child Neurol 2002;17:891–5.

[35] Pegelow CH, Macklin EA, Moser FG, et al. Longitudinal changes in brain magnetic resonance imaging findings in children with sickle cell disease. Blood 2002;99:3014–8.

[36] Adams RJ. Lessons from the stroke prevention trial in sickle cell anemia (STOP) study. J Child Neurol 2000;15:344–9.

[37] Abboud MR, Cure J, Granger S, et al. Magnetic resonance angiography in children with sickle cell disease and abnormal transcranial Doppler ultrasonography findings enrolled in the STOP study. Blood 2004;103:2822–6.

[38] Vermeer SE, Prins ND, den Heijer T, et al. Silent brain infarcts and the risk of dementia and cognitive decline. N Engl J Med 2003;348:1215–22.

[39] Moran CJ, Siegel MJ, DeBaun MR. Sickle cell disease: imaging of cerebrovascular complications. Radiology 1998;206:311–21.

[40] Mullins ME, Schaefer PW, Sorensen AG, et al. CT and conventional and diffusion-weighted MR imaging in acute stroke: study in 691 patients at presentation to the emergency department. Radiology 2002;224(2):356–60.

[41] Moritani T, Numaguchy Y, Lemer NB, et al. Sickle cell cerebrovascular disease: usual and unusual findings on MR imaging and MR angiography. Clin Imag 2004;28:173–86.

[42] Steen RG, Reddick WE, Mulhern RK, et al. Quantitative MRI of the brain in children with sickle cell disease reveals abnormalities unseen by conventional MRI. J Magn Reson Imaging 1998;8:535–43.

[43] Crisostomo RA, Garcia MM, Tong DC. Detection of diffusion-weighted MRI abnormalities in patients with transient ischemic attack: correlation with clinical characteristics. Stroke 2003;34:932–7.

[44] Schaefer PW, Ozsunar Y, He J, et al. Assessing tissue viability with MR diffusion and perfusion imaging. AJNR Am J Neuroradiol 2003;24(3):436–43.

[45] Kandeel AY, Zimmerman RA, Ohene-Frempong K. Comparison of magnetic resonance angiography and conventional angiography in sickle cell disease: clinical significance and reliability. Neuroradiology 1996;38:409–16.

[46] Adams RJ, Brambilla DJ, Granger S, et al. Stroke and conversion to high risk in children screened with transcranial Doppler ultrasound during the STOP study. Blood 2004; 103:3689–94.

[47] Venketasubramanian N, Prohovnik I, Hurlet A, et al. Middle cerebral artery velocity changes during transfusion in sickle cell anemia. Stroke 1994;25:2153–8.

[48] Noguchi K, Ogawa T, Inugami A, et al. Acute subarachnoid hemorrhage: MR imaging with fluid-attenuated inversion recovery pulse sequences. Radiology 1995;196:773–7.

[49] Witt O, Monkemeyer S, Ronndahl G, et al. Induction of fetal hemoglobin expression by the histone-deacetylase inhibitor apicidin. Blood 2003;101:2001–7.

[50] Rogers ZR, Buchanan GR. Expanding the role of hydroxyurea in children with sickle cell disease. J Pediatr 2004;145:287–8.

[51] Brott T, Bogousslavsky J. Treatment of acute ischemic stroke. N Engl J Med 2000;343: 710–22.

[52] Scheidtmann K, Fries W, Muller F, et al. Effect of levodopa in combination with physio-therapy on functional motor recovery after stroke: a prospective, randomized, double-blind study. Lancet 2001;358:787–90.

[53] Schoning M, Hartig B. Age dependence of total cerebral blood flow volume from childhood to adulthood. J Cereb Blood Flow Metab 1996;16:827–33.

[54] Huttenlocher PR, Moohr JW, Johns L, et al. Cerebral blood flow in sickle cerebrovascular disease. An Pediatr (Barc) 1984;73(5):615–21.

[55] Raj A, Bertolone SJ, Mangold S, et al. Assessment of cerebral tissue oxygenation in patients with sickle cell disease: effect of transfusion therapy. J Pediatr Hematol Oncol 2004;26:279–83.

[56] Buchanan GR, Bowman WP, Smith SJ. Recurrent cerebral ischemia during hypertransfusion therapy in sickle cell anemia. J Pediatr 1983;103:921–3.

[57] Pegelow CH, Adams RJ, McKie V, et al. Risk of recurrent stroke in patients with sickle cell disease treated with erythrocyte transfusions. J Pediatr 1995;126(6):896–9.

[58] Russell MO, Goldberg HI, Hodson A, et al. Effect of transfusion therapy on arteriographic abnormalities and on recurrence of stroke in sickle cell disease. Blood 1984;63(1):162–9.

[59] Cohen AR, Martin MB, Silber JH, et al. A modified transfusion program for prevention of stroke in sickle cell disease. Blood 1992;79:1657–61.

[60] Olivieri NF. Progression of iron overload in sickle cell disease. Semin Hematol 2001; 38:57–62.

[61] Ware RE, Zimmerman SA, Schultz WH. Hydroxyurea as an alternative to blood transfusions for the prevention of recurrent stroke in children with sickle cell disease. Blood 1999;94:3022–6.

[62] Sumoza A, de Bisotti R, Sumoza D, et al. Hydroxyurea (HU) for prevention of recurrent stroke in sickle cell anemia (SCA). Am J Hematol 2002;71:161–5.

[63] Zimmerman SA, Schultz WH, Davis JS, et al. Sustained long-term hematologic efficacy of hydroxyurea at maximum tolerated dose in children with sickle cell disease. Blood 2004; 103:2039–45.

[64] Steinberg MH, Barton F, Castro O, et al. Effect of hydroxyurea on mortality and morbidity in adult sickle cell anemia: risks and benefits up to 9 years of treatment. JAMA 2003; 289:1645–51.

[65] Rana S, Houston PE, Surana N, et al. Discontinuation of long-term transfusion therapy in patients with sickle cell disease and stroke. J Pediatr 1997;131:757–60.

[66] Ware RE, Zimmerman SA, Sylvestre PB, et al. Prevention of secondary stroke and resolution of transfusional iron overload in children with sickle cell anemia using hydroxyurea and phlebotomy. J Pediatr 2004;145:346–52.

[67] Wang WC, Wynn LW, Rogers ZR, et al. A two-year pilot trial of hydroxyurea in very young children with sickle-cell anemia. J Pediatr 2001;139:790–6.

[68] Jackson PL, Lafleur MF, Malouin F, et al. Functional cerebral reorganization following motor sequence learning through mental practice with motor imagery. Neuroimage 2003; 20:1171–80.

[69] Stevens JA, Stoykov ME. Using motor imagery in the rehabilitation of hemiparesis. Arch Phys Med Rehabil 2003;84:1090–2.

[70] Taub E, Uswatte G, Pidikiti RD. Constraint-induced movement therapy: a new family of techniques with broad application to physical rehabilitation. A clinical review. J Rehab Res Dev 1999;36:237–51.

[71] Winstein CJ, Wing AM, Whitall J. Motor control and learning principles for rehabilitation of upper limb movements after brain injury. In: Grafman J, Robertson I, editors. Plasticity and rehabilitation. 2nd edition. (Handbook of neuropsychology, vol. 9). Amsterdam: Elsevier Science BV; 2003. p. 77–137.

[72] van der Lee J, Wagenaar R, Lankhorst G, et al. Forced use of the upper extremity in chronic stroke patients: results from a single-blind randomized clinical trial. Stroke 1999;30: 2369–75.

[73] Gladstone DJ, Black SE. Enhancing recovery after stroke with noradrenergic pharmacotherapy: a new frontier? Can J Neurol Sci 2000;27:97–105.

Hematol Oncol Clin N Am 19 (2005) 857–879

HEMATOLOGY/ONCOLOGY CLINICS
OF NORTH AMERICA

The Acute Chest Syndrome

Cage S. Johnson, MD

Comprehensive Sickle Cell Center, Keck School of Medicine, University of Southern California, RMR 304, 2025 Zonal Avenue, Los Angeles, CA 90033, USA

The sickling disorders, sickle cell anemia and its variants, are inherited hemoglobinopathies due to at least one substitution of valine for glutamic acid at position 6 of the beta globin chain. Following deoxygenation of the erythrocyte, hemoglobin (Hb) S undergoes intracellular polymerization with the associated morphologic transformation to the sickled shape. Repeated cycles of Hb S polymerization induce a series of erythrocyte abnormalities, including cytoplasmic and membrane rigidity and cellular dehydration with an increase in intracellular Hb concentration. The circulating erythrocyte population is thus composed of a heterogeneous population of cells, including low-density reticulocytes, very dense discocytes, and irreversibly sickled cells. These dense, poorly deformable cells are ultimately responsible for the elevated whole blood viscosity and microvascular occlusion seen in this disease [1,2]. The clinical features of the disease result from Hb S polymerization and consist of chronic hemolytic anemia, frequent infections, and, most importantly, microvascular obstruction producing acute and chronic ischemia, resulting in organ damage from infarction and fibrosis [3].

Sickle cell anemia is the homozygous form of the disease (Hb SS); it is the most common variant and generally has the most severe clinical manifestations. Other variants are due to the inheritance of compound heterozygous states for Hb S and another Hb that interacts with Hb S and participates in polymer formation, causing disease. Heterozygosity for both Hb S and Hb C results in sickle-C disease, whereas combinations of Hb S with $beta^0$ or $beta^+$ thalassemia are known as sickle-thalassemia. Combinations of Hb S with other variants (eg, D, E, O-Arab) are rare.

Acute pulmonary disease is a common complication of the sickling diseases, with a frequency estimated at several hundred times that of the general population [4], and is the second most common cause of hospital admission in these patients, resulting in considerable morbidity and mortality [5,6]. Nearly half of all patients will have at least one episode, and a subset will have multiple events.

This work was supported by National Institutes of Health grants HL 15162, HL 48484, and HL 070595.
E-mail address: cagejohn@email.usc.edu

The term "acute chest syndrome" was introduced by Charache and colleagues [7] and reflects the difficulty of establishing a definitive cause for these acute pulmonary episodes, particularly in distinguishing infection from pulmonary infarction by microvascular occlusion. The terminology is potentially misleading, because it includes those cases with a relatively benign course as well as those that develop progressive disease with a picture similar to that of adult respiratory distress syndrome (ARDS). The acute chest syndrome (ACS) in sickle cell disease (SCD) is currently defined as a new infiltrate on chest radiograph associated with one or more symptoms, such as fever, cough, sputum production, tachypnea, dyspnea, or new-onset hypoxia [8]. The illness clinically and radiographically resembles bacterial pneumonia, with fever, leucocytosis, pleuritic chest pain, pleural effusion, and cough with purulent sputum. However, the clinical course in SCD is considerably different from that in hematologically normal individuals. Multiple lobe involvement and recurrent infiltrates are more common in SCD, and the duration of clinical illness and of radiologic clearing of infiltrates is prolonged to 10 to 12 days [5,8–10].

EPIDEMIOLOGY

In the seminal reports by Barrett-Connor [4,11], 84 of 169 episodes of ACS had evidence of bacterial infection on culture of blood or sputum. Because there was no difference in the clinical course between culture-positive and culture-negative cases, Barrett-Connor concluded that all cases were most likely due to infection, most commonly to *Streptococcus pneumoniae*. Her conclusion was supported by the known propensity to bacterial infection in SCD and was widely accepted. However, since that time, numerous epidemiologic studies in people with normal Hb type have indicated a changing epidemiology for pneumonia. For example, studies [12] in armed forces personnel indicate that the attack rate of pneumonia in the 1990s (77.6/100,000/year) was one fourth that of the 1970s (307.6/100,000/year). Furthermore, the frequency of *S pneumoniae* has declined substantially while that of *Mycoplasma pneumoniae* and other atypical organisms has increased. Moreover, a definite cause is not established by culture in 65% to 75% of cases. More recent data indicate that viruses, particularly rhinovirus at 45%, account for the majority of events in children, and that infection with *M pneumoniae* at 35% continues to rise in frequency [13]. Moreover, in adult populations, *M pneumoniae* and *Chlamydia pneumoniae* are the leading causes of pulmonary infection outside the hospital setting [14]. In as many as 55% of episodes, no definite causative agent can be identified. Thus, the epidemiology of pneumonia in the general population continues to evolve over time, and the spectrum of pulmonary microbial infection is likely to undergo further changes in both the general and SCD populations.

These secular changes in microbial flora were first demonstrated in SCD by Poncz and colleagues [15], who studied 102 episodes of ACS in 70 patients with careful culture techniques and found that they could document bacterial infection in only 12 episodes. The single most common cause found was *Mycoplasma* (16%), and viral disease at 8% was almost as frequent as the common bacterial agents. In 66% of the episodes, no cause was established. Nearly identical findings were reported by Sprinkle and colleagues [16] in their study of 100 episodes of ACS in 57 patients. By contrast, in Curacao [17], 43% of sputum cultures were positive in 81 episodes seen in 53 patients. The most common bacterium was *Haemophilus influenzae*, and both *Staphylococcus aureus* and *Klebsiella* were more common than *S pneumoniae*. Other reports have stressed the evolving importance of *C pneumoniae* and *Legionella pneumophilia*. Viral agents causing ACS include influenza, respiratory syncytial virus, cytomegalovirus, parvovirus, adenovirus, and parainfluenza virus.

The publication of data from two large cooperative groups in recent years has provided a clearer picture of ACS and its impact on SCD. The Cooperative Study of Sickle Cell Disease (CSSCD) reported on 1722 episodes of ACS in 939 patients with a new infiltrate on chest radiograph. Data from this study indicate that ACS occurs with an overall incidence of 10.5 per 100 patient-years [5,10], most often as a single episode, but certain patients have multiple episodes. A past history of ACS was associated with earlier mortality than that found in patients who had never had an episode. The disorder is most common in the 2- to 4-year age group, with a peak incidence of 25.3 per 100 patient-years, and gradually declines in incidence with age to 8.8 per 100 patient-years in those more than 20 years old. It is believed that the slower decline of Hb F concentration compared with normals exerts a protective effect in those patients less than 2 years of age. The decline in the incidence of ACS observed in older age groups is believed to be related to at least two factors: (1) excess mortality in the group that had an ACS and (2) fewer viral episodes in adults because of acquired immunity. The incidence of ACS is related to genotype: the frequency in Hb SS is slightly greater than that in Hb S beta° thalassemia, but the frequency is much lower in Hb SC and Hb S beta$^+$ thalassemia. Additional data showed that a lower hematocrit or a higher Hb F was associated with a reduced incidence of ACS, whereas a high white blood cell count was associated with a higher incidence.

The National Acute Chest Syndrome Study Group (NACSSG) [8] employed a more stringent definition of ACS: its inclusion criteria were a new infiltrate plus one or more pulmonary signs or symptoms, such as fever, cough, sputum production, tachypnea, dyspnea, or new-onset hypoxia. Viral culture techniques and acute and convalescent serologies were employed, as well as careful examination of deep sputum cytology for fat-laden macrophages indicative of fat embolism. In this study, there were 671 episodes of ACS in 538 patients. In 48% of the episodes, ACS developed during hospitalization for acute pain or other causes. A definite cause was established in 256 (38%) of these episodes, but incomplete data precluded full assessment in 306 episodes (46%). Of the 27 pathogens identified, the most common infectious agents were *Chlamydia* (7.2%), *Mycoplasma* (6.6%), and viruses (6.4%), particularly respiratory syncytial virus. Pulmonary infarction was diagnosed by exclusion and found in 16.1% of episodes, whereas fat embolism was found in 8.8%. *S pneumoniae* was recovered in only 11 episodes. A variety of bacterial and viral agents were identified in the remainder of cases. Mechanical ventilation was required in 13% of patients and was associated with extensive lobar involvement, a platelet count of less than 200,000/μL, or a preceding history of cardiac disease. Eighteen deaths occurred (2.7%), primarily as the consequence of pulmonary embolism with bone marrow, fat, or thrombi.

CLINICAL PRESENTATION

The clinical characteristics of ACS in both children and adults have been more clearly defined by large clinical studies in recent years. The CSSCD reported on 1722 episodes of ACS in 939 subjects [10], and the NACSSG study [8] described the findings in 671 cases of ACS in 538 subjects (Table 1). Fever of greater than 38.5°C and cough were the most common presenting symptoms and were significantly more common in children than in adolescents or adults. Tachypnea and bronchospasm, particularly in children, were the common physical findings; however, a normal physical examination was found in 35% of the cases, and additional data support the unreliability of the physical examination in the detection of ACS [18]. Chest, rib, and extremity pain were more common in older adolescents and adults. Isolated upper and middle

Table 1

Age-related clinical presentation percentages for the acute chest syndrome in the Cooperative Study of Sickle Cell Disease and National Acute Chest Syndrome Study Group studies

	Age <10 y*		Age >10 y*	
	CSSCD	NACSSG	CSSCD	NACSSG
Presentation	n = 483	n = 264	n = 454	n = 273
Fever	90	86	70	74
Cough	81	69	66	56
Chest pain	26	27	81	61
Rib pain	NA	14	NA	27
Extremity pain	NA	22	NA	51
Dyspnea	17	31	38	50
Temperature >39°C	44	86	12	74
Respiratory rate >40/min	28	NA	7	NA
Pulse >140/min	27	NA	7	NA
ACS not present on admission	39	NA	59	NA
Mechanical ventilation	10	NA	15	NA
Reactive airway disease	NA	17	NA	9
Length of stay (d)	9.7	NA	11.3	NA
Mortality	<1	NA	5	NA

Abbreviation: NA, not available.

   * The differences between young children and adolescents/adults were significant, at $P \leq .006$ or better, for all variables except for length of stay, where $P \leq .04$.

   Data from Vichinsky EP, Neumayr LD, Earles AN, et al, National Acute Chest Syndrome Study Group. Causes and outcomes of the acute chest syndrome in sickle cell disease. N Engl J Med 2000;342:1855–65; and Vichinsky EP, Styles LA, Colangelo LH, et al, The Cooperative Study of Sickle Cell Disease. Acute chest syndrome in sickle cell disease: clinical presentation and course. Blood 1997;89:1787–92.

lobe involvement were more common in children, with isolated lower lobe disease more common in adults. Pleural effusions were more common in adults. Bacteremia was more common in children aged 2 to 4 years; *S pneumoniae* was detected in 78% of those children but found in only 25% of adults with bacteremia. Moreover, in nearly half the cases, ACS developed several days after hospitalization for another reason. In both series, the hospital stay was longer for adults than for children. The longer duration of hospital stay in the NACSSG study reflects the enrollment of a more acutely ill population because of more stringent inclusion criteria. These criteria included a new pulmonary infiltrate involving at least one complete lung segment, excluding atelectasis, together with at least one of the following: chest pain, fever greater than 38.5°C, tachypnea, wheezing, or cough. Additional data supporting the greater severity of clinical illness in the NACSSG study were the more frequent use of transfusions and the higher mortality. Mortality in both studies was four- to ninefold greater in adults than in children and was due to respiratory failure, cor pulmonale, hypovolemic shock, or sepsis.

These features of ACS indicate that infection is its most frequent cause in young children. In adults, the strong association with bone pain and less frequent identification of microbial infection suggest that vascular occlusion is the cause of ACS in most cases.

PATHOPHYSIOLOGY

The pathophysiology of acute lung injury in the sickling disorders is complex. Microbial infection, in-situ vaso-occlusion, fat embolism from ischemic/necrotic bone marrow, or thromboembolism may initiate this process, and establishing a specific cause is often difficult.

Patients who have SCD have increased susceptibility to infection that is not fully understood but appears related to functional asplenia, decreased opsonic activity in their serum, and a relatively poor antibody response to the polysaccharide component of the bacterial capsule. Splenic hypofunction correlates with the increased susceptibility to infection [19]. Defective activation of the alternate pathway has been demonstrated [20,21] and correlates with a past history of pneumococcal infection [22]. This same defect in alternate pathway activation has been described in sickle-C disease and presumably extends to the other sickle variants; serial studies show that the defect is persistent for at least 1 year [23]. Serotype-specific IgG antibody responses to pneumococcal reimmunization are generally mediocre to poor. This poor response is not surprising, because pneumococcal polysaccharides are T lymphocyte–independent antigens [24] and are not thought to induce immunologic memory in either children or adults [25]. The occurrence of pneumococcal bacteremia is associated with low IgG antibody concentrations to the infecting serotype. The most prevalent pneumococcal serotypes causing disease in this era of prophylactic antibiotics and vaccination include types 6, 14, 18, 19, and 23; these same serotypes were most frequently involved in previously reported "vaccine failures" [26]. Aside from evidence supporting an immune defect related to pneumococcal infections and the phagocytic defect, there is little evidence to suggest that impaired immunity has substantial clinical relevance to the spectrum of the ACS. However, recent evidence for impaired lymphocyte blastogenic response and γ-interferon production in patients with ACS suggests that these immunologic abnormalities may contribute to the clinical severity of acute pulmonary disease in this patient population [27].

Progression of pulmonary disease to an ARDS-like picture is often attributed to vaso-occlusion (reviewed by Chiang and Frenette elsewhere in this issue), in which Hb S–containing cells interact with microvascular endothelium or endothelial matrix. This interaction occurs through a variety of adhesive proteins expressed on the sickle erythrocyte and corresponding molecules on the endothelial cell; these interactions are mediated by plasma ligands, such as thrombospondin and von Willebrand factor (vWF) [28,29]. Adhesogenic molecules on the sickle reticulocyte include the integrin $\alpha_4\beta_1$ (very late activation antigen–4 or VLA-4), CD36, CD47, phosphatidyl serine, basal cell adhesion molecule, Lutheran blood group, and sulfated glycans. Other endothelial cell receptors, such as the integrin $\alpha_v\beta_3$ and P-selectin, may also play substantial roles. Matrix components participating in adhesion include fibronectin, thrombospondin, vWF, and laminin [28,29]. Hb S polymerization generates reactive oxygen species [30], which activate the transcription factor NF-κB. NF–κB upregulates expression of the adhesion molecule VCAM-1 on endothelium, which facilitates the endothelial adhesion of sickle erythrocytes by means of erythrocyte $\alpha_4\beta_1$ [28,31,32]. VCAM-1 is also upregulated by hypoxia and by inflammatory cytokines such as interleukin-1 and tumor necrosis factor (TNF)–α, both of which are elevated in ACS over the steady-state levels [28].

A growing body of evidence indicates that granulocytes and monocytes play an important role in microvascular occlusion (see Chiang and Frenette elsewhere in this issue). Elevated leukocyte counts in SCD are associated with an increased risk for mortality and with cerebral infarction [6,33]. In addition, leukocyte counts are indicative of overall disease severity [34,35]. Reduction in leukocyte counts on hydroxyurea correlated with the improvement in frequency of both acute painful events and ACS [36]. Several recent reports appear to establish a link between severe vaso-occlusive events and the administration of G-CSF for hematopoietic stem cell mobilization, including apparent induction of an ACS [37–39]. Moreover, intravital microscopy of a transgenic sickle mouse model demonstrated adherence of circulating sickle erythrocytes to granulocytes already adherent to venular endothelium [40]. This interaction increased after administration of TNF-α and resulted in complete vaso-occlusion.

Additional vasoactive components may play a role in the ACS process. Endothelin-1 (ET-1) is a potent vasoconstrictor of the pulmonary vascular bed; its levels are increased with hypoxemia [41]. In patients who have SCD, ET-1 levels are increased during the steady state and rise sharply just before and during ACS [42]. Nitric oxide (NO) is a potent vasodilator that is generated from the amino acid L-arginine by means of NO synthase [43]. When administered by inhalation in low concentration, NO causes selective pulmonary vasodilatation, improving ventilation/perfusion ratios. Systemic vasodilatation does not occur, because NO is rapidly inactivated by Hb binding. Inhaled NO decreases PAP and PVR in acute lung injury and improves oxygenation in neonates with pulmonary hypertension [43–45]. L-arginine levels are low in adults with SCD and decrease during acute pain episodes and in ACS [46], whereas NO metabolites [47,48] are increased, suggesting accelerated metabolism and possible depletion of NO in these acute illnesses. NO is important in counteracting the upregulation of VCAM-1. It has been shown to reduce cytokine-induced endothelial cell activation by repression of VCAM-1 gene transcription [49]. Furthermore, NO inhibits the adherence of normal and sickle erythrocytes to vascular endothelium and prolongs survival in a transgenic mouse model of SCD exposed to hypoxia [50–52]. Alterations in the balance between ET-1 vasoconstriction and NO vasodilatation can affect capillary transit time, endothelial cell expression of VCAM-1, and its attendant adherence characteristics, altering intrapulmonary flow and enhancing microvascular obstruction. However, trapping of dense erythrocytes may occur on a mechanical basis in areas of hypoxic lung aside from the mechanisms of cellular adhesion [52,53].

Thus, microvascular occlusion in the sickling diseases may occur as the result of a complex series of reactions involving activation of the endothelium by oxygen radicals from the erythrocytes, or it may occur by means of infectious processes that induce the secretion of inflammatory cytokines. Adherence of less-dense sickle erythrocytes or leukocytes to endothelium and adherence of dense sickle erythrocytes to leukocytes follows, leading to partial obstruction of microcirculatory flow. Prolonged transit time allows extensive polymerization of Hb S with its resultant erythrocyte rigidity. Trapping of poorly deformable sickle erythrocytes results in transient or prolonged obstruction of microvascular flow. The subsequent ischemia further induces endothelial activation, leading to a vicious cycle of adherence, trapping, and prolonged ischemia that is responsible for the signs and symptoms of ACS in this disease.

LABORATORY FEATURES

The chest radiographic findings are variable and may include segmental, lobar, or multilobar consolidation. In nearly half the cases, the initial chest radiograph is negative, showing only the characteristic findings of cardiomegaly with redistribution of blood flow to the upper lobes resulting from the chronic anemia. Infiltrates may not appear until 2 or 3 days later [8,10,18,54]. The chest radiograph findings vary by age; children have isolated upper or middle lobe disease significantly more often than adults, whereas adults have lower lobe or multilobe disease more often [8,10]. Pleural effusions are seen in more than half the episodes and are more common in adults [8,10,54]. The chest radiograph underestimates the degree of pulmonary involvement, as has been shown by simultaneous high-resolution CT scan or perfusion scintigraphy. Thin-section (3-mm) CT scans have shown consolidation, hypoperfusion, a paucity of arterioles and venules, and areas of ground-glass attenuation in areas both involved and uninvolved on plain radiograph [55]. Perfusion lung scans have also shown defects in areas that were normal on radiograph [56,57]. These imaging findings are consistent with vascular occlusion of large vessels as an important component of ACS.

Typically, the Hb declines by 0.7 g/dL, and the white blood cells increase by 70% on average [5,8,10]. Bacteremia is more common in children, with *S pneumoniae and H influenzae* found most often. Sputum and blood cultures are insensitive means of detecting bacterial pneumonia and most likely underestimate its frequency. There is a growing trend toward the use of bronchoscopy to obtain high quality material for culture. In one study, bacterial disease was detected by bronchoalveolar lavage in 20% of adult cases [58], a substantially higher frequency than that reported in the multi-institutional group studies, despite an aggressive approach to obtaining deep sputum for culture. Bronchoscopy has been extremely successful in detecting lipid-laden macrophages for the diagnosis of fat embolism [59,60]. Bronchoscopy has the additional advantage of detecting plastic bronchitis, a complication with branching bronchial cast formation that can produce worsening hypoxemia from ventilation/perfusion mismatch [61]. Plastic bronchitis was detected in 21 of 29 episodes of ACS (72%) in one study where bronchoscopy was performed in patients with worsening lung consolidation and progressive hypoxemia [61]; it was associated with improvement in chest radiograph findings after the procedure. This high frequency of plastic bronchitis may not be representative of all cases of ACS, because the procedure tends to be performed in the most seriously ill group of patients [59,61].

Secretory phospholipase A_2 ($sPLA_2$) is a potent inflammatory mediator that has been implicated in the pathophysiology of multiple conditions, including sepsis, multiorgan failure, arthritis, and ARDS [62–64]. $sPLA_2$ hydrolyzes phospholipids to produce free fatty acids and lysophospholipids, both of which cause acute lung injury. Additional inflammatory hydrolysis products, such as leukotrienes, thromboxanes, and prostaglandins, are produced when arachadonic acid is the fatty acid product of $sPLA_2$ [62]. $sPLA_2$ is modestly elevated in sickle cell patients at baseline and increases dramatically with ACS; the degree of elevation correlates with measures of the severity of the lung injury, such as A-a gradient [65,66]. Because nearly half of ACS episodes occur in patients presenting with acute pain and because $sPLA_2$ rises 24 to 48 hours before the onset of ACS in preliminary studies [65,66], $sPLA_2$ in combination with fever may have predictive value for the development of ACS in patients presenting with pain. It may indicate the fat embolism syndrome, in which free fatty acids and eicosanoids may be generated from the fat particles lodged in the pulmonary circulation.

Measurement of oxygen saturation in Hb S disorders is confounded by the lower oxygen affinity of Hb S (Fig. 1) [67,68] and by elevations of carboxyhemoglobin and methemoglobin consequent to the hemolytic anemia. The oxygen saturation as assessed by automated blood gas analyzers calculates the saturation from the measured PaO_2 against a standard oxygen dissociation curve for Hb A; consequently, this method overestimates the saturation for samples containing

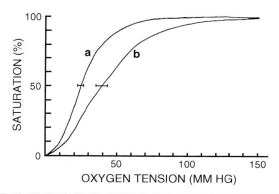

Fig. 1. Representative oxygen saturation curves (by association) in (a) 41 normals (mean p50 = 26.3 mm Hg, standard error of the mean [sem] = 1.1) and in (b) 53 subjects with sickle cell anemia (mean p50 = 37.8, sem = 4.1). Note that for any given pO2, the saturation for Hb SS cells is less than that for normal erythrocytes. (*Artwork by* SL Johnson. *Modified from* Johnson CS, Verdegem TV. Pulmonary complications of sickle cell disease. Semin Resp Med 1988; 9:291; with permission.)

Hb S [68]. Co-oximetry uses multiple wavelengths to distinguish oxyhemoglobin from deoxyhemoglobin, carboxyhemoglobin, and methemoglobin and is the most accurate method [69,70]. Pulse oximetry measurements may overestimate the oxygen saturation by including methemoglobin and carboxyhemoglobin, which are often slightly increased in Hb S disorders; pulse oximetry is further affected by conditions that reduce the pulse amplitude, such as hypotension, hypothermia, and vasoconstriction [70]. In one study comparing the three methods, the co-oximetry and pulse oximetry showed near agreement (pulse oximetry only 2% greater than co-oximetry), but the calculated saturation overestimated the co-oximetry measurement by nearly 7% on average [68]. A subsequent study confirmed that pulse oximetry overestimates co-oximetry by only 1.1% [71].

DIAGNOSIS

The causes of ACS are multiple (Box 1) and include disorders directly or indirectly related to the sickling process as well as causes distinct from sickling. *Chlamydia*, *Mycoplasma*, and viral infections are now the infectious agents most commonly identified [8,15,16]. *Chlamydia* was found more commonly in adolescents and adults, whereas *Mycoplasma* and viral infections were more common in young children. Sputum and blood culture should be performed, despite the historically low yield, so as to identify bacterial agents when present. Cultures positive for nonrespiratory pathogens must be carefully interpreted [72]. Negative cultures are often explained by problems in contamination, collection, storage, or handling or by prior antibiotic administration [73,74]. Serologic studies for *Mycoplasma*, *Chlamydia*, and parvovirus are helpful in the diagnosis of these infections. Nasopharyngeal samples for viral cultures should

---

Box 1: Specific causes for the acute chest syndrome

The frequencies of specific diagnoses are listed as described by the NACSSG.

1. *Hb S–Related*
   a. *Direct consequences of Hb S*
      - Pulmonary vaso-occlusion (16.1%)
      - Fat embolism from bone marrow ischemia/infarction (8.8%)
      - Hypoventilation secondary to rib/sternal bone infarction or to narcotic administration
      - Pulmonary edema induced by narcotics or fluid overload
   b. *Indirect consequences of Hb S*
      - Infection
         Atypical bacterial
            Chlamydia pneumoniae (7.2%)
            Mycoplasma pneumoniae (6.6%)
            Mycoplasma hominis (1.0%)
         Bacterial
            Staphylococcus aureus, coagulase-positive (1.8%)
            Streptococcus pneumoniae (1.6%)
            Haemophilus influenzae (0.7%)
         Viral
            Respiratory syncytial virus (3.9%)
            Parvovirus B19 (1.5%)
            Rhinovirus (1.2%)
2. *Unrelated to Hb S*
   a. *Fibrin thromboembolism*
   b. *Other common pulmonary diseases (eg, aspiration, trauma, asthma)*

(*Data from* Refs. [8,67].)

---

be included, especially in children, where viral disease is increasingly recognized [13]. Recent data indicate that fiber optic bronchoscopy and bronchoalveolar lavage (BAL) provide higher-quality specimens for culture and microscopic examination and a higher yield, thus improving confidence in a negative result [58–60].

However, all studies stress that, as in the general population [14], most ACS episodes in this patient population cannot be proved to be of infectious origin, and noninfectious causes must be sought carefully. Vichinsky and colleagues [75] published a study in which 12 of 27 episodes of ACS had evidence of fat embolism as the cause; subsequent reports indicate an even higher prevalence of fat embolism in ACS [59,60]. Data from the NACSSG indicate that fat embolism, at 8.8%, was the most common diagnosis established and was found more often in adults [8]. Fat and bone marrow elements within the circulation, released from necrotic marrow sites of ischemic vaso-occlusion, can produce embolic phenomena involving the lungs and other tissues. The spectrum of disease in fat embolism varies widely, from isolated pulmonary fat embolism to a fulminant multiorgan failure syndrome with high fever, severe tachypnea, hypoxemia, bilateral alveolar infiltrates, tachycardia, neurologic changes, thrombocytopenia, worsening anemia, and altered renal or liver function [76,77]. Laboratory findings in the fat embolism syndrome include a dramatic rise in LDH, uric acid, and nucleated red blood cells and a decline in serum Ca^{++}. Serum lipase and $sPLA_2$ increase. None of these biochemical tests are specific for the diagnosis, so that clinical suspicion remains its mainstay. Examination of deep sputum or BAL specimens for fat-laden macrophages [59,60] is useful in the diagnosis of the fat embolism syndrome, as is examination for trunkal petechiae and lipemia retinalis; fat globules may be found in the blood and urine. Severe bone pain and relative thrombocytopenia may provide clues to this diagnosis in sickle cell patients.

Vascular occlusion by sickle cells and pulmonary infarction appear to be important causes of ACS, as suggested by the lack of positive bacterial or viral cultures in carefully studied patients and by the data indicating that antibiotic therapy produces no faster resolution than treatment with supportive care alone [7,8,10,72]. The results from the Multi-Institutional Study of Hydroxyurea in SCD, which indicate a significant reduction in ACS in those patients who are on hydroxyurea, further suggest that a substantial number of ACS episodes are secondary to vascular obstruction [36]. Hence our focus on infection as the most prevalent cause may have been misplaced.

Fibrin thromboembolism appears to occur at a rate similar to that in the general population [78], but distinguishing thromboemboli from sickle cell vaso-occlusion by chest tomography or scintigraphy is extremely difficult; recent data indicate nearly identical findings with these modalities [55,57]. Evidence for concomitant venous thrombosis, comparison of current lung scintigraphy with baseline data or angiography may be helpful in establishing a diagnosis [79]. In those cases of ACS where pulmonary angiography has been performed, the findings were most consistent with vascular occlusion [80]. Exchange transfusion before angiography is recommended to prevent vaso-occlusion due to sickling induced by hyperosmolar contrast media [81].

Hypoventilation can lead to regional pulmonary hypoxia and initiate the sequence of events that leads to adhesion-related vascular occlusion. The recognition that splinting due to the pain of rib infarction was frequently associated with atelectasis and evolved into ACS led to the use of incentive spirometry for prevention [82,83]. More recently, it was found that patients receiving oral sustained-release morphine for pain control during a vaso-occlusive crisis (VOC) developed an ACS at a rate threefold that of patients randomized to continuous-intravenous morphine [84]. The difference was attributed to an area under the curve for sustained-release morphine that was two- to threefold greater than that for intravenous morphine and was associated with a significant decrease in SaO_2 for those on oral morphine, related to hypoventilation.

MANAGEMENT

In the absence of a specific causative diagnosis, treatment of ACS is primarily supportive and can be approached from three general directions: prophylaxis, standard management, and treatment of evolving respiratory failure. Prophylactic penicillin and the use of the pneumococcal and *H influenza* vaccines may have had a role in the changing epidemiology of ACS in SCD. Although specific studies of vaccine impact on the frequency of pneumococcal pneumonia have not been reported, the reduced frequency of this organism in the ACS, as reported in recent studies, may be extrapolated from vaccine use and from the effect of prophylactic penicillin on the frequency of pneumococcal sepsis [85,86]. The HiB vaccine may have had a similar effect on the previously reported high frequency of pulmonary infection with this organism in SCD. Parvovirus B19 infection has been associated with a particularly severe form of ACS, so vaccination for this virus, as well as influenza and respiratory syncytial virus, should be considered, depending on future availability [87]. Treatment with hydroxyurea reduces the incidence of ACS by approximately 40% and is indicated for those who have had two or more episodes of ACS, independent of its indication for recurrent VOC [36]. Because of the relationship between ACS and premature mortality, prevention of ACS and its associated complications with hydroxyurea is a possible factor in the reduction of mortality recently reported for hydroxyurea-treated patients [88].

In an episode of ACS, the immediate goals of therapy are prevention of alveolar collapse, maintenance of gas exchange, and prevention of further pulmonary injury leading to a progressive downhill course. Serial determination of arterial blood gases can be quite useful in assessing progress. Charache and colleagues [7] first noted that an increase in arterial oxygen tension is the first sign of improvement, before a change in chest radiograph, and that a PaO_2 of less than 75 mm Hg (approximately equal to an SaO_2 of 85% to 90% [see Fig. 1]) is associated with a poor prognosis.

The chest radiograph lags behind the physiologic changes by a substantial margin and is not as useful for prognostication, although Davies and colleagues [72] noted that the duration of fever and degree of tachycardia were related to the extent of chest radiograph involvement. However, Charache and colleagues [7] did not find a difference in PaO_2 among patients with more extensive radiographic changes. The arterial blood gas data should be carefully interpreted relative to the fraction of inspired oxygen required to achieve adequate oxygenation [89] and in view of the reduced oxygen affinity of Hb S (see Fig. 1) [67]. SaO_2 should be maintained with supplemental oxygen at 92% or greater, because the effect of moderate arterial desaturation on the microvascular rheology of sickle erythrocyte is adversely affected by partial polymerization of intracellular Hb S [90,91], with its attendant risk for pulmonary trapping of poorly deformable erythrocyte [52,53]. In patients who have partial nasal obstruction, oxygen by mask may provide superior efficacy over delivery by nasal cannula.

Serial chest radiographs are needed to assess the extent and course of the pulmonary changes. However, serial arterial blood gas determinations on an FiO_2 of 0.21 provide a clearer picture of ongoing pulmonary function, because the chest radiograph often lags behind physiologic events. Arterial blood gas measurements may be replaced by continuous pulse oximetry monitoring, especially when there have been simultaneous determinations in the patient to establish the correlation between the two. Oxygen saturation or the alveolar-arterial oxygen gradient, rather than oxygen tension, provide more relevant information [92]. Careful attention to clinical parameters—vital signs, respiratory effort, and overall status—is the key ingredient in overall assessment.

Antibiotics are generally administered, although the studies of Charache [7] and Davies [72] and their colleagues indicate that antibiotic treatment may not shorten the clinical course. The choice of antibiotic coverage must be made on clinical grounds, considering the well-described secular changes in microbial flora as well as geographic effects on the microbial spectrum [8,12,17]. In view of recent epidemiologic studies, the current recommendation is to use a third- or fourth-generation cephalosporin and a macrolide [8], but the decision should be guided by knowledge of local bacterial patterns and by the results of sputum smear analysis and should be modified as culture results become available. Alternative regimens include a quinolone or a macrolide plus a betalactam. Progression of disease should prompt a reassessment of antibiotic coverage because of the occasional gram-negative organism and the high frequency of viral agents.

Pain management often requires narcotic analgesia, which can produce respiratory depression with its attendant risk of hypoxia and its potential for acceleration of pulmonary vaso-occlusion [84]. Pleuritic chest pain is a particular problem, because splinting reduces ventilation and may predispose to atelectasis. Intercostal nerve block with a long-acting local anesthetic, such as bupivacaine, can alleviate chest wall pain and splinting and has the additional advantage of reducing the amount of systemic analgesia needed to control pain and lessening the consequent risks of respiratory depression, hypoxia and atelectasis. A nerve block may provide relief for 18 to 24 hours and can be repeated as needed to control symptoms [67].

Limiting intravenous fluid administration to a rate of 1.5 to 2.0 times maintenance is the standard practice, because overly aggressive hydration, as well as opioid administration, can lead to pulmonary edema and cause ACS [16,93]. It appears unlikely that fluid overload alone could be a common cause of ACS, given the large numbers of patients treated with this modality, unless those affected had a subtle underlying cardiopulmonary pathologic condition that was unmasked by high-volume saline administration. Because the objective is rehydration of erythrocytes [91], a hypotonic infusion, such as half-normal saline (0.25 normal for children) with or without dextrose, is preferred over normal saline, which might be responsible for the reported cases of pulmonary edema [16,93].

Incentive spirometry (maximum of 10 inspirations every 2 hours while awake) has been shown significantly to reduce the development of atelectasis and the risk for ACS and should be instituted for all hospitalizations for pain as well as for those with ACS [94]. The high frequency of reactive airway disease with wheezing reported in SCD supports the universal use of bronchodilators as an important adjunctive therapy [8,10,95,96]. Mechanical ventilation is indicated, as for other causes of progressive respiratory insufficiency. Both high-frequency ventilation and extracorporeal membrane oxygenation have been successfully employed in severe cases of respiratory failure in ACS [97–101].

The role of transfusion support is not clearly defined, although there are sporadic case reports of rapid reversal of chest radiograph findings and symptoms immediately posttransfusion [72,102,103]. At least two broad indications for transfusion clearly appear to exist. Simple transfusion of one or two units may be given to raise the Hb level whenever there is a need for an increase in oxygen-carrying capacity. The therapeutic objectives are to make the patient more comfortable and to reduce the cardiac workload; the indications include moderately severe anemia, high cardiac output, tachycardia, and easy fatigability. Whenever the clinical situation indicates impending respiratory failure such that mechanical ventilation might be required, exchange transfusion should be considered on an urgent basis. Exchange transfusion should be used early, at the first hint of difficulty, rather than later, when the situation may no longer be reversible. Exchange transfusion may produce rapid resolution of ACS, which justifies its early use and suggests that vascular occlusion is readily reversible, at least in the early stages [72,102,103]. This rapid improvement after transfusion is further evidence for microvascular occlusion as a part of ACS, but it could also indicate another reversible lung disease, such as fat embolism.

The indications for exchange transfusion in ACS have not been fully defined, but extrapolation from the pneumonia severity index identifies poor prognostic factors that are applicable to SCD (Box 2) [104]. The pneumonia severity index has not yet been applied to ACS but has features that are intuitively attractive. In clinical practice, transfusions are recommended whenever there is evidence of worsening pulmonary function, as evidenced by a progressive decrease in SaO_2, a decrease in PaO_2, an increase in $A-aO_2$ gradient, worsening infiltrates on chest radiograph, or increasing tachycardia or work of breathing. In addition to these indications, exchange transfusion may have a specific therapeutic action in the fat embolism syndrome, where normal red cells may bind the free fatty acids, preventing further pulmonary damage. Finally, exchange should be considered whenever there is general clinical evidence of a declining course or when indicators of poor prognosis are present. Exchange transfusion dilutes the proportion of sickle cells, improves the blood rheology and flow, reduces the risk of further organ damage from either intrapulmonary or peripheral sickle vaso-occlusion, and improves oxygenation (see the article by Wanko and Telen elsewhere in this issue for further exploration of this topic) [8]. The objective of

Box 2: Clinical features that imply poor prognosis and are potential indications for exchange transfusion in the acute chest syndrome

Physical Examination Findings

- Altered mental status and other acute neurologic findings
- Persistent tachycardia >125/min
- Persistent respiratory rate >30/min or increased work of breathing (nasal flaring, use of accessory muscles, sternal retractions)
- Temperature >40°C
- Hypotension compared with baseline

Laboratory and Radiographic Findings

- Arterial pH <7.35
- Arterial oxygen saturation persistently <88%, despite aggressive ventilatory support
- Serial decline in pulse oximetry or increasing A-a gradient
- Hemoglobin concentration falling by 2 g/dL or more
- Platelet count <200,000/μL
- Evidence for multiorgan failure
- Pleural effusion
- Progression to multilobe infiltrates

(Data from Refs. [8,67,104].*)*

transfusion in these situations is life saving, because progressive worsening of clinical status is associated with high mortality.

Transfusion carries two risks that are particularly relevant to the sickle cell patient: alloimmunization and acute hyperviscosity. Alloimmunization data from the preoperative transfusion study indicate a 10% rate of new alloantibody formation from a transfusion intervention [105]. Subsequent transfusion therapy has an increased risk for delayed hemolytic transfusion reaction [106]; such reactions are extremely difficult to treat, because further transfusion is usually ineffective in maintaining the hematocrit. An extended phenotype match can reduce the incidence of alloimmunization [107,108] and should include Rh, C, E, and Kell antigens at a minimum [108] (see the article by Johnson elsewhere in this issue for further exploration of this topic). The hyperviscosity syndrome may occur with mixtures of A and S cells at near-normal hematocrits [109,110]. The syndrome is characterized by hypertension and altered mental status or seizure activity. Screening donor units for sickle cell trait and maintaining the posttransfusion hematocrit at levels less than 35% may prevent this syndrome. It is widely believed that a posttransfusion level of Hb S of less than 10% is therapeutically superior to one of 20% or 30%. Data in support of this contention are lacking. However, the hypothesis is intuitively attractive. The simplest method of monitoring the posttransfusion Hb S level is to determine the percentage of sickled cells in a meta-bisulfite preparation. Alternatively, Hb S can be measured by one of the common column chromatography methods.

Recurrent episodes of ACS may lead to sickle cell chronic lung disease, characterized by diffuse interstitial fibrosis on chest radiograph, abnormal pulmonary function tests, symptomatic hypoxia, pulmonary hypertension, and sudden death [111–113]. The further association of recurrent ACS with premature mortality in the CSSCD [5] provides justification for aggressive secondary prevention approaches in patients with recurrent episodes, including hydroxyurea, chronic transfusion therapy, and stem cell transplantation [114].

FUTURE DIRECTIONS

Despite the recent advances in our understanding of the pathophysiology and epidemiology of ACS, there are still needs for better methods of distinguishing vaso-occlusion from fibrin or fat embolism, for rapid diagnostic tests to identify microbial infection positively, for adjunctive therapies that would affect prognosis, and for identification of factors that influence prognosis and might predict which patients will recover with supportive care alone and which will progress to pulmonary failure. Documentation of the clinical utility of $sPLA_2$ for ACS and its relationship to the fat embolism syndrome would be useful as an early marker for the ACS and, perhaps, for clinical severity. Potential therapies for $sPLA_2$ inhibition are under development, and clinical trials examining the predictive capability of $sPLA_2$ are under way [115].

In a recent study, dexamethasone, 0.3 mg/kg, was administered to patients who had ACS at 12-hour intervals for four doses and produced significant reductions in the treated group versus placebo with respect to duration of fever, analgesic use, supplemental oxygen therapy, transfusion requirements, and hospital stay (reduced by 40%) [116]. The beneficial effect was attributed to inhibition of $sPLA_2$ and inhibition of inflammation; however, this steroid also prevents cytokine induction of VCAM-1 on endothelial cells and could ameliorate the course of ACS by this mechanism as well [117]. Prolonged infusion (240 mg/d for 7 days) of glucocorticoid has been reported in studies of community-acquired pneumonia in the general population; beneficial effects on chest radiograph, oxygenation, indices of inflammation, length of hospital stay, and mortality have been shown [118]. In addition, beneficial effects of high-dose steroid in the fat embolism syndrome have been reported in small controlled trials in trauma patients [119,120] and could have produced benefit in sickle ACS, where fat embolism is common, owing to inhibition of inflammation. These results indicate the need for further studies of the efficacy of steroid use in ACS.

A beneficial effect of nitric oxide (NO) has been reported in small numbers of patients who had ACS, where inhaled NO at 80 ppm for 47 to 92 hours rapidly improved A-a gradient, reduced PAP and PVR, and was believed to have accelerated recovery [121–123]. Inhaled NO could benefit patients who have

ACS by pulmonary vascular dilation, reducing pulmonary vascular resistance and improving intrapulmonary blood flow. Further studies are needed to define the therapeutic utility and potential for methemoglobin toxicity of this agent, but its use has the potential to reduce the need for more aggressive therapies and to improve prognosis.

Purified polaxamer 188 is a nonionic surfactant that reduces blood viscosity and inhibits erythrocyte adhesion to endothelium [124]. A recent clinical trial of this agent showed a modest effect on the duration of VOC [125]. The results of the polaxamer 188 study suggest that blocking sickle cell adhesion to endothelium may be beneficial for vascular occlusive events in SCD, such as ACS. A further step in this process is the development of a recombinant P-selectin glycoprotein ligand that binds to P-selectin and, to a lesser degree, to E- and L-selectin [126]. Recent studies using monoclonal antibodies and knock-out mice have shown that P-selectin mediates the initial interaction of sickle erythrocytes and leukocytes with activated endothelial cells [127,128]. Thus, blockade of P-selectin using this fusion protein could provide clinical benefit in ACS by inhibiting the adhesion of leukocytes and sickle erythrocytes to pulmonary endothelium in the vaso-occlusive process. Additional agents that inhibit other adhesogenic proteins involved in the vaso-occlusive process, such as the integrin $\alpha_V\beta_3$ and VLA-4, are also under study [129–131].

SUMMARY

The recent large clinical studies of ACS have improved our understanding of the pathophysiology and epidemiology of ACS. However, there are still needs for better methods of distinguishing vaso-occlusion from fibrin or fat embolism, for rapid diagnostic tests to make positive identifications of microbial infection, for adjunctive therapies that would affect prognosis, and for identification of factors that influence prognosis. The difference in clinical course and severity between children and adults supports the results of current studies indicating multiple causes for ACS. Infectious causes are more common in children, as suggested by the shorter and milder course, seasonal variation, upper lobe disease, and higher rate of bacteremia. In adults, severe bone pain and lower lobe or multilobe disease point to vascular occlusion as the common cause of ACS, much as Barrett-Connor indicated in her initial reports [4,11]. The mainstay of successful treatment remains high-quality supportive care. Consultation with pulmonary, infectious disease, and intensive care specialists is a necessary part of management. Fluid management, oxygenation, bronchodilators, and incentive spirometry are essential elements of supportive care management. The judicious use of transfusion therapy has a major role in preventing mortality in the absence of a specific therapy that consistently improves the clinical course.

References

[1] Kaul DK, Fabry ME, Nagel RL. The pathophysiology of vascular obstruction in the sickle syndromes. Blood Rev 1996;10:29–44.

[2] Steinberg MH, Rodgers GP. Pathophysiology of sickle cell disease: role of cellular and genetic modifiers. Semin Hematol 2001;38:299–306.

[3] Serjeant GR. Sickle cell disease. 3rd edition. Oxford (UK): Oxford University Press; 2001.

[4] Barrett-Connor E. Acute pulmonary disease and sickle cell anemia. Am Rev Respir Dis 1971;104:155–65.

[5] Castro O, Brambilla DJ, Thorington B, et al, The Cooperative Study of Sickle Cell Disease. The acute chest syndrome in sickle cell disease: incidence and risk factors. Blood 1994; 84:643–9.

[6] Platt OS, Brambilla DJ, Rosse WF, et al. Mortality in sickle cell disease. Life expectancy and risk factors for early death. N Engl J Med 1994;330:1639–44.

[7] Charache S, Scott JC, Charache P. Acute chest syndrome in adults with sickle cell anemia: microbiology, treatment and prevention. Arch Intern Med 1979;139:67–9.

[8] Vichinsky EP, Neumayr LD, Earles AN, et al, National Acute Chest Syndrome Study Group. Causes and outcomes of the acute chest syndrome in sickle cell disease. N Engl J Med 2000;342:1855–65.

[9] Petch MC, Serjeant GR. Clinical features of pulmonary lesions in sickle-cell anaemia. BMJ 1970;3:31.

[10] Vichinsky EP, Styles LA, Colangelo LH, et al, The Cooperative Study of Sickle Cell Disease. Acute chest syndrome in sickle cell disease: clinical presentation and course. Blood 1997;89:1787–92.

[11] Barrett-Connor E. Pneumonia and pulmonary infarction in sickle cell anemia. JAMA 1973;224:997–1000.

[12] Gray GC, Mitchell BS, Tueller JE, et al. Pneumonia hospitalizations in the US Navy and Marine Corps: rates and risk factors for 6,522 admissions, 1981–1991. Am J Epidemiol 1994;139:793–802.

[13] Tsolia MN, Psarras S, Bossios A, et al. Etiology of community-acquired pneumonia in hospitalized school-age children: evidence for high prevalence of viral infections. Clin Infect Dis 2004;39:681–6.

[14] Apisarnthanarak A, Mundy LM. Etiology of community-acquired pneumonia. Clin Chest Med 2005;26:47–55.

[15] Poncz M, Kane E, Gill FM. Acute chest syndrome in sickle cell disease: etiology and clinical correlates. J Pediatr 1985;107:861–6.

[16] Sprinkle RH, Cole T, Smith S, et al. Acute chest syndrome in children with sickle cell disease: a retrospective analysis of 100 hospitalized cases. Am J Pediatr Hematol Oncol 1986;8:105–10.

[17] van Agtmael MA, Cheng JD, Nassent HC. Acute chest syndrome in adult Afro-Caribbean patients with sickle cell disease. Arch Intern Med 1994;154:557–61.

[18] Morris C, Vichinsky E, Styles L. Clinician assessment for acute chest syndrome in febrile patients with sickle cell disease: is it accurate enough? Ann Emerg Med 1999;34:64–9.

[19] Falter ML, Robinson MG, Kim OS, et al. Splenic function and infection in sickle cell anemia. Acta Hematol 1973;59:154–61.

[20] Wilson WA, Thomas EJ, Sissons JGP. Complement activation in asymptomatic patients with sickle cell anaemia. Clin Exp Immunol 1979;36:130–9.

[21] Larcher VF, Wyke RJ, Davies LR, et al. Defective yeast opsonisation and functional deficiency of complement in sickle cell disease. Arch Dis Child 1982;57:343–6.

[22] Bjornson AB, Lobel JS, Harr KS. Relation between serum opsonic activity for Streptococcus pneumoniae and complement function in sickle cell disease. J Infect Dis 1985;152: 701–9.

[23] Bjornson AB, Lobel JS. Direct evidence that decreased serum opsonization of Streptococcus pneumoniae via the alternative complement pathway in sickle cell disease is related to antibody deficiency. J Clin Invest 1987;79:388–98.

[24] Bjornson AB, Falletta JM, Verter JI, et al. Serotype-specific immunoglobulin G antibody responses to pneumococcal polysaccharide vaccine in children with sickle cell anemia: effects of continued penicillin prophylaxis. J Pediatr 1996;129:828–35.

[25] Siber GR. Pneumococcal disease: prospects for a new generation of vaccines. Science 1994;265:1385–7.

[26] Wang WC, Wong WY, Rogers ZA, et al. Antibiotic-resistant pneumococcal infection in children with sickle cell disease in the United States. J Pediatr Hematol Oncol 1996;18:140–4.
[27] Taylor SC, Shacks SJ, Mitchell RA. In vitro lymphocyte blastogenic responses and cytokine production in sickle cell disease patients with acute pneumonia. Pediatr Infect Dis J 1996;15:340–4.
[28] Frenette P. Sickle cell vaso-occlusion: multistep and multicellular paradigm. Curr Opin Hematol 2002;9:101–6.
[29] Setty BNY, Stuart MJ. Vascular cell adhesion molecule–1 is involved in mediating hypoxia induced sickle red blood cell adherence to endothelium: potential role in sickle cell disease. Blood 1996;88:2311–20.
[30] Browne P, Shalev O, Hebbel RP. The molecular pathobiology of cell membrane iron: the sickle red cell as a model. Free Radic Biol Med 1998;24:1040–8.
[31] Shiu Y-T, Udden MM, McIntire LV. Perfusion with sickle erythrocytes up-regulates ICAM-1 and VCAM-1 gene expression in cultured human endothelial cells. Blood 2000;95: 3232–41.
[32] Kunsch C, Medford RM. Oxidative stress as a regulator of gene expression in the vasculature. Circ Res 1999;85:753–66.
[33] Kinney TR, Sleeper LA, Wang WC, et al, The Cooperative Study of Sickle Cell Disease. Silent cerebral infarcts in sickle cell anemia: a risk factor analysis. Pediatrics 1999; 103:640–5.
[34] Miller ST, Sleeper LA, Pegelow CH, et al. Prediction of adverse outcomes in children with sickle cell disease. N Engl J Med 2000;342:83–9.
[35] Anyaegbu CC, Okplal IE, Aken'Ova AY, et al. Peripheral blood neutrophil count and candicidal activity correlate with the clinical severity in sickle cell anaemia. Eur J Hematol 1998;60:267–8.
[36] Charache S, Terrin ML, Moore RD, et al. Effect of hydroxyurea on the frequency of painful crises in sickle cell anemia. N Engl J Med 1995;332:1317–22.
[37] Abgboud M, Laver J, Blau CA. Granulocytosis causing sickle-cell crisis. Lancet 1998; 351:959.
[38] Adler BK, Salzman DE, Carabasi MH, et al. Fatal sickle cell crisis after granulocyte colony–stimulating factor administration. Blood 2001;97:3313–4.
[39] Grigg AP. Granulocyte colony–stimulating factor–induced sickle cell crisis and multiorgan dysfunction in a patient with compound heterozygous sickle cell/beta+ thalassemia. Blood 2001;97:3998–9.
[40] Turhan A, Weiss LA, Mohandas N, et al. Primary role for adherent leukocytes in sickle cell vascular occlusion: a new paradigm. Proc Natl Acad Sci U S A 2002;99:3047–51.
[41] Yuan X-J, Wang J, Juhaszova M, et al. Attenuated K+ channel gene transcription in primary pulmonary hypertension. Lancet 1998;351:726–7.
[42] Hammerman SI, Kourembanas S, Conca TJ, et al. Endothelin-1 production during the acute chest syndrome in sickle cell disease. Am J Respir Crit Care Med 1997;156:280–5.
[43] Moncada S, Higgs A. Mechanisms of disease: the L-arginine-nitric oxide pathway. N Engl J Med 1993;329:2002–12.
[44] Rossaint R, Falke KJ, Lopez F, et al. Inhaled nitric oxide for the adult respiratory distress syndrome. N Engl J Med 1993;328:399–405.
[45] Clark RH, Kueser TJ, Walker MW, et al, The Clinical Inhaled Nitric Oxide Research Group. Low-dose nitric oxide therapy for persistent pulmonary hypertension of the newborn. N Engl J Med 2000;342:469–74.
[46] Morris CR, Kuypers FA, Larkin S, et al. Patterns of arginine and nitric oxide in patients with sickle cell disease with vaso-occlusive crisis and acute chest syndrome. J Pediatr Hematol Oncol 2000;22:515–20.
[47] Morris CR, Kuypers FA, Larkin S, et al. Arginine therapy: a novel strategy to induce nitric oxide production in sickle cell disease. Br J Haematol 2000;111:498–500.
[48] Rees DC, Cervi P, Grimwade D, et al. The metabolites of nitric oxide in sickle-cell disease. Br J Haematol 1995;91:834–7.

[49] De Caterina R, Libby P, Peng H, et al. Nitric oxide decreases cytokine-induced endothelial activation: nitric oxide selectively reduces endothelial expression of adhesion molecules and proinflammatory cytokines. J Clin Invest 1995;96:60–8.

[50] Space SL, Lane PA, Pickett CK, et al. Nitric oxide attenuates normal and sickle red blood cell adherence to pulmonary endothelium. Am J Hematol 2000;63:200–4.

[51] Martinez-Ruiz R, Montero-Huerta P, Hromi J, et al. Inhaled nitric oxide improves survival rates during hypoxia in a sickle cell (SAD) mouse model. Anesthesiology 2001;94:1113–8.

[52] Aldrich TK, Dhuper SK, Patwa NS, et al. Pulmonary entrapment of sickle cells: the role of regional alveolar hypoxia. J Appl Physiol 1996;80:531–9.

[53] Haynes Jr J, Taylor AE, Dixon D, et al. Microvascular hemodynamics in the sickle red blood cell perfused isolated rat lung. Am J Physiol 1993;264:H484–9.

[54] Martin L, Buonomo C. Acute chest syndrome of sickle cell disease: radiographic and clinical analysis of 70 cases. Pediatr Radiol 1997;27:637–41.

[55] Bhalla M, Abboud MR, McLoud TC, et al. Acute chest syndrome in sickle cell disease: CT evidence of microvascular occlusion. Radiology 1993;187:45–9.

[56] Lisbona R, Derbekyan V, Novales-Diaz JA. Scintigraphic evidence of pulmonary vascular occlusion in sickle cell disease. J Nucl Med 1997;38:1151–3.

[57] Babiker MA, Obeid HA, Ashong EF. Acute reversible pulmonary ischemia. A cause of the acute chest syndrome in sickle cell disease. Clin Pediatr 1985;24:716–8.

[58] Kirkpatrick MB, Haynes J, Bass Jr JB. Results of bronchoscopically obtained lower airway cultures from adult sickle cell disease patients with the acute chest syndrome. Am J Med 1991;90:206–10.

[59] Godeau B, Schaeffer A, Bachir D, et al. Bronchoalveolar lavage in adult sickle cell patients with the acute chest syndrome: value for diagnostic assessment of fat embolism. Am J Respir Crit Care Med 1996;153:1691–6.

[60] Maitre B, Habibi A, Roudot-Thoraval F, et al. Acute chest syndrome in adults with sickle cell disease: therapeutic approach, outcome, and results of BAL in a monocentric series of 107 episodes. Chest 2000;117:1386–92.

[61] Moser C, Nussbaum E, Cooper DM. Plastic bronchitis and the role of bronchoscopy in the acute chest syndrome of sickle cell disease. Chest 2001;120:608–13.

[62] Schuster DP. ARDS: clinical lessons from the oleic acid model of acute lung injury. Am J Respir Crit Care Med 1994;149:245–60.

[63] Green J-A, Smith GM, Buchta R, et al. Circulating phospholipase A$_2$ activity associated with sepsis and septic shock is indistinguishable from that associated with rheumatoid arthritis. Inflammation 1991;15:355–67.

[64] Rae D, Porter J, Beechey-Newman N, et al. Type I phospholipase A$_2$ propeptide in acute lung injury. Lancet 1994;344:1472–3.

[65] Styles LA, Schalkwijk CG, Aarsman AJ, et al. Phospholipase A$_2$ levels in acute chest syndrome of sickle cell disease. Blood 1996;87:2573–8.

[66] Styles LA, Aarsman AJ, Vichinsky EP, et al. Secretory phospholipase A$_2$ predicts impending acute chest syndrome in sickle cell disease. Blood 2000;96:3276–8.

[67] Johnson CS, Verdegem TV. Pulmonary complications of sickle cell disease. Semin Resp Med 1988;9:287–93.

[68] Kress JP, Pohlman AS, Hall JB. Determination of hemoglobin saturation in patients with acute sickle chest syndrome: a comparison of arterial blood gases and pulse oximetry. Chest 1999;115:1316–20.

[69] Forte Jr VA, Malconian MK, Burse RL, et al. Operation Everest II: comparison of four instruments for measuring blood O$_2$ saturation. J Appl Physiol 1989;67:2135–40.

[70] Barker SJ, Tremper KK. Pulse oximetry: applications and limitations. Int Anesthesiol Clin 1987;25:155–75.

[71] Ortiz FO, Aldrich TK, Nagel RL, et al. Accuracy of pulse oximetry in sickle cell disease. Am J Respir Crit Care Med 1999;159:447–51.

[72] Davies SC, Luce PJ, Win AA, et al. Acute chest syndrome in sickle-cell disease. Lancet 1984;1:36–8.

[73] Barrett-Connor E. The nonvalue of sputum culture in the diagnosis of pneumococcal pneumonia. Am Rev Respir Dis 1971;103:845–8.

[74] Dean D, Neumayr L, Kelly DM, et al, Acute Chest Syndrome Study Group. Chlamydia pneumoniae and acute chest syndrome in patients with sickle cell disease. J Pediatr Hematol Oncol 2003;25:46–55.

[75] Vichinsky E, Williams R, Das M, et al. Pulmonary fat embolism: a distinct cause of severe acute chest syndrome in sickle cell anemia. Blood 1994;83:3107–12.

[76] Dang NC, Johnson C, Eslami-Farsani M, et al. Bone marrow embolism in sickle cell disease: a review. Am J Hematol 2005;79:61–7.

[77] Hassell KL, Eckman JR, Lane PA. Acute multiorgan failure syndrome: a potentially catastrophic complication of severe sickle cell pain episodes. Am J Med 1994;96:155–62.

[78] Haupt HM, Moore GW, Bauer TW, et al. The lung in sickle cell disease. Chest 1982; 81:332–7.

[79] Walker BK, Ballas SK, Burka ER. The diagnosis of pulmonary thromboembolism in sickle cell disease. Am J Hematol 1979;7:219–32.

[80] Bashour TT, Lindsay Jr J. Hemoglobin S-C disease presenting as acute pneumonitis with pulmonary angiographic findings in two patients. Am J Med 1975;58:559–62.

[81] Richards D, Nulsen FE. Angiographic media and the sickling phenomenon. Surg Forum 1971;22:403–4.

[82] Rucknagel DL, Kalinyak KA, Gelfand MJ. Rib infarcts and acute chest syndrome in sickle cell diseases. Lancet 1991;337:831–3.

[83] Gelfand MJ, Daya SA, Rucknagel DL, et al. Simultaneous occurrence of rib infarction and pulmonary infiltrates in sickle cell disease patients with acute chest syndrome. J Nucl Med 1993;34:614–8.

[84] Kopecky EA, Jacobson S, Joshi P, et al. Systemic exposure to morphine and the risk of acute chest syndrome in sickle cell disease. Clin Pharmacol Ther 2004;75:140–6.

[85] Ammann AJ, Addiego J, Wara DW, et al. Polyvalent pneumococcal-polysaccharide immunization of patients with sickle-cell anemia and patients with splenectomy. N Engl J Med 1977;297:897–900.

[86] Gaston MH, Verter JI, Woods G, et al, The Prophylactic Penicillin Study Group. Prophylaxis with oral penicillin in children with sickle cell anemia. A randomized trial. N Engl J Med 1986;314:1593–9.

[87] Lowenthal EA, Wells A, Emanuel PD, et al. Sickle cell acute chest syndrome associated with parvovirus B19 infection: case series and review. Am J Hematol 1996;51:207–13.

[88] Steinberg MH, Barton F, Castro O, et al. Effect of hydroxyurea on mortality and morbidity in adult sickle cell anemia: risks and benefits up to 9 years of treatment. JAMA 2003;289:1645–51.

[89] Gilbert R, Keighley JF. The arterial/alveolar oxygen tension ratio: an index of gas exchange applicable to varying inspired oxygen concentrations. Am Rev Respir Dis 1974;109:142–5.

[90] Stuart J, Johnson CS. Rheology of the sickle cell disorders. Bailliere's Clin Haematol 1987;1:747–75.

[91] Sowter MC, Green MA, Keidan AJ, et al. Filtration of sickle cells is sensitive to factors that enhance polymerization of haemoglobin S. Clin Hemorheol 1988;8:223–36.

[92] Emre U, Miller ST, Rao SP, et al. Alveolar-arterial oxygen gradient in acute chest syndrome of sickle cell disease. J Pediatr 1993;123:272–5.

[93] Haynes Jr J, Allison RC. Pulmonary edema: complication of the management of sickle cell pain crisis. Am J Med 1986;80:833–40.

[94] Bellet PS, Kalinyak KA, Shukla R, et al. Incentive spirometry to prevent acute pulmonary complications in sickle cell diseases. N Engl J Med 1995;333:699–703.

[95] Leong MA, Dampier C, Varlotta L, et al. Airway hyperreactivity in children with sickle cell disease. J Pediatr 1997;131:278–83.

[96] Koumbourlis AC, Zar HJ, Hurlet-Jensen A, et al. Prevalence and reversibility of lower airway obstruction in children with sickle cell disease. J Pediatr 2001;138:188–92.

[97] Wratney AT, Gentile MA, Hamel DS, et al. Successful treatment of acute chest syndrome with high-frequency oscillatory ventilation in pediatric patients. Respir Care 2004;49: 263–9.

[98] Baird JS, Johnson JL, Escudero J, et al. Combined pressure control/high frequency ventilation in adult respiratory distress syndrome and sickle cell anemia. Chest 1994;106: 1913–6.

[99] Pelidis MA, Kato GJ, Resar LM, et al. Successful treatment of life-threatening acute chest syndrome of sickle cell disease with venovenous extracorporeal membrane oxygenation. J Pediatr Hematol Oncol 1997;19:459–61.

[100] Trant Jr CA, Casey JR, Hansell D, et al. Successful use of extracorporeal membrane oxygenation in the treatment of acute chest syndrome in a child with severe sickle cell anemia. ASAIO J 1996;42:236–9.

[101] Gillett DS, Gunning KE, Sawicka EH, et al. Life threatening sickle chest syndrome treated with extracorporeal membrane oxygenation. Br Med J (Clin Res Ed) 1987;294: 81–2.

[102] Emre U, Miller ST, Gutierez M, et al. Effect of transfusion in acute chest syndrome of sickle cell disease. J Pediatr 1995;127:901–4.

[103] Mallouh AA, Asha M. Beneficial effect of blood transfusions in children with sickle cell disease. Am J Dis Child 1988;142:178–82.

[104] Fine MJ, Auble TE, Yealy DM, et al. A prediction rule to identify low-risk patients with community-acquired pneumonia. N Engl J Med 1997;336:243–50.

[105] Vichinsky EP, Haberkern CM, Neumayr L, et al, The Preoperative Transfusion in Sickle Cell Disease Study Group. A comparison of conservative and aggressive transfusion regimens in the perioperative management of sickle cell disease. New Engl J Med 1995;333:206–13.

[106] Petz LD, Calhoun L, Shulman I, et al. The sickle cell hemolytic transfusion reaction syndrome. Transfusion 1997;37:382–92.

[107] Sosler SD, Jilly BJ, Saporito C, et al. A simple, practical method for reducing alloimmunization in patients with sickle cell disease. Am J Hematol 1993;43:103–6.

[108] Rosse WF, Gallagher D, Kinney TR, et al, The Cooperative Study of Sickle Cell Disease. Transfusion and alloimmunization in sickle cell disease. Blood 1990;76:1431–7.

[109] Rackoff WR, Ohene-Frempong K, Month S, et al. Neurologic events after partial exchange transfusion for priapism in sickle cell disease. J Pediatr 1992;120:882–5.

[110] Schmalzer EA, Lee JO, Brown AK, et al. Viscosity of mixtures of sickle and normal red cells at varying hematocrit levels, implications for transfusion. Transfusion 1987;27: 228–33.

[111] Powars D, Weidman JA, Odom T, et al. Sickle cell chronic lung disease: prior morbidity and the risk of pulmonary failure. Medicine (Baltimore) 1988;67:66–76.

[112] Castro O, Hoque M, Brown BD. Pulmonary hypertension in sickle cell disease: cardiac catheterization results and survival. Blood 2003;101:1257–61.

[113] Gladwin MT, Sachdev V, Jison ML, et al. Pulmonary hypertension as a risk factor for death in patients with sickle cell disease. N Engl J Med 2004;350:886–95.

[114] Walters MC, Patience M, Leisenring W, et al, Multicenter Investigation of Bone Marrow Transplantation for Sickle Cell Disease. Stable mixed hematopoietic chimerism after bone marrow transplantation for sickle cell anemia. Biol Blood Marrow Transplant 2001;7: 665–73.

[115] Franson RC, Rosenthal MD. PX-52, a novel inhibitor of 14 kDa secretory and 85 kDa cytosolic phospholipases A2. Adv Exp Med Biol 1997;400A:365–73.

[116] Bernini JC, Rogers ZR, Sandler ES, et al. Beneficial effect of intravenous dexamethasone in children with mild to moderately severe acute chest syndrome complicating sickle cell disease. Blood 1998;92:3082–9.

[117] Aziz KE, Wakefield D. Modulation of endothelial cell expression of ICAM-1, E-selectin and VCAM-1 by ß-estradiol, progesterone, and dexamethasone. Cell Immunol 1996; 167:79–85.

[118] Confalonieri M, Urbino R, Potena A, et al. Hydrocortisone infusion for severe community-acquired pneumonia. Am J Respir Crit Care Med 2005;171:242–8.

[119] Lindeque BG, Schoerman HS, Dommisse GF, et al. Fat embolism and the fat embolism syndrome: a double-blind therapeutic study. J Bone Joint Surg Br 1987;69:128–31.

[120] Schonfeld SA, Ploysongsang Y, DiLisio R, et al. Fat embolism prophylaxis with corticosteroids. A prospective study in high-risk patients. Ann Intern Med 1983;99: 438–43.

[121] Sullivan KJ, Goodwin SR, Evangelist J, et al. Nitric oxide successfully used to treat acute chest syndrome of sickle cell disease in a young adolescent. Crit Care Med 1999;27: 2563–8.

[122] Atz AM, Wessel DL. Inhaled nitric oxide in sickle cell disease with acute chest syndrome. Anesthesiology 1997;87:988–90.

[123] Oppert M, Jorres A, Barckow D, et al. Inhaled nitric oxide for ARDS due to sickle cell disease. Swiss Med Wkly 2004;134:165–7.

[124] Carter C, Fisher TC, Hamai H, et al. Hemorheological effects of a nonionic copolymer surfactant (poloxamer 188). Clin Hemorheol 1992;12:109–20.

[125] Orringer EP, Casella JF, Ataga KI, et al. Purified poloxamer 188 for treatment of acute vaso-occlusive crisis of sickle cell disease: a randomized controlled trial. JAMA 2001; 286:2099–106.

[126] Khor SP, McCarthy K, Dupont M, et al. Pharmacokinetics, pharmacodynamics, allometry, and dose selection of rPSGL-Ig for phase I trial. J Pharmacol Exp Ther 2000;293: 618–24.

[127] Matsui NM, Borsig L, Rosen SD, et al. P-selectin mediates the adhesion of sickle erythrocytes to the endothelium. Blood 2001;98:1955–62.

[128] Hicks AER, Nolan SL, Ridger VC, et al. Recombinant P-selectin glycoprotein ligand-1 directly inhibits leucocyte rolling by all 3 selectins in vivo: complete inhibition of rolling is not required for anti-inflammatory effect. Blood 2003;101:3249–56.

[129] Kumar A, Eckman JR, Wick TM. Inhibition of plasma-mediated adherence of sickle erythrocytes to microvascular endothelium by conformationally constrained RGD-containing peptides. Am J Hematol 1996;53:92–8.

[130] Kaul DK, Tsai HM, Liu XD, et al. Monoclonal antibodies to $\alpha_V\beta_3$ (7E3 and LM609) inhibit sickle red blood cell–endothelium interactions induced by platelet-activating factor. Blood 2000;95:368–74.

[131] Lutty GA, Taomoto M, Cao J, et al. Inhibition of TNF-alpha–induced sickle RBC retention in retina by a VLA-4 antagonist. Invest Ophthalmol Vis Sci 2001;42:1349–55.

Hematol Oncol Clin N Am 19 (2005) 881–896

HEMATOLOGY/ONCOLOGY CLINICS
OF NORTH AMERICA

.SEVIER
.UNDERS

Pulmonary Hypertension in Sickle Cell Disease: Mechanisms, Diagnosis, and Management

Oswaldo Castro, MD[a,b,*], Mark T. Gladwin, MD[b,c]

[a]Howard University College of Medicine, Center for Sickle Cell Disease, HURB-1, 1840 7th Street NW, Washington, DC 20001, USA
[b]Critical Care Medicine Department, Clinical Center Building 10-CRC, Room 5-5142, National Institutes of Health, Bethesda, MD 20892, USA
[c]Vascular Therapeutics Section, Cardiovascular Branch, National Heart, Lung, and Blood Institute, National Institutes of Health, Bethesda, MD 20892, USA

In the last decade, pulmonary arterial hypertension (PAH) has emerged as one of the most frequent and serious complications in patients with sickle cell disease (SCD) [1–5]. The Sickle-Cell Pulmonary Hypertension Screening Study documented prospectively a 32% frequency of PAH in adult patients and its association with high mortality [4]. This and other prospective series [6,7] validated retrospective reports of the high frequency and mortality of PAH in SCD [1,2]. It is not known why early reviews of the complications of SCD did not emphasize PAH, even though chronic lung disease and cor pulmonale were documented [8,9]. Although it is possible that the diagnosis was not recognized, it seems more likely that the high frequency of PAH in the current population of older SCD patients reflects the success in preventing the high mortality of severely affected children and young adults.

The pathophysiology of PAH in SCD is unknown and probably multifactorial. All of the clinical manifestations of SCD ultimately derive from the tendency of deoxygenated HbS to polymerize and aggregate. Intracellular HbS polymerization increases the mechanic fragility of red blood cells, resulting in their premature mechanical destruction, that is, hemolytic anemia. In addition to mechanical stress on the erythrocyte membrane and cytoskeleton, inflammation and oxidant stress impair erythrocytic reductive potential and deplete ATP, contributing to energetic failure and increased surface phosphatidyl serine exposure [10], and marking the red cell for premature clearance. Polymerization also markedly reduces red blood cell deformability. That effect along with the increased tendency for sickle red blood cells to adhere to endothelium predis-

* Corresponding author. Howard University College of Medicine, Center for Sickle Cell Disease, HURB-1, 1840 7th Street NW, Washington, DC 20001. E-mail address: olcastro@aol.com (O. Castro).

0889-8588/05/$ – see front matter
doi:10.1016/j.hoc.2005.07.007

poses to episodes of vascular occlusion and ischemic damage to vital organs. All basic and clinical evidence obtained thus far indicates that intravascular hemolysis, which occurs in SCD [11,12], is an important contributing factor to the development of PAH. Intravascular hemolysis interferes with the nitric oxide (NO) vasodilating system in two ways. It releases red blood cell arginase into the plasma, lowering the synthesis of NO [13]. At the same time, hemolysis increases the level of free plasma hemoglobin, which directly scavenges endothelial-derived NO [14,15]. This effect produces a state of endothelial dysfunction characterized by a resistance to NO, vasoconstriction, and secondary increases in the vasoconstrictor and mitogen endothelin 1. Hemolysis also activates the thrombotic system via direct effects on platelet activation through release of red cell ADP and indirectly by plasma hemoglobin-mediated NO scavenging and increased phosphatidyl serine exposure, which activate platelets and tissue factor [16]. The NO scavenging and prothrombotic effects of the damaged erythrocyte membrane, plasma red cell microvesicles, and plasma hemolysate likely produce progressive vascular pathologic remodeling, including intimal and smooth muscle proliferation and in situ thrombosis of the pulmonary arteries.

PAH must be added to the classically recognized complications of hemolysis in SCD—anemia, cholelithiasis, and leg ulcers. It is unknown to what extent the endothelial dysfunction and NO resistance may contribute to the common vaso-occlusive manifestations of SCD (acute chest syndrome, painful events, priapism) and, in particular, to the proliferative cerebral vasculopathy that develops during childhood. This SCD vasculopathy bears similarities to PAH in its risk factors (low hemoglobin, high systolic blood pressure [17]) and pathologic features (large and medium sized vessel intimal and smooth muscle proliferation [18,19]). Nolan and colleagues showed in the journal, Blood (June 28, 2005, Epub ahead of print), that markers of hemolysis (anemia, LDH, bilirubin, reticulocyte count) are significant risk factors for sickle cell-priapism. This provides additional support for the role of hemolysis and the NO system in SCD complications.

In view of the mechanistic role of hemolysis in SCD-related pulmonary hypertension, it is not surprising that pulmonary hypertension also complicates thalassemia intermedia [20,21], hereditary spherocytosis [22], and other chronic hemolytic anemias [23–27]. The concept that the anemia, per se, is not involved in the genesis of PAH is supported by the absence of PAH reports in hypoproliferative nonhemolytic anemias such as iron deficiency, end-stage renal disease, and Fanconi anemia (Table 1). PAH is prevented in well-transfused patients with thalassemia major, in whom the anemia, ineffective erythropoiesis, and intramedullary hemolysis are largely suppressed [28].

HEMODYNAMICS AND RISK FACTORS

The pulmonary vascular resistance (PVR) is directly related to the pulmonary artery pressure and inversely related to the cardiac output. In patients without SCD with idiopathic PAH, the hypertension is defined by high pulmonary artery pressure, usually associated with low cardiac output and a high PVR (from about 500 to 1000 $dyn/s/cm^5$) [29]. The mean PVR in patients with SCD

Table 1		
Association between chronic hemolysis and pulmonary hypertension		
Hematologic condition	Hemolysis	Pulmonary hypertension
Sickle cell anemia (HbSS)	+ + +	+ + +
Hemoglobin SC disease (HbSC)	+	+
Homozygous HbC disease	+ +	?
Thalassemia intermedia	+ + +	+ + +
Thalassemia major (adequately transfused)	–	–
Unstable hemoglobins	+	+
Hereditary spherocytosis	+	+
Hereditary stomatocytosis	+ + +	+
Pyruvate kinase deficiency	+ +	+ +
Congenital dyserythropoietic anemia (neonates)	+ +	+
Paroxysmal nocturnal hemoglobinuria	+ + +	+ +
Anemia of renal disease	–	–
Fanconi anemia	–	–
Iron deficiency anemia	–	–

Hemolysis ranges from none (–) to severe (+++).
  Pulmonary hypertension frequency ranges from absent (–) to very common (+++).

who do not have pulmonary hypertension (83 ± 46 dyn/s/cm^5 [Table 2]) is within the normal range [30]. The cardiac output is high in SCD owing to the high stroke volume that compensates for the anemic state. Furthermore, the precapillary pulmonary microcirculation in SCD needs to adapt to the flow of the most deoxygenated and most HbS-polymer laden and sickled erythrocytes, which are those reaching the lungs [31,32]. Pulmonary vascular adaptation to a high cardiac output, particularly one associated with sickle-related high viscosity blood, requires an optimal vasodilated state. Any interference with this system will raise pulmonary pressure. A chronic increase in pulmonary pressure develops in many patients who have SCD. Because the high cardiac output is maintained and necessary for survival in the face of severe anemia, the high pulmonary pressures are associated with relatively low PVR values when compared with those in patients with idiopathic PAH or other forms of secondary PAH (see Table 2).

Although the degree of pulmonary hypertension is mild, with mean pulmonary artery pressures of approximately 36 mm Hg, patients with sickle cell anemia do not appear to tolerate this pulmonary vascular disease, because 2-year mortality rates range from 16% to 50% [1–4]. Accordingly, in adult patients with SCD, pulmonary hypertension estimated using the tricuspid regurgitant jet velocity (TRV) measured by Doppler echocardiography is a major independent prospective risk factor for death (relative risk of 10.1; CI, 2.7–44) [4].

A statistical association between high pulmonary pressures and systemic systolic hypertension, renal insufficiency, and iron overload suggests that pulmonary hypertension is a marker for systemic vasculopathy [4]; however, a high pulmonary artery pressure is independently associated with mortality, even after adjustment for systemic hypertension and creatinine. The authors believe that

Table 2
Pulmonary hemodyamics in normal individuals, patients with idiopathic pulmonary hypertension, and sickle cell disease patients with and without pulmonary hypertension

Parameter	Normal mean (range) [30] (N = 55)	Idiopathic PAH, males [29] (mean ± SD) (N = 69)	Idiopathic PAH, females [29] (mean ± SD) (N = 118)	SCD, no PAH (mean ± SD) (N = 22)	SCD and PAH (mean ± SD) (N = 39)
Mean pulmonary arterial pressure (mm Hg)	13 (7–19)	60.7 ± 19.7	60.3 ± 16.5	19 ± 4.5	36 ± 8
Cardiac output (L/min)	6.4 (4.4–8.4)	2.35 ± 1.0[a]	2.21 ± 0.9[a]	9 ± 3	8.6 ± 2
Pulmonary vascular resistance (dyn/s/cm⁵)	55 (11–99)	1025[b]	1097[b]	83 ± 46	205 ± 112

[a] Cardiac index. Assuming a body surface area of 1.73 m^2, the values would be 4.06 L/min for males and 3.82 L/min for females.
[b] *Calculated from data in* Rich S, Dantzker DR, Ayres SM, et al. Primary pulmonary hypertension: a national prospective study. Ann Intern Med 1987;107:216–23.

patients with severe hemolytic anemia and multiorgan dysfunction secondary to SCD simply do not survive substantial increases in pulmonary pressures. In support of this, patients with β-thalassemia intermedia present with higher pulmonary pressures and seem to develop prominent right heart failure before death [20]. The authors have also observed significant increases in pulmonary pressure during exercise and vaso-occlusive crisis in sickle cell patients [33]. It is possible that acute-on-chronic increases in pulmonary artery pressure might lead to acute right heart failure, atrial or ventricular dysrhythmia, and sudden death.

The extremely high mortality in patients with SCD despite moderate elevations in pulmonary pressures supports a unique definition of pulmonary hypertension in this disease. In patients with primary pulmonary hypertension, a tricuspid regurgitant jet velocity of greater than 3.0 m/s or evidence of right heart failure on echocardiography would be required for this diagnosis. In the authors' patients, the relationship between tricuspid regurgitant jet velocity and mortality is linear, with a dramatic logistic increase in the risk of death around a value of 2.5 m/s. Even patients with mild increases in tricuspid regurgitant jet velocity (2.5–2.9 m/s) should be considered for intensive therapy.

INCIDENCE AND PREVALENCE

Incidence in Adult Patients

Although the high prevalence of PAH in SCD has been shown in most cross-sectional studies, data on its incidence are only now being collected. The Sickle-

Table 3
Tricuspid regurgitant jet velocity at baseline and at 2-year follow-up in 74 sickle cell disease patients

Baseline diagnosis	TRV increased	TRV decreased	TRV unchanged	
PAH (N=28)	12 (42.9%)	10 (35.7%)	6 (21.4%)	TRV normal, 4 (14.3%)[a]
No PAH (N=46)	27 (58.7%)	14 (30.4%)	5 (10.9%)	TRV ≥2.5 m/s, 8 (17.4%)[b]

   [a] Included in the group of 10 patients with decreased TRV.
   [b] Included in the group of 27 patients with increased TRV.

Cell Pulmonary Hypertension Screening Study started in 2001 [4] used echocardiographic measurements of the tricuspid regurgitant jet velocity to screen 195 unselected adult sickle cell patients for PAH and is now in its third year of prospective follow-up. At the end of March 2004, 134 patients had been followed up for at least 2 years, and 74 of these patients had echocardiographic examinations 1.5 to 2.6 years after study enrollment. Table 3 lists the number of patients according to their baseline diagnosis and the tricuspid regurgitant jet velocity changes observed at the 2-year echocardiographic study.

Forty-six patients did not have PAH at study enrollment (mean tricuspid regurgitant jet velocity, 1.95 m/s), and, as a group, the velocity at the 2-year follow-up had not increased significantly (mean, 2.1; $P=.08$). Nevertheless, eight of the patients (17.4%) with initially normal velocities (mean, 2.01; range, 1.3–2.4 m/s) had PAH at 2 years (mean tricuspid regurgitant jet velocity, 2.74; range, 2.5–2.9 m/s). The age, sex, Hb phenotype, and hydroxyurea treatment status of the eight patients who had PAH at the 2-year follow-up were not significantly different from the findings in patients who did not. These preliminary results suggest that the incidence of PAH in adults with SCD could be as high as 8% per year [34]. Although there are not enough data to comment on the frequency of screening, the authors recommend that all adults be screened at least once every 5 years with transthoracic Doppler echocardiography so that the absolute value of the tricuspid regurgitant jet velocity can be determined.

Prevalence in Pediatric Patients

Prospective studies of the prevalence of pulmonary hypertension in younger patients with SCD are not yet available. The Cooperative Study of SCD obtained echocardiograms for 191 individuals (71% children or young adults) and found no evidence that these patients had elevated pulmonary artery pressure. The mean right ventricular systolic time interval was normal [35]; however, the right ventricular wall thickness and tricuspid regurgitant jet velocities were not reported, and it is possible that some of the patients could have had elevated pulmonary artery pressure. In a Jamaican study, echocardiograms were obtained in 40 adolescents with SCD aged 11 to 18 years. The pulmonary artery systolic pressure ranged from 17 to 39 mm Hg [36]. Because the central venous pressure was assumed to be 14 mm Hg, one can infer that the tricuspid regurgitant jet velocities were all within the normal range.

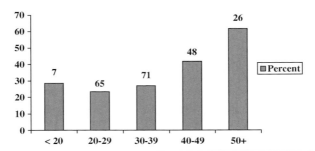

Fig. 1. Percentage of sickle cell disease patients with pulmonary arterial hypertension by decade of life. The abscissa shows age groups in years. The numbers of patients tested for each age group are shown on top of the columns.

The prospective PAH screening study enrolled only adult patients (18 years of age or older). Fig. 1, which shows the prevalence of PAH by age group, suggests a prevalence of 28% in 18-year-old subjects (all seven patients in the <20 years column were 18 years old).

The prevalence of PAH in 40 SCD adolescents (mean age, 16 years) with history of pulmonary disorders (acute chest syndrome, obstructive sleep apnea, or reactive airway disease) was determined recently by echocardiography [37]. Twenty-three of these patients (57.5%) had PAH defined by a tricuspid regurgitant jet velocity of 2.5 m/s or greater, and five patients (12.5%) had a velocity greater than 3 m/s. As is true in adult patients, adolescents with high tricuspid regurgitant jet velocity had significantly higher serum lactate dehydrogenase and bilirubin levels and lower Hb levels, suggesting the association of hemolysis with PAH in this age group.

Another recent (although nonprospective) study presented in abstract form suggested a 25% prevalence of echocardiogram-defined PAH in 110 children [38]. When compared with children without this complication, affected children were more likely to have a history of acute chest syndrome, asthma, and surgery, and less likely to have a history of stroke. Because most children with stroke are treated with chronic transfusions, the researchers postulated that early transfusions may protect against the development of PAH in this age group.

Prevalence in Non-United States Populations with Sickle Cell Disease
No reports of PAH in sickle cell patients from Sub-Saharan Africa are available, and the absence of PAH in Jamaican adolescents has been mentioned previously [36]. No increases in pulmonary pressures were detected in 25 Brazilian patients (aged 14 to 45 years) when compared with those in 25 control subjects [39]. A recent communication reported a 26% prevalence of PAH in a group of 75 Brazilian HbSS patients (aged 15 to 74 years) but did not specify diagnostic criteria [40].

The question of whether high fetal hemoglobin (HbF) levels or hydroxyurea treatment protect SCD patients from the development of pulmonary hypertension has not been settled [4,6]. It would seem important to examine the frequency of PAH in Arab or Indian sickle cell patient populations, who characteristically have a high (approximately 20%) level of HbF even without hydroxyurea treatment. In a single study from the Middle East, none of the 36 children with SCD undergoing cardiovascular evaluation had evidence of PAH [41]. One would also expect that if HbF were to have a protective effect, the lowest PAH frequency in African patients would be observed in patients who are homozygous for the Senegal haplotype (associated with higher HbF levels), and the highest frequency in those who are homozygous for the Bantu haplotype (with the lowest HbF levels). Considering the proposed role of hemolysis in the pathogenesis of PAH, it will be interesting to explore the effect of chronic and intermittent malaria infection on the risk for PAH in SCD patients from areas where malaria is endemic.

DIAGNOSIS

Doppler Echocardiography

The current gold standard for screening is transthoracic Doppler echocardiographic assessment of tricuspid regurgitant jet velocity [4]. This simple noninvasive test should be performed in all adults with SCD and the absolute value for the velocity reported. Cost should not be an issue considering that all pregnant women in the United States are screened by ultrasound despite the fact that little outcome data support this routine screening. It is important to screen subjects as outpatients in their steady state more than 2 weeks after a vaso-occlusive crisis and at least 1 month from an episode of acute chest syndrome. These prerequisites are important because both conditions can increase tricuspid regurgitant jet velocity. It is also important to have subjects sit and rest for 20 minutes before the study, because even mild exertion will dramatically increase pulmonary pressures in this population.

The patient with SCD has an excellent Doppler window owing to thin body habitus. Approximately 87% of patients with SCD have a detectable regurgitant jet, allowing for the measure of jet velocity. The authors spend most of the echocardiographic time on assessment of the tricuspid regurgitant jet velocity using three views. The best jet velocity estimate is used, and the highest value of seven consecutive measurements is used to calculate the tricuspid regurgitant velocity. The screening cardiologist should be asked to report the actual velocity (in m/s), because this value is the most objective piece of information available and is highly associated with prospective risk. Additional information on left ventricular systolic function (wall motion, ejection fraction), left ventricular diastolic function (E/A ratio, deceleration time), right atrial and right ventricular size and function, paradoxical septal motion of the intraventricular septum, and pericardial effusions should be documented.

The tricuspid regurgitant jet velocity is used to estimate pulmonary artery systolic pressure using the modified Bernoulli equation, that is, $4(TRV)^2 + CVP$, where TRV is the velocity and CVP is the estimated central venous pressure. The authors use a technique to estimate CVP by monitoring inferior vena cava collapse during a deep inspiration [42,43]. A value of 5 mm Hg is assigned for a collapse of greater than 50% and a value of 15 mm Hg for a collapse of less than 50%. The estimated pulmonary artery systolic pressure by Doppler echocardiography correlated with the actual measurement at the time of right heart catheterization with an R value of 0.77 [4].

It is unlikely that patients with significant pulmonary hypertension will not have a detectable tricuspid regurgitant jet [42]. This statement appears to be validated by the low mortality observed in the authors'cohort with low tricuspid regurgitant jet velocity and by the fact that no deaths were observed in the 13% of cohort subjects with undetectable tricuspid regurgitant jet velocity.

Right Heart Catheterization

In patients with a tricuspid regurgitant jet velocity greater than 2.9 m/s, the authors recommend right heart catheterization to rule out left ventricular systolic and diastolic dysfunction. The authors have catheterized more than 60 patients at the National Institutes of Health (NIH) and Howard University over the last 5 years [3,4]. The hemodynamics are summarized in Table 2. Remarkably similar profiles have been observed at both institutions, with a mean pulmonary artery pressure of 37 mm Hg and a high cardiac output and relatively high pulmonary capillary wedge pressure. Although the wedge pressure is typically high (mean value, 17 mm Hg), this result may be an overestimate because it is very difficult to obtain an accurate wedge position in these patients with cardiac outputs of greater than 8 L/min.

In half of patients, the pulmonary hypertension hemodynamics are classic for PAH, that is, a high mean pulmonary artery pressure, high pulmonary arterial diastolic pressure, and low wedge pressure. These patients have a gradient from the wedge pressure (left atrial pressure) to the pulmonary vasculature of greater than 10 mm Hg and a high calculated PVR. They represent approximately 5% of the total SCD population and will likely respond favorably to classic pulmonary vasodilator drugs, such as bosentan, prostacyclin, sildenafil, and NO gas. The other half of patients (also 5% of the total sickle cell adult population) has a mixture of diastolic dysfunction and PAH. These subjects have a high mean pulmonary arterial pressure but also a high pulmonary capillary wedge pressure (>18 mm Hg). They maintain a wedge-to-pulmonary artery diastolic gradient of 10 mm Hg or greater, suggesting that they have PAH in addition to left heart diastolic dysfunction. In the authors' experience, in only 10% of catheterized patients (1% to 2% of entire population) is the pulmonary hypertension purely secondary to left ventricular diastolic or systolic dysfunction. Such patients have high wedge pressures (>25 mm Hg) and no gradient between wedge and pulmonary artery diastolic pressure, and they respond to diuretics with large and rapid decreases in all pressures. The authors manage these patients according to standard practices for patients with diastolic or systolic dysfunction using diuretics, angiotensin-converting enzyme inhibitors, and beta-blockers.

The high prevalence of a mixed etiology for SCD-related pulmonary hypertension (ie, pulmonary arterial remodeling and diastolic left ventricular dysfunction) raises questions about the risks and efficacies of certain pulmonary vaso-dilators. In particular, prostacyclin and bosentan are known to increase wedge pressure and do not help patients with congestive heart failure with secondary pulmonary hypertension. This observation is an important reason to perform pretreatment right heart catheterization, and these agents must be used judi-ciously until randomized placebo-controlled trials can be performed.

Exercise Measurements of Pulmonary Pressure

Because pulmonary hypertension is defined by a mean pulmonary artery pressure of greater than 25 mm Hg at rest and 30 mm Hg or greater during exercise [44], the authors routinely ask patients to exercise during right heart catheterization. A substantial increase in pressures of greater than 10 mm Hg has been observed with exercise in almost all patients with a minimal increase in pulmonary capillary wedge pressure (Dr. Roberto Machado, Dr. Mark Gladwin, unpublished observations, 2005). Exercise in the catheterization laboratory can be performed simply by "bench pressing" 1 L bags of saline in each hand and measuring hemodynamics after 1 and 5 minutes of exertion.

PROGNOSIS

In patients with idiopathic (primary) pulmonary hypertension, survival is clearly related to the severity of the hemodynamic abnormalities. Higher pulmonary pressure and lower cardiac output predict a short survival [45]. In this group of patients, the prognosis is also predicted by the responsiveness of the pulmonary vasculature to vasodilators [46]. The median survival in untreated idiopathic PAH is 2.8 years [45]. Retrospective studies of SCD-related PAH estimated median survivals of 60% at 22 months [1] and 50% at 25 months [3]. For each 10-mm increase in mean pulmonary pressure, the mortality risk increased by a factor of 1.7 [3]. Nevertheless, in all likelihood, these studies were biased for inclusion of the most severely affected patients. The survival of patients in the prospective Sickle Cell Pulmonary Hypertension screening study was clearly and independently affected by the presence of pulmonary hypertension [4]. The authors are still following this patient cohort, and the association of high pulmonary pressures and death remains impressive. Although the median survival of patients with a tricuspid regurgitant jet velocity of 2.5 m/s or higher has not yet been reached, only 60% are still alive at 40 months since the echocardiographic diagnosis, and their relative risk for death is 7.4 (CI, 2.4–22.6; $P < .001$) [5].

The risk of death is significant by linear regression as well as by logistic analysis of velocities greater and less than 2.5 m/s. Even mild increases in tricuspid regurgitant jet velocity between 2.5 and 2.9 m/s are associated with substantial risk. A more definitive evaluation of the relative risk of different jet velocities will require a larger study of the magnitude of the STOP cohort [47]. Such a cohort will likely develop as registries are formed by centers participating in randomized placebo-controlled trials targeting pulmonary hypertension in the near future.

The mortality in the authors' sickle cell PAH cohort remains high despite the fact that all patients with high pulmonary pressures are being prospectively and intensively managed. Interventions include those that optimize the clinical course of SCD (hydroxyurea, transfusions) as well as those that specifically lower pulmonary pressures. Another important corollary of the mortality data is that patients with SCD do not appear to tolerate even moderate increases in pulmonary artery pressure. It is not yet known whether the deaths in this group of patients are due to the effects of PAH, per se, or to a PAH-related increase in the frequency or severity of life-threatening SCD complications (eg, acute chest syndrome, multiorgan failure), or whether PAH is simply a marker of a severe sickling-related vasculopathy, which would result in a high mortality independent of PAH. Even if a median survival of as long as 4 to 5 years could be documented for SCD patients with PAH, it would be no better than that of patients with chronic granulocytic leukemia before the era of bone marrow transplantation and more effective chemotherapeutic agents such as imatinib.

MANAGEMENT
Intensifying Sickle Cell Disease Treatment
Fig. 1 shows that the highest frequencies of PAH are seen in patients aged 40 years or older. This age group is at a high risk for frequent and severe vaso-occlusive events, such as acute chest syndrome [48] and pain events [49], including chronic pain. They are also at high risk for worsening anemia and cumulative vital organ damage owing to the long-term effects of sickle cell–related injury to kidneys [50], lungs [8,51], and brain [17], which are compounded by iron overload [52]. Furthermore, vaso-occlusive events and particularly acute chest syndrome can result in transient increases in pulmonary pressure [33], which would be even more deleterious in SCD patients with PAH. The first goal in the treatment of PAH in all SCD patients, but particularly in older patients, is to intensify sickle cell–specific management to minimize the direct or indirect effects of SCD.

Hydroxyurea
Patients (HbSS or HbSC) who are not on hydroxyurea should be given a trial of this drug. Those already on hydroxyurea should have a gradual dose escalation (250 mg/day increments every 8 weeks with monitoring for myelotoxicity every 2 weeks up to a maximum of 30 mg/kg/day) unless there is documentation of such a dose escalation in the past.

Many older patients with severe anemia also have reductions in renal function, which are typically mild [50]. These patients usually require administration of parenteral erythropoietin before or during hydroxyurea treatment. Because they are relatively reticulocytopenic, hydroxyurea cannot be started or needs to be discontinued. Because pulmonary hypertension and renal insufficiency are statistically associated with each other [4], it is common to find mild renal insufficiency in patients with a high screening tricuspid regurgitant jet velocity. It is vital to remember that the HbSS patient without any renal impairment has a high renal plasma flow, a supernormal measured creatinine clearance [50], and low plasma creatinine (0.3–0.7 mg/dL) [53]. If an HbSS patient has a "normal" creatinine clearance and creatinine level, he or she likely has relative renal insufficiency and might require erythropoietin for maximal HbF induction with hydroxyurea. In fact, an analysis of the Multicenter Study of Hydroxyurea follow-up cohort has revealed that patients with low reticulocyte counts and mild renal insufficiency respond poorly to hydroxyurea [54]. Furthermore, the patients with highest reticulocyte counts evidence the best responses.

Theoretically, even patients with severe renal insufficiency (creatinine clearance < 60 mL/min) may be able to tolerate hydroxyurea at a low starting dose (7.5 mg/kg/day) [55], particularly with the addition of erythropoietin.

The erythropoietin doses required in sickle cell anemia patients with renal insufficiency are larger [56,57] than those given to azotemic patients without SCD. Many of the authors' HbSS patients are given starting doses of about 300 units/kg three times per week. Because in SCD these high erythropoietin doses could raise the hematocrit to levels that increase blood viscosity (and cause potentially serious vaso-occlusion), patients who are not on hydroxyurea should have their hemoglobin levels monitored at weekly intervals. This practice generally allows a safe escalation of the erythropoietin dose if no hemoglobin increase occurs. In HbSS patients with hemoglobin levels greater than 10 g/dL, erythropoietin should be temporarily held and then restarted at a lower dose. Phlebotomy should also be considered to manage these erythropoietin-induced "polycythemic" levels (relative to those usual for HbSS), particularly if the patient is not on an effective dose of hydroxyurea. The goal of erythropoietin treatment in patients at a stable hydroxyurea dose is to maintain the hemoglobin level at 9 to 11 g/dL.

It is the authors' practice to start hydroxyurea and erythropoietin simultaneously in patients with pulmonary hypertension and mild renal insufficiency (creatinine values of 0.8 or higher). This practice has allowed patients to tolerate 15 mg/kg/day of hydroxyurea and ensures that increases in hematocrit are accompanied by increases in HbF and F cells.

Transfusions

Long-term treatment with monthly transfusions, or better, exchange transfusions, is indicated in SCD when patients experience ischemic stroke, when a hydroxyurea trial (with or without erythropoietin) is ineffective in preventing frequent vaso-occlusive events, particularly acute chest syndrome, or when hydroxyurea is contraindicated because of pregnancy, end-stage renal disease, or hepatic insufficiency. Considering the high associated mortality rate, transfusions should be considered in patients with severe pulmonary hypertension (tricuspid regurgitant jet velocity ≥ 2.9 m/s) who do not respond to hydroxyurea therapy. There are three advantages of regular transfusions in SCD. First, they can prevent painful events and acute chest syndrome [58], comorbid complications that increase pulmonary pressures. Second, they increase oxygen-carrying capacity and mixed venous oxygen saturation, which will improve global cardiopulmonary function and exercise capacity. Third, they may reduce reticulo-cytosis and the hemolytic rate.

The authors have found that many sickle cell patients with pulmonary hypertension have "hyperhemolysis" with very high absolute reticulocytosis and lactate dehydrogenase values. In these patients, it is often difficult to suppress erythropoiesis and lower the hemolytic rate using traditional targets for red blood cell transfusion (hemoglobin of 10 g/dL). In some of these patients, the authors have increased the transfusion target to 12 g/dL and even added hydroxyurea in an attempt to decrease the hemolytic rate.

Iron chelation therapy

Iron overload was independently associated with pulmonary hypertension in the authors' patient cohort [4]. Although it is not know whether hemosiderosis contributes to the development of pulmonary hypertension, efforts to chelate seem prudent. Iron chelation is indicated not only in patients on long-term transfusions but also in any patient who has clinically significant iron overload [59]. If a reliable transfusion history is available, the amount of body iron can be estimated by the number of red blood cell transfusions. Although a high serum ferritin concentration is consistent with iron overload, the only reliable way of determining clinically significant hemosiderosis is to measure hepatic iron by noninvasive magnetic susceptometry [60], or by quantitative analysis of iron in liver tissue obtained at biopsy. The guidelines for initiating iron chelation and monitoring liver iron in thalassemia major are applicable to patients with SCD [61]. Iron chelation is difficult to achieve because of poor adherence to daily subcutaneous infusions with deferoxamine, the only Food and Drug Administration (FDA)–approved iron chelator. Preliminary results of trials with orally effective iron chelators are promising [62].

Anticoagulation

Patients with primary and other forms of secondary PAH are at risk for in situ pulmonary thrombosis and are generally prescribed long-term warfarin treatment [63]. Pulmonary thrombosis is a frequent autopsy finding in SCD-related PAH [64] and may have a role in its pathogenesis [65]; therefore, anticoagulation may benefit these patients.

Pulmonary Vasodilating and Remodeling Medications

During the last decade, the FDA has approved multiple new selective pulmonary vasodilator and remodeling agents. The first agent to be approved was intravenous epoprostenol (Flolan), a prostacyclin, which was shown to improve exercise capacity (6-minute walk distance) and hemodynamics and to lower mortality in patients with primary pulmonary hypertension and that associated with scleroderma [66,67]. At Howard University, eight patients were given test doses of prostacyclin at the time of cardiac catheterization, with reductions in PVR from 271 to 170 dyn/s/cm^5 [3]. The use of prostacyclin requires continuous infusion by central venous access, a cooled delivery unit, and is extremely expensive. In addition, patients with SCD seem to be at high risk for catheter-related thrombosis and line sepsis [68].

Another prostacyclin is treprostinil (Remodulin), approved for subcutaneous and intravenous infusion in primary PAH [69]. Its longer half-life and stability offer advantages in that it can be used without an iced unit, and the risk of discontinuation may be less. Subcutaneous delivery is associated with injection site pain and redness that often limits dosing increases and leads to reduced compliance. There are no reports of the use of this drug in SCD.

Bosentan (Tracleer) is a dual endothelin A and B receptor antagonist that has been shown to increase the 6-minute walk distance and improve hemodynamics in patients with PAH [70]. Similar results have been reported recently in HIV-infected patients with PAH [71]. Enthusiasm for bosentan use in the sickle cell population, owing to its oral dosing and the known increases in plasma endothelin-1 levels [72], must be tempered by potential side effects of this drug, namely, transaminase elevation, anemia, and increases in plasma volume.

Sildenafil (Viagra) is a phosphodiesterase-5 inhibitor that prevents the catabolism of cGMP, a second messenger of NO-dependent signaling. Phosphodiesterase-5 levels are high in the corpora cavernosa as well as in the pulmonary vasculature, explaining the drug's efficacy in treating erectile dysfunction and PAH. The SUPER-1 phase III placebo-controlled trial of sildenafil for the treatment of PAH has been completed and data presented at the American College of Chest Physicians in 2004. The study demonstrated a significant increase in the 6-minute walk distance and improvement in hemodynamics. Preliminary data from the authors' group [73] and from recently published case series [74] suggest remarkable efficacy in open label studies in patients with SCD and PAH. The authors have observed a significant reduction in tricuspid regurgitant jet velocity and an increase in 6-minute walk distance. There remains concern over the potential for priapism in men with SCD using sildenafil, and additional meticulous clinical studies will be required to establish safety and efficacy.

References

[1] Sutton LL, Castro O, Cross DJ, et al. Pulmonary hypertension in sickle cell disease. Am J Cardiol 1994;74:626–8.

[2] Castro O. Systemic fat embolism and pulmonary hypertension in sickle cell disease. Hematol Oncol Clin North Am 1996;10:1289–303.

[3] Castro O, Hoque M, Brown BD. Pulmonary hypertension in sickle cell disease: cardiac catheterization results and survival. Blood 2003;101:1257–61.

[4] Gladwin MT, Sachdev V, Jison ML, et al. Pulmonary hypertension as a risk factor for death in patients with sickle cell disease. N Engl J Med 2004;350:886–95.

[5] Machado RF, Gladwin MT. Chronic sickle cell lung disease: new insights into the diagnosis, pathogenesis and treatment of pulmonary hypertension. Br J Haematol 2005;129: 449–64.

[6] Ataga KI, Sood N, De Gent G, et al. Pulmonary hypertension in sickle cell disease. Am J Med 2004;117:665–9.

[7] De Castro LM, Jonassiant JC, Graham FL, et al. Pulmonary hypertension in SS, SC and S thalassemia: prevalence, associated clinical syndromes, and mortality [abstract]. Blood 2004;104(Suppl):462.

[8] Powars D, Weidman JA, Odom-Maryon T, et al. Sickle cell chronic lung disease: prior morbidity and the risk of pulmonary failure. Medicine 1988;67:66.

[9] Powars D. Sickle cell anemia: ßS-gene-cluster haplotypes as prognostic indicators of vital organ failure. Semin Hematol 1991;28:202.

[10] Choe HR, Schlegel RA, Rubin E, et al. Alteration of red cell membrane organization in sickle cell anaemia. Br J Haematol 1986;63:761–73.

[11] Bensinger TA, Gillette PN. Hemolysis in sickle-cell disease. Arch Intern Med 1974; 133:624–31.

[12] Washington R, Boggs DR. Urinary iron in patients with sickle cell anemia. J Lab Clin Med 1975;86:17–23.

[13] Schnog JJ, Jager EH, van der Dijs FP, et al. Evidence for a metabolic shift of arginine metabolism in sickle cell disease. Ann Hematol 2004;83:371–5.

[14] Reiter CD, Wang X, Tanus-Santos JE, et al. Cell-free hemoglobin limits nitric oxide bioavailability in sickle-cell disease. Nat Med 2002;8:1383–9.

[15] Jison ML, Gladwin M. Hemolytic anemia-associated pulmonary hypertension of sickle cell disease and the nitric oxide/arginine pathway. Am J Respir Crit Care Med 2003; 168:3–4.

[16] Rother RP, Bell L, Hillmen P, et al. The clinical sequelae of intravascular hemolysis and extracellular plasma hemoglobin: a novel mechanism of human disease. JAMA 2005;293:1653–62.

[17] Ohene-Frempong K, Weiner SJ, Sleeper LA, et al. Cerebrovascular accidents in sickle cell disease: rates and risk factors. Blood 1998;91:288–94.

[18] Rothman SM, Fulling KH, Nelson JS. Sickle cell anemia and central nervous system infarction: a neuropathological study. Ann Neurol 1986;20:684–90.

[19] Koshy M, Thomas C, Goodwin J. Vascular lesions in the central nervous system in sickle cell disease (neuropathology). J Assoc Acad Minor Phys 1990;1:71–8.

[20] Aessopos A, Stamatelos G, Skoumas V, et al. Pulmonary hypertension and right heart failure in patients with ß-thalassemia intermedia. Chest 1995;107:50–3.

[21] Aessopos A, Farmakis D, Karagiorga M, et al. Cardiac involvement in thalassemia intermedia: a multicenter study. Blood 2001;97:3411–6.

[22] Verresen D, De Backer W, Van Meerbeeck J, et al. Spherocytosis and pulmonary hypertension: coincidental occurrence or causal relationship? Eur Respir J 1991;4:629–31.

[23] Jais X, Till SJ, Cynober T, et al. An extreme consequence of splenectomy in dehydrated hereditary stomatocytosis: gradual thrombo-embolic pulmonary hypertension and lung-heart transplantation. Hemoglobin 2003;27:139–47.

[24] Chou R, DeLougherty TG. Recurrent thromboembolic disease following splenectomy for pyruvate kinase deficiency. Am J Hematol 2001;67:197–9.

[25] Shalev H, Moser A, Kapelushnik J, et al. Congenital dyserythropoietic anemia type I presenting as persistent pulmonary hypertension in the newborn. J Pediatr 2000;136: 553–5.

[26] Heller PG, Grinberg AR, Lencioni M, et al. Pulmonary hypertension in paroxysmal nocturnal hemoglobinuria. Chest 1992;102:642.

[27] Jubelirer SJ. Primary pulmonary hypertension: its association with microangiopathic hemolytic anemia and thrombocytopenia. Arch Intern Med 1991;151:1221–3.

[28] Aessopos A, Farmakis D, Hatziliami A, et al. Cardiac status in well-treated patients with thalassemia major. Eur J Hematol 2004;73:359–66.

[29] Rich S, Dantzker DR, Ayres SM, et al. Primary pulmonary hypertension: a national prospective study. Ann Intern Med 1987;107:216–23.

[30] Naeije R. Pulmonary vascular function. In: Peacock AJ, Rubin LJ, editors. Pulmonary circulation. 2nd edition. London: Edward Arnold Limited; 2004. p. 3–13.

[31] Jensen WN, Rucknagel DL, Taylor WJ. In vivo study of the sickle cell phenomenon. J Lab Clin Med 1960;56:854–65.

[32] Serjeant GR, Petch MC, Serjeant BE. The in vivo sickle phenomenon: a reappraisal. J Lab Clin Med 1973;81:850–6.

[33] Kato GJ, Martyr S, Machado R, et al. Acute on chronic pulmonary hypertension in patients with sickle cell disease [abstract]. Blood 2004;104(Suppl 1, Part 1):464.

[34] Castro O, Kato G, Sachdev V, et al. The sickle cell–pulmonary hypertension screening study: ECHO findings at two-years of follow up [abstract]. Presented at the 27th Annual Meeting of the National Sickle Cell Disease Program. Los Angeles (CA), April 18–21, 2004.

[35] Covitz W, Espeland M, Gallagher D, et al. The heart in sickle cell anemia: the Cooperative Study of Sickle Cell Disease (CSSCD). Chest 1995;108:1214–9.

[36] Denbow CE, Chung EE, Serjeant GR. Pulmonary artery pressure and the acute chest syndrome in homozygous sickle cell disease. Br Heart J 1993;69:536–8.

[37] Onyekwere OC, Campbell A, Teshome M, et al. Prevalence of pulmonary hypertension (PHTN) in sickle cell disease (SCD) adolescents with pulmonary complications [abstract]. Presented at the 28th Annual Meeting of the National Sickle Cell Disease Program, Cincinnati, 2005.

[38] Morris CR, Gardner J, Hagar W, et al. Pulmonary hypertension in sickle cell disease: a common complication for both adults and children [abstract]. Presented at the 27th Annual Meeting of the National Sickle Cell Disease Program. Los Angeles (CA), April 18–21, 2004.

[39] de Andrade Martins W, Tinoco Mesquita E, Maria da Cunha D, et al. Doppler echocardiographic study of adolescents and young adults with sickle cell anemia. Arq Bras Cardiol 1999;73:469–74.

[40] Vicari P, Rosario Cavalheiro RC, de Gouveia A, et al. Echocardiographic abnormalities in Brazilian sickle cell patients. Am J Hematol 2005;78:160–1.

[41] Wali YA, Venugopalan P, Rivera E, et al. Cardiovascular function in Omani children with sickle cell anaemia. Ann Trop Paediatr 2000;20:243–6.

[42] Berger M, Haimowitz A, Van Tosh A, et al. Quantitative assessment of pulmonary hypertension in patients with tricuspid regurgitation using continuous wave Doppler ultrasound. J Am Coll Cardiol 1985;6:359–65.

[43] Kircher BJ, Himelman RB, Schiller NB. Noninvasive estimation of right atrial pressure from the inspiratory collapse of the inferior vena cava. Am J Cardiol 1990;66:493–6.

[44] Rubin LJ. Primary pulmonary hypertension. N Engl J Med 1997;336:111–7.

[45] D'Alonzo GE, Barst RJ, Ayres SM, et al. Survival in patients with primary pulmonary hypertension: results form a national prospective registry. Ann Intern Med 1991;115:343–9.

[46] Raffy O, Azarian R, Brenot F, et al. Clinical significance of the pulmonary vasodilator response during short-term infusion of prostacyclin in primary pulmonary hypertension. Circulation 1996;93:484–8.

[47] Adams RJ, Brambilla DJ, Granger S, et al. Stroke and conversion to high risk in children screened with transcranial Doppler ultrasound during the STOP study. Blood 2004;103:3689–94.

[48] Castro O, Brambilla DJ, Thorington B, et al. The acute chest syndrome in sickle cell disease: incidence and risk factors. The Cooperative Study of Sickle Cell Disease. Blood 1994;84:643–9.

[49] Platt OS, Thorington BD, Brambilla DJ, et al. Pain in sickle cell disease: rates and risk factors. N Engl J Med 1991;325:11–6.

[50] Ataga KI, Orringer EP. Renal abnormalities in sickle cell disease. Am J Hematol 2000;63:205–11.

[51] Powars DR. Beta s-gene-cluster haplotypes in sickle cell anemia: clinical and hematologic features. Hematol Oncol Clin North Am 1991;5:475–93.

[52] Olivieri NF. Progression of iron overload in sickle cell disease. Semin Hematol 2001;38(1 Suppl 1):57–62.

[53] West MS, Wethers D, Smith J, et al, and the Cooperative Study of Sickle Cell Disease. Laboratory profile of sickle cell disease: a cross-sectional analysis. J Clin Epidemiol 1992;45:893–909.

[54] Steinberg MH, Barton F, Castro O, et al. Effect of hydroxyurea on mortality and morbidity

in adult sickle cell anemia: risks and benefits up to 9 years of treatment. JAMA 2003; 289:1645–51.

[55] Yan J-H, Ataga K, Kaul S, et al. The influence of renal function on hydroxyurea pharmacokinetics in adults with sickle cell disease. J Clin Pharmacol 2005;45:434–45.

[56] Tomson CR, Edmunds ME, Chambers K, et al. Effect of recombinant human erythropoietin on erythropoiesis in homozygous sickle-cell anaemia and renal failure. Nephrol Dial Transplant 1992;7:817–21.

[57] Claster S, Lewis B, Vichinsky E. High dose erythropoietin in sickle cell anemia patients with renal disease. Blood 1996;88(Suppl 1, Part 1):11.

[58] Miller ST, Wright E, Abboud M, et al. Impact of chronic transfusion on incidence of pain and acute chest syndrome during the Stroke Prevention Trial (STOP) in sickle-cell anemia. J Pediatr 2001;139:785–9.

[59] Kwiatkowski JL, Cohen AR. Iron chelation therapy in sickle-cell disease and other transfusion-dependent anemias. Hematol Oncol Clin North Am 2004;18:1355–77.

[60] Brittenham GM, Sheth S, Allen CJ, et al. Noninvasive methods for quantitative assessment of transfusional iron overload in sickle cell disease. Semin Hematol 2001;38(1 Suppl 1): 37–56.

[61] Olivieri NF, Brittenham GM. Iron-chelating therapy and the treatment of thalassemia. Blood 1997;89:739–61.

[62] Porter J, Vichinsky E, Rose C, et al. A phase II study with ICL670 (Exjade), a once-daily oral iron chelator, in patients with various transfusion-dependent anemias and iron overload. Blood 2004;104(Suppl 1):827.

[63] Humbert M, Sitbon O, Simonneau G. Treatment of pulmonary arterial hypertension. N Engl J Med 2004;351:1425–36.

[64] Adedeji MO, Cespedes J, Allen K, et al. Pulmonary thrombotic arteriopathy in patients with sickle cell disease. Arch Pathol Lab Med 2001;125:1436–41.

[65] Yung GL, Channick RN, Fedullo PF, et al. Successful pulmonary thromboendarterectomy in two patients with sickle cell disease. Am J Respir Crit Care Med 1998;157:1690–3.

[66] Barst RJ, Rubin LJ, Long WA, et al. Primary Pulmonary Hypertension Group: a comparison of continuous intravenous epoprostenol (prostacyclin) with conventional therapy for primary pulmonary hypertension. N Engl J Med 1996;334:296–301.

[67] Badesch DB, Tapson VF, McGoon MD, et al. Continuous intravenous epoprostenol for pulmonary hypertension due to the scleroderma spectrum of disease: a randomized, controlled trial. Ann Intern Med 2000;132:425–34.

[68] Wagner SC, Eschelman DJ, Gonsalves CF, et al. Infectious complications of implantable venous access devices in patients with sickle cell disease. J Vasc Interv Radiol 2004; 15:375–8.

[69] McLaughlin VV, Gaine SP, Barst RJ, et al. Efficacy and safety of treprostinil: an epoprostenol analog for primary pulmonary hypertension. J Cardiovasc Pharmacol 2003; 41:293–9.

[70] Rubin LJ, Badesch DB, Barst RJ, et al. Bosentan therapy for pulmonary arterial hypertension. N Engl J Med 2002;346:896–903.

[71] Sitbon O, Gressin V, Speich R, et al. Bosentan for the treatment of human immunodeficiency virus-associated pulmonary arterial hypertension. Am J Respir Crit Care Med 2004;170:1212–7.

[72] Rybicki AC, Benjamin LJ. Increased levels of endothelin-1 in plasma of sickle cell anemia patients. Blood 1998;92:2594–6.

[73] Machado RT, Martyr SE, Anthi A, et al. Pulmonary hypertension in sickle cell disease: cardiopulmonary evaluation and response to chronic phosphodiesterase 5 inhibitor therapy. Br J Haematol 2005;130:445–53.

[74] Derchi G, Forni GL, Formisano F, et al. Efficacy and safety of sildenafil in the treatment of severe pulmonary hypertension in patients with hemoglobinopathies. Haematologica 2005;90:452–8.

Hematol Oncol Clin N Am 19 (2005) 897–902

HEMATOLOGY/ONCOLOGY CLINICS
OF NORTH AMERICA

Surgery in Sickle Cell Disease

Jackie Buck, RGN, BSc Hons, MSc[a],
Sally C. Davies, MBBS, PhD, FRCP, FRCPCh, FMedSci[b],*

[a]John Walls Renal Unit, Leicester General Hospital, Gwendolen Road, Leicester, LE5 4PW, England, UK
[b]Imperial College Faculty of Medicine, Central Middlesex Hospital, Acton Lane, London, NW10 7NS, England, UK

Because of the nature of the complications of sickle cell disease (SCD), persons with this illness are more likely to undergo surgery than are the general population during their lifetime. For example, cholecystectomy as a consequence of gallstones is more frequent in persons with SCD, as is hip arthroplasty in younger people as a result of avascular necrosis of the femoral head. Because surgery exposes patients to many of the factors that are known to precipitate red blood cell sickling, persons with SCD undergoing surgery require meticulous clinical care to prevent perioperative sickle cell–related complications. Even with meticulous care, approximately 25% to 30% of patients will have a postoperative complication [1,2]. This article provides readers with information about the role of surgery in SCD and the measures that should be taken to ensure patients are well cared for in the perioperative period.

COMMON SURGICAL PROCEDURES IN PATIENTS WHO HAVE SICKLE CELL DISEASE

Adenotonsillectomy

Adenotonsillectomy is a common surgical procedure in children with SCD owing in part to adenotonsillar hypertrophy, probably associated with early functional hyposplenism [2]. Obstructive sleep apnea secondary to enlarged adenoids is frequently observed in children with SCD and often precipitates the need for adenotonsillectomy [3]. Clinicians should be aware that postoperative complications may be greater if obstructive sleep apnea is present [4]. Age is also thought to have an effect on the likelihood of postoperative complications, with children younger than 4 years more prone to postoperative complications [4].

Cholecystectomy and Splenectomy

Abdominal operations, particularly cholecystectomy and splenectomy, are the most frequent type of surgery in patients with SCD [5]. Cholecystectomy is often

* Corresponding author. E-mail address: sally.davies@dh.gsi.gov.uk (S.C. Davies).

0889-8588/05/$ – see front matter
doi:10.1016/j.hoc.2005.07.004

necessary as a result of cholelithiasis, a condition more frequent in patients with SCD than in the general population owing to chronic hemolytic anemia. Splenectomy is often performed in children following sequestration events [6]. During the early 1990s, laparoscopic cholecystectomy superseded open chole-cystectomy, and the procedure is now widely used in patients with SCD. Although the laparoscopic approach may expose the patient to longer anesthesia [7], the recovery time postoperatively may be shorter, resulting in a reduced stay in hospital [8], although this is not always true [7]. Abdominal surgery has long been classified as a medium-risk surgery [1] based on the 20% risk for postoperative complications. The laparoscopic approach does not reduce the rate of postoperative acute chest syndrome [7,9]; therefore, practitioners must remain vigilant. Another important aspect when considering cholecystectomy in patients with SCD is the timing of the surgery. Patients presenting with acute cholelithiasis are inherently different from patients who have asymptomatic gallstones. There is an increasing trend toward elective cholecystectomy when-ever possible, because the risks of operating on a surgically well-prepared individual are clearly less than in a patient already acutely unwell [10]. Never-theless, with adequate preoperative preparation, it is possible to perform laparo-scopic cholecystectomy safely in a patient who has acute cholecystitis [11].

Hip Arthroplasty

Osteonecrosis of the hip occurs in as many as 50% of adults with SCD [12]. Hip arthroplasty is a common procedure in young persons with SCD, who often undergo the surgery in their twenties and thirties [13]. The use of a tourniquet during orthopedic procedures is not recommended because the combined con-ditions of circulatory stasis, acidosis, and hypoxia underneath the cuff provide the ideal conditions for sickling to occur. In a study performed in Nigeria, the use of a tourniquet led to an increase in postoperative complications [14]; however, a recent study in Saudi Arabia reported a successful operation on a patient using tourniquets [15].

CARE MEASURES

Preoperative Blood Transfusion

In many parts of the developed world, patients with SCD often have a blood transfusion before surgery, because it is believed this will lower their risk for postoperative complications. This procedure may be an exchange transfusion, which is given to lower the level of HbS, usually to around 30%, or a simple transfusion of 1 or 2 units of blood to raise the overall hemoglobin level to approximately 10 g/dL [16], improving the overall oxygen-carrying capacity. In a large randomized controlled trial of simple versus exchange transfusion performed preoperatively [1], the conservative approach of simple transfusion was as safe as exchange transfusion in relation to the frequency of postoperative complications. This finding has led many centers to adopt a less aggressive approach to preoperative blood transfusion. Subsequent publications from the same study showed that this observation was true in hip arthroplasty [17] and adenotonsillectomy [18].

Although preoperative blood transfusion is routine practice in many centers, the role of blood transfusion before surgery remains a topic of debate among clinicians caring for patients with SCD because it has never been fully researched [19]. In areas of the world where the blood supply is less safe, preoperative transfusion is rarely given [20,21]. Furthermore, many practitioners rarely give a transfusion preoperatively [22] before certain procedures and report few complications as a result.

The case for preoperative transfusion is based on improving oxygen delivery, because most patients with SCD are chronically anemic, although they develop compensatory mechanisms to ensure reasonable functioning at low hemoglobin levels. In addition, by lowering the level of HbS and the number of sickled red blood cells, whole blood viscosity should fall, reducing the risk of vaso-occlusion. Some reports have suggested a low perioperative complication rate among transfused patients [23].

The case against preoperative blood transfusion focuses on the risks, albeit, low. Blood transfusion carries a risk of transmission of bloodborne infectious agents such as hepatitis and parvovirus [24], as well as variant Creutzfeldt-Jakob disease. The first two agents are recognized to cause problems in persons with SCD. Furthermore, the incidence of red blood cell alloimmunization among patients with SCD ranges from 8% to 50% and increases with the number of transfusions [25], whereas iron overload is a direct consequence of multiple transfusions. In the developed world, antigen-matched red blood cells may be in short supply. In the developing world, transfusion services are often unstable and the blood supply unsafe.

In reality, many hospitals and sickle cell centers have policies that err on the side of caution and advocate giving a transfusion to patients before surgery. Many centers have adopted a more conservative policy following the publication of the study by the Preoperative Transfusion in Sickle Cell Disease Group [1], which showed that this policy was as safe as exchange transfusion. Some centers do not routinely transfuse patients before surgery but rely heavily on the delivery of excellent care from a wide multidisciplinary team to prevent the development of postoperative sickle cell events [22]. In a recent national survey of practice in the United Kingdom, it was shown that most patients undergoing cholecystectomy and adenoidectomy do so without preoperative blood transfusion, whereas almost all patients undergoing hip arthroplasty are prepared by an exchange transfusion [13]. There was no difference in the rate of postoperative complications in patients who received a transfusion and those who did not, suggesting a growing trend in the United Kingdom to avoid transfusion when possible.

When patients are transfused preoperatively, leukocyte-depleted blood should always be used to minimize side effects and the risks of infection from blood products. In the United Kingdom and United States, the use of leukocyte-depleted blood for patients with SCD is now required by regulatory bodies.

The authors advocate an individualized approach to preoperative blood transfusion as follows:

> Assess every case individually. If it is absolutely necessary to transfuse (benefits outweigh the risks), ensure that (1) the patient understands the risks of blood transfusion and (2) leukocyte-depleted blood is used.
> Assess the need for transfusion based on the type of surgery (low, moderate, high risk), the length of time of surgery, the transfusion history, the history of sickle cell–related complications, and the general health state of the patient.

Surgical risk categories are as follows:

> Low: eyes, skin, nose, ears, distal extremities, and dental, perineal, and inguinal areas
> Medium: throat, neck, spine, proximal extremities, genitourinary system, intra-abdominal areas
> High: intracranial, cardiovascular, intrathoracic

Surgical risk is believed to be related to changes in ventilatory function postoperatively. Until a fully randomized trial comparing preoperative transfusion with no preoperative transfusion is performed, the decision to transfuse will never be completely evidence based.

Pain

As is true for any patient undergoing surgery, one should assess pain and provide prompt relief. For patients who have SCD, this control is of utmost importance for two reasons. First, painful crisis is a common complication of SCD that can be brought on as a result of the physiologic stress of surgery [26] or infection; therefore, adequate baseline measurements are essential to determine the origin and nature of any pain events. Second, patients with SCD often experience some degree of chronic pain and may be on a regular analgesia regimen before having an operation.

Pain management strategies that may work in other people may not be as effective in this patient group owing to tolerance to analgesics developed over many years. Increasingly, patients with SCD who experience acute pain crisis are treated with a patient-controlled analgesia pump delivery system for opiates; therefore, it is likely that patients will have experience with the use of these agents. It is recommended that a recognized pain assessment scale, such as the visual analogue scale, be used for all patients with SCD and that pain be regularly assessed. The type of pain relief given will vary with local policy, the situation, cause, and severity, although it must be remembered that patients with SCD may have developed tolerance to some analgesia and may require greater doses than other patients.

Hydration

Dehydration is a recognized cause of sickle cell–related complications. Patients with SCD are particularly prone to this condition owing to an inability to concentrate urine. For this reason, patients are encouraged to drink clear fluids freely until as close to surgery as possible before intravenous fluids are commenced for the duration of the surgery and until they can tolerate an adequate input of oral fluids. During surgery, fluids should be increased to compensate for volume loss.

Oxygenation

A decrease in oxygenation as well as ventilation perfusion mismatching can increase the risk of pulmonary infarction or infection in patients with SCD, increasing the risk of acute chest syndrome. The acute chest syndrome is the most common cause of death in young adults with SCD [27]. Patients should be well oxygenated before surgery, throughout the procedure, and until fully awake. Hyperoxygenation is recommended at induction of anesthesia. Careful monitoring of oxygen saturation is a key aspect of perioperative nursing care for patients with SCD. Decreasing oxygen saturations should be promptly assessed by the physician to detect mucous plugging, evolution of the acute chest syndrome, or pulmonary embolism as the cause.

Temperature

Hypothermia can cause vasoconstriction and red blood cell sludging, leading to an increase in capillary transit time and the risk of vaso-occlusion [28]; therefore, the use of hypothermia in patients with SCD undergoing surgery remains controversial. During most surgical procedures, patients should be kept warm. The operative ambient temperature should also be maintained.

Infection Control

Patients with SCD are generally immunocompromised at a young age as a result of splenic infarction [29]. Because infection is often a precursor to sickle cell complications, it is extremely important to prevent infection in perioperative patients with SCD. Standard measures such as good hydration, early mobilization, and meticulous hand washing are important and relatively easy to implement. Prophylactic antibiotics should be commenced intraoperatively and continued until after discharge from the hospital.

References

[1] Vichinsky EP, Haberkern CM, Neumayr L, et al. A comparison of conservative and aggressive transfusion regimens in the perioperative management of sickle cell disease: the Preoperative Transfusion in Sickle Cell Disease Study Group [see comment]. N Engl J Med 1995;333:206–13.

[2] Wali YA, al Okbi H, al Abri R. A comparison of two transfusion regimens in the perioperative management of children with sickle cell disease undergoing adenotonsillectomy. Pediatr Hematol Oncol 2003;20:7–13.

[3] Kemp JS. Obstructive sleep apnea and sickle cell disease [comment]. J Pediatr Hematol Oncol 1996;18:104–5.

[4] Halvorson DJ, McKie V, McKie K, et al. Sickle cell disease and tonsillectomy: preoperative management and postoperative complications. Arch Otolaryngol Head Neck Surg 1997; 123:689–92.

[5] Koshy M, Weiner SJ, Miller ST, et al. Surgery and anesthesia in sickle cell disease: Cooperative Study of Sickle Cell Diseases. Blood 1995;86:3676–84.

[6] Minkes RK, Lagzdins M, Langer JC. Laparoscopic versus open splenectomy in children. J Pediatr Surg 2000;35:699–701.

[7] Wales PW, Carver E, Crawford MW, et al. Acute chest syndrome after abdominal surgery in children with sickle cell disease: is a laparoscopic approach better? J Pediatr Surg 2001;36:718–21.

[8] Haberkern CM, Neumayr LD, Orringer EP, et al. Cholecystectomy in sickle cell anemia patients: perioperative outcome of 364 cases from the National Preoperative Transfusion Study. Preoperative Transfusion in Sickle Cell Disease Study Group. Blood 1997;89: 1533–42.

[9] Delatte SJ, Hebra A, Tagge EP, et al. Acute chest syndrome in the postoperative sickle cell patient. J Pediatr Surg 1999;34:188–91 [discussion: 191–82].

[10] Suell MN, Horton TM, Dishop MK, et al. Outcomes for children with gallbladder abnormalities and sickle cell disease [see comment]. J Pediatr 2004;145:617–21.

[11] Al-Mulhim AS, Al-Mulhim FM, Al-Suwaiygh AA. The role of laparoscopic cholecystectomy in the management of acute cholecystitis in patients with sickle cell disease. Am J Surg 2002;183:668–72.

[12] Firth PG, Head CA. Sickle cell disease and anesthesia. Anesthesiology 2004;101: 766–85.

[13] Buck J, Casbard A, Llewelyn C, et al. Preoperative transfusion in sickle cell disease: a survey of practice in England. Eur J Haematol 2005;75:14–21.

[14] Oginni LM, Rufai MB. How safe is tourniquet use in sickle-cell disease? Afr J Med Med Sci 1996;25:3–6.

[15] Abdulla Al-Ghamdi A. Bilateral total knee replacement with tourniquets in a homozygous sickle cell patient [see comment]. Anesth Analg 2004;98:543–4.

[16] Ohene-Frempong K. Indications for red cell transfusion in sickle cell disease. Semin Hematol 2001;38:5–13.

[17] Vichinsky EP, Neumayr LD, Haberkern C, et al. The perioperative complication rate of orthopedic surgery in sickle cell disease: report of the National Sickle Cell Surgery Study Group. Am J Hematol 1999;62:129–38.

[18] Waldron P, Pegelow C, Neumayr L, et al. Tonsillectomy, adenoidectomy, and myringotomy in sickle cell disease: perioperative morbidity. Preoperative Transfusion in Sickle Cell Disease Study Group. J Pediatr Hematol Oncol 1999;21:129–35.

[19] Riddington C, Williamson L. Preoperative blood transfusions for sickle cell disease. Cochrane Database Syst Rev 2001;3:CD003149.

[20] Homi J. General anaesthesia in sickle-cell disease. BMJ 1979;2:739.

[21] Thame JR, Hambleton IR, Serjeant GR. RBC transfusion in sickle cell anemia (HbSS): experience from the Jamaican Cohort Study. Transfusion 2001;41:596–601.

[22] Griffin TC, Buchanan GR. Elective surgery in children with sickle cell disease without preoperative blood transfusion. J Pediatr Surg 1993;28:681–5.

[23] Adams DM, Ware RE, Schultz WH, et al. Successful surgical outcome in children with sickle hemoglobinopathies: the Duke University experience. J Pediatr Surg 1998;33: 428–32.

[24] Vichinsky EP. Current issues with blood transfusions in sickle cell disease. Semin Hematol 2001;38:14–22.

[25] Davies SC. Blood transfusion in sickle cell disease. Curr Opin Hematol 1996;3:485–91.

[26] Dix HM. New advances in the treatment of sickle cell disease: focus on perioperative significance. AANA J 2001;69:281–6.

[27] Platt OS, Brambilla DJ, Rosse WF, et al. Mortality in sickle cell disease: life expectancy and risk factors for early death [see comment]. N Engl J Med 1994;330:1639–44.

[28] Marchant WA, Walker I. Anaesthetic management of the child with sickle cell disease. Paediatr Anaesth 2003;13:473–89.

[29] Tobin JR, Butterworth J. Sickle cell disease: dogma, science, and clinical care [comment]. Anesth Analg 2004;98:283–4.

Hematol Oncol Clin N Am 19 (2005) 903–916

HEMATOLOGY/ONCOLOGY CLINICS
OF NORTH AMERICA

Pregnancy and Sickle Cell Disease

Kathryn Hassell, MD

Colorado Sickle Cell Treatment and Research Center, University of Colorado Health Sciences Center, 4200 East Ninth Avenue, C-222, Denver, CO 80262, USA

With advances in management, men and women with sickle cell disease are enjoying an improved quality of life well into adulthood, when they may elect to plan a family. Pregnancy has been associated with exacerbation of sickle cell disease and may place women, especially those with sickle cell anemia (HbSS), at an additional risk for obstetric complications. Appropriate management by health care providers familiar with sickle cell diseases and high-risk obstetric care can result in a successful pregnancy for most women with sickle cell disease.

POTENTIAL PATHOPHYSIOLOGIC INTERACTION BETWEEN SICKLE CELL DISEASE AND PREGNANCY
Red Blood Cell Sickling

Hemoglobin S polymerization and subsequent red blood cell sickling is associated with hypoxia, changes in red blood cell ion content, hydration, and hemoglobin concentration. Physiologic changes in pregnancy include increased cardiac output in response to decreased systemic vascular resistance [1]. Increased tidal volume, minute ventilatory volume, and minute oxygen uptake, reduced functional residual capacity and residual volume, and the increased total pulmonary resistance associated with progesterone [1] may potentially compromise oxygen delivery. A study of 15 women with sickle cell disease revealed an accentuated increase in cardiac output by an increase in left ventricular end-diastolic volume without associated tachycardia, increased fractional shortening, or decompensation of cardiac function [2]. Nevertheless, previously asymptomatic underlying chronic cardiopulmonary dysfunction might be revealed in some women with sickle cell disease by physiologic stressors in pregnancy. Respiratory alkalosis also develops, which optimizes placental gas exchange but may affect red blood cell sickling. Increased plasma renin and aldosterone activity lead to increased plasma volume and decreased plasma osmolality, which might diminish the risk of red cell dehydration [1]. The cumulative

E-mail address: kathryn.hassell@uchsc.edu

0889-8588/05/$ – see front matter
doi:10.1016/j.hoc.2005.07.003

impact of these pregnancy-related changes on hemoglobin S polymerization and sickling has not been explored.

Vascular Occlusion

A variety of factors contribute to vaso-occlusion and chronic organ injury in sickle cell disease. They include the adhesion of red blood cells, increased inflammatory, adhesion, and coagulation proteins, endothelial dysfunction, and the dysregulation of vascular tone. Increased release of adhesion and coagulation proteins, including von Willebrand factor, fibrinogen, and factor VIII, during pregnancy [3] may exacerbate red blood cell adhesion. The maternal placental circulation is susceptible to vaso-occlusion, which may account for the areas of fibrosis, villous necrosis, and infarction observed in the placenta from pregnancies in women with sickle cell disease [4–6]. Doppler ultrasound studies have demonstrated evidence of restricted uteroplacental blood flow [7,8], indicative of possible vessel injury, narrowing, or vasoconstriction. Fetal circulation is not directly impacted by sickle red blood cells, and blood flow in the umbilical artery and vein seems to be relatively less affected as assessed by Doppler ultrasound [9]. There is little evidence of inflammation in the fetal circulation, with minimal leukocyte recruitment in the umbilical vessel walls from pregnancies in women with sickle cell disease. Interleukin-8 (IL-8) and IL-6 levels are not increased in cord blood [5]; however, increased von Willebrand factor staining and vascular endothelial growth factor, as well as redistribution of CD31 (PECAM-1), suggest a response to hypoxia in the fetal circulation [5]. A reduction of endothelial nitric oxide synthase is also noted, which may impact the compensatory increase in placental nitric oxide production that occurs in response to pre-eclampsia and eclampsia [10]. Restricted uteroplacental circulation is associated with low birth weight and intrauterine growth retardation in pregnant women with sickle cell disease [7,8], although acute changes in umbilical artery blood flow do not occur during sickle cell pain events [9]. Abnormal uteroplacental flow does not improve after acute or chronic transfusion therapy with reduction in anemia or sickle red blood cells [11].

Maternal Anemia

The expanded plasma volume in pregnancy is associated with dilutional anemia, but there are no data documenting to what extent baseline anemia is exacerbated in women with sickle cell disease who may have a chronically expanded plasma volume before pregnancy [12]. Anemia does not correlate with adverse fetal outcomes, including intrauterine growth retardation and low birth weight, or maternal complications, even in women with HbSS and low baseline hemoglobin values of 6.0 to 7.0 g/dL [13–16].

STUDIES OF PREGNANCY IN WOMEN WITH SICKLE CELL DISEASE

In women with sickle cell disease, statistics collected before 1975 report remarkably worse pregnancy outcomes when compared with more recent data [17]. Contemporary data are predominately gathered from retrospective single-institution case series. The largest of these series [18–23] are listed in Table 1.

Table 1
Studies of pregnancy in women with sickle cell disease

Study [reference]	Study years	Total no. of pregnancies	Hemoglobinopathy		
			HbSS	HbSC	HbSßthal
Retrospective—single institution					
Koshy and Burd [18]	1979–1984	117	28	66	23
Morrison et al [20]	1981–1990	131	101	30	0
Koshy et al [19]	1986–1990	54	39	9	6
Seoud et al [21]	1981–1991	58	36	22	0
Sun et al [22]	1989–1999	127	69	58	0
Retrospective— multi-institution					
Howard et al [23]	1991–1993	81	39	33	5
Cohort studies					
Smith et al (Cooperative Study) [13]	1979–1986	445	320	77	48
Serjeant et al [14]	NR	94	94	0	0
Randomized trial					
Koshy et al [24]	1979–1984	72	72	0	0

Abbreviation: NR, not reported.

Pregnancy outcomes for women enrolled in the Cooperative Study of Sickle Cell Disease were tracked, and available data from 1979 to 1986 have been reported [13]. The results of pregnancy in a cohort of Jamaican women with sickle cell anemia established through a newborn screening program and followed up for at least 25 years have been compared with those in a matched birth cohort of persons without hemoglobinopathies [14]. A single prospective randomized trial of transfusion support in pregnancy has been conducted in 72 women with sickle cell anemia [24]. In aggregate, these data represent information from over 1100 pregnancies in women with sickle cell disease, although each series is generally too small to discern statistical differences between many of the outcomes in patients and controls. Treatment recommendations are based on the interpretation of retrospective data, and the benefits and consequences of specific management, other than transfusion therapy, have not been systematically evaluated.

MATERNAL ISSUES IN SICKLE CELL DISEASE
Maternal Mortality
Retrospective data from limited numbers of patients in the 1960s and 1970s suggested the rate of maternal mortality in sickle cell disease was increased when compared with that of women without sickle cell disease [17]. Since 1975, there have been at least 11 series in which the maternal death rate was 0% to 2%, representing one to two deaths in most series [13,14,17,20,21]. In several series and in the prospective transfusion study there were no maternal deaths [17–19,22,24]. The reported timing and causes of death are listed in Table 2. Most of the reported deaths occurred in women with HbSS, and three of seven

Table 2
Reported causes of maternal mortality in women with sickle cell disease

Study [reference]	Timing of death	Maternal hemoglobinpathy	Cause of death (time)	Prenatal care	Transfusion
Smith et al (Cooperative Study) [13]	Prepartum	HbSS	Fatal PE (4 mo)	Yes	NR
Seoud et al [21]		HbSS	PE versus ACS (33 wk)	Yes	Yes
Seoud et al [21]		HbSS	Pneumonia/ACS?/GI bleeding	Yes	Limited by alloimmunization
Koshy et al [19]		HbSC	Stroke/HELLP	No	Yes
Serjeant et al [14]	Peripartum	HbSS	Hemorrhage/DIC with toxemia	No	No
Smith et al (Cooperative Study) [13]	Postpartum	HbSS	ACS, acute renal failure (3 wk)	NA	NR
Serjeant et al [14]		HbSS	Fatal PE (14 wk)	NA	No

Abbreviations: ACS, acute chest syndrome; DIC, disseminated intravascular coagulation; GI, gastrointestinal; HELLP, hemolysis, elevated liver enzymes, and low platelet count; NA, not applicable; NR, not reported; PE, pulmonary embolism.

were related to documented or suspected thromboembolic events, as seen in other pregnant populations.

Miscarriage

The rate of spontaneous abortions in women with sickle cell disease is unclear. It seems to be higher than in African American women without sickle cell disease, but the older literature suggesting high rates reflected retrospective data from 1950 to 1980. The prospective transfusion study performed from 1979 to 1986 demonstrated that 55% to 65% of women with HbSS, hemoglobin SC disease (HbSC), and hemoglobin $S\beta^{+/o}$-thalassemia (HbSβ-thalassemia) had a history of spontaneous or elective abortion compared with 41% of healthy African American women [24]. A study of 94 pregnancies in 52 women from the Jamaican cohort with HbSS reported a spontaneous abortion rate of 35% compared with a 10.4% rate in controls [14]. The Cooperative Study reported a miscarriage rate of 6.5% in women with HbSS, HbSC disease, $HbS\beta^o$-thalassemia, and $HbS\beta^+$-thalassemia in 445 pregnancies [13].

Intrapartum Complications

Some obstetric complications, including placental abruption, pre-eclampsia, toxemia, and preterm labor, have been reported more frequently in women with HbSS than in healthy African American women without sickle cell anemia or those with HbSC disease. Table 3 summarizes the observed incidences from the prospective transfusion study [24] and the experience of the Cooperative Study [13] in a comparison of African American women without hemoglobin-opathies. The rate of placental abruption was higher in patients in the randomized trial [24], but this was not noted in the Jamaican cohort [14] or the retrospective series reported by Sun and coworkers [22]. More recent data from a retrospective review of a single institution's experience [22] and from the Jamaican cohort [14] have found no increase in the risk of pre-eclampsia or hypertensive disorders in women with HbSS or HbSC disease when compared with controls. Preterm labor was reported to occur in 38% to 45% of patients with HbSS and 20% of patients with HbSC in other retrospective case series [19,21,22]. The prospective transfusion trial [24] and the Cooperative Study [13]

Table 3 Frequency of obstetric complications in women with sickle cell disease					
	Transfusion study, 1979–1984 [24]				Cooperative study, 1979–1986 [13]
Parameter	Control	HbSS	HbSC	HbSβthal	
Number of pregnancies	8981	100	66	23	225
Gestational age at delivery (wk)	40	37.5	38.6	37.1	37.7
Preterm labor (%)	17	26	15	22	9
Placenta previa (%)	0.4	1	2	4	NR
Abruptio placenta (%)	0.5	3	2	4	NR
Pre-eclampsia/toxemia (%)	4	18	9	13	11
Cesarean section (%)	14	29	30	26	NR

Abbreviation: NR, not reported.

did not find statistically different rates of preterm labor in a comparison with normal African American controls. Some observations suggest that patients who require transfusion therapy for sickle cell complications may be at increased risk for preterm labor or toxemia [21]. This transfusion requirement may be indicative of patients who are more severely affected by chronic and acute vascular injury from sickle cell disease and at increased risk for obstetric complications.

The mode of delivery and cesarean section rate have not been demonstrated to be statistically different for women with sickle cell disease when compared with normal controls, with 15% to 20% of deliveries performed by cesarean section across several studies [13,14,17,22].

Postpartum Complications

Ante- and postpartum hemorrhage does not seem to be more common in women with sickle cell disease [14]. Retained placenta was noted to be slightly more prevalent in the Jamaican cohort of women with HbSS [14], and one study noted the development of postpartum endometritis in 10% of pregnancies [21].

Overall, there are no consistent data suggesting that antepartum, intrapartum, and postpartum complications are significantly more common in women with sickle cell disease when compared with unaffected women. Nevertheless, because various studies have demonstrated an increased tendency toward these complications in these women, especially those with HbSS, access to high-risk obstetric care, patient education, and close follow-up are important to minimize maternal morbidity and mortality.

FETAL IMPLICATIONS OF MATERNAL SICKLE CELL DISEASE
Perinatal Mortality

Historically, perinatal mortality has been reported to be as high as 53% for infants born to women with HbSS [17]. The rate has decreased dramatically over the last three decades as obstetric and neonatal care has improved. Since 1980, the reported neonatal mortality rate has ranged from 0% to 10% but is generally less than 5% [17,19,22], and Apgar scores at 5 minutes average 9 in infants born to women with all types of sickle cell disease [6,13]. In infants affected by sickle cell disease, there are no manifestations antenatally, perinatally, or in the immediate postpartum period [6] until the production of fetal hemoglobin is replaced by the production of hemoglobin S.

Intrauterine Growth Retardation/Low Birth Weight

Factors in women with sickle cell disease that might affect fetal growth include chronic anemia and placental damage owing to vascular occlusion. Birth weights for infants born to women with HbSS average 2.5 to 2.8 kg compared with 2.7 to 3.0 kg for infants born to women with hemoglobin HbSC disease, HbSβ^{+}-thalassemia, and healthy African American women [13,19,24]. These data have been confirmed in subsequent studies [14,22]. At least four reports have found no correlation between birth weight and the degree of anemia in women with sickle cell disease [13–16]. There is an increased frequency of abnormal placentas in women with sickle cell disease, often showing infarcted areas with fibrosis

[4,6]. This observation suggests the presence of hypoxic or vaso-occlusive stresses, although in the Jamaican cohort, birth weight did not correlate with antepartum or peripartum episodes of acute chest syndrome, an acute complication of sickle cell disease characterized by acute hypoxia [14]. Despite concerns about diminished blood flow to the placenta during sickle cell pain episodes owing to increased red blood cell adherence and vascular occlusion, studies have demonstrated no change in umbilical artery flow during these episodes, despite apparent increased uterine vascular resistance [9]. It is likely that chronic vascular occlusion, even in the absence of clinically overt pain crisis or acute chest syndrome, contributes to placental injury and adversely affects fetal growth. In a study of 15 pregnancies, third-trimester Doppler flow velocimetry demonstrated a correlation between decreased uterine flow and birth weight [7]. Third-trimester Doppler analysis, when combined with ultrasound findings (the "ultradop index"), had an 89% sensitivity and 89% positive predictive value for small-for-gestational-age births in one series of 27 pregnant women with HbSS [8]. Measurement of uteroplacental Doppler velocimetry showed no change after transfusion therapy despite a significant reduction in sickle hemoglobin [11]; therefore, altered vascular flow rather than anemia may account for low birth weights in infants and women with HbSS, which is not improved with transfusion support.

Fetal Monitoring During Pain Events

Assessment of fetal well being during a pain episode is complicated by the use of opiates to treat sickle cell pain, which transiently affect nonstress testing and biophysical profile scores [9]. Caution must be used when interpreting the results of these tests during an acute pain episode, because they may not be predictive of increased perinatal morbidity and mortality in the absence of other findings.

OBSTETRIC MANAGEMENT RECOMMENDATIONS

Appropriate management of pregnant patients with sickle cell disease depends on recognition of the specific type of disease (eg, HbSS, HbSC, HbSβ-thalassemia), the expected steady-state hemoglobin value, and potential associated complications. Hemoglobin electrophoresis should be performed if diagnosis of the specific type of sickle cell disease is uncertain.

Obstetric/Fetal Monitoring

Pregnant women with sickle cell disease should be followed closely and collaboratively by medical personnel familiar with high-risk obstetrics and sickle cell disease. Prenatal diagnosis of sickle cell disease, which may be appropriate if the fetus is at risk, can be made by amniocentesis or chorionic villous sampling, even though the fetus does not yet produce sickle hemoglobin [25].

In the first trimester, prevention of dehydration and control of nausea may reduce the risk of sickle cell pain episodes. In the first and second trimester, biweekly visits to educate the patient about and monitor for placenta previa, placental abruption, preterm labor, and assessment of sickle cell disease activity will facilitate early detection and treatment of these potential complications. A complete blood count and reticulocyte count should be obtained at each visit. Prenatal vitamins, without iron in chronically transfused patients, and additional folate (1.0 mg) are recommended [2,17]. Patients on chronic pain medications, including methadone, should be discouraged from abrupt discontinuation of these medications resulting in maternal withdrawal symptoms, which may significantly affect the fetus [26,27].

Starting at 24 to 28 weeks, monthly ultrasonography is recommended to assess fetal growth, and patients should be instructed in daily fetal movement counts. Nonstress testing and biophysical profile testing should be considered weekly beginning at 32 to 34 weeks. Doppler ultrasound, performed at 28 to 30 weeks to assess umbilical artery flow and systolic/diastolic ratios as a predictor of intrauterine growth retardation, may be a useful adjunct [7,8].

Baseline blood pressure values are generally lower in HbSS patients when compared with the general population. Relatively modest changes in blood pressure may be an early indication of pregnancy-induced hypertension or pre-eclampsia in these women, warranting close monitoring. A specific threshold blood pressure for predicting this complication has not been established for pregnant women with HbSS, although a value of 125/75 mm Hg has been suggested by some authorities [18].

Labor and Delivery

Unless otherwise obstetrically indicated, pregnancy should be allowed to go to term, with spontaneous onset of labor [17–19]. During labor, adequate hydration and oxygenation should be maintained. Doses of analgesia may exceed those usually required for obstetric pain owing to an increased tolerance to pain medications [28]. Epidural analgesia may provide excellent pain control [29] and is well tolerated, although the use of an epidural blood patch has been deferred in lieu of injection of colloid material for spinal headache [30]. Vaginal delivery is preferred, reserving cesarean section for obstetric indications. If a cesarean section is planned in an untransfused patient with HbSS, transfusion should be considered first, if possible, to avoid perioperative sickle cell complications [19].

OTHER ISSUES RELATED TO SICKLE CELL DISEASE

Urinary Tract Infections

Women with sickle cell disease have an increased risk of asymptomatic bacteriuria, lower urinary tract infection, and pyelonephritis, which is exacerbated during pregnancy. Lower urinary tract infections have been noted in 30% to 40% of pregnancies [21] and pyelonephritis in 7% to 9% [22]. Studies in the 1960s associated these infections with low birth weights [23], an observation confirmed by the recent Jamaican cohort study in women with HbSS [14].

Treatment of Sickle Cell Pain Episodes

During pregnancy, women with sickle cell disease may experience an increase in the frequency and severity of painful episodes and acute chest syndrome, although the extent to which this occurs has not been well characterized.

None of the studies document the pre-pregnancy rate of pain events, which makes interpretation of reported pain rates during pregnancy difficult. The Cooperative Study noted an average of one to two episodes of significant pain during 445 pregnancies [13].

Treatment of sickle cell crisis during pregnancy should proceed as for the nonpregnant patient, with a goal of reducing sickling, limiting red blood cell adherence to vessels, and controlling pain. Intravenous fluids and oxygen therapy are used to maintain normal intravascular volume and oxygenation. Recognition and treatment of infection reduces inflammatory stimuli. Opiates are not associated with teratogenicity, congenital malformations, or toxic effects other than transient suppression of movement and variability in fetal heart tones [19]. Chronic exposure to opiates, such as in women who require methadone or other medications to control severe chronic pain, can result in neonatal abstinence syndrome after birth, although the rate was relatively low (11%) in women who received methadone for pain management [31] and was not related to the maternal medication dosage [32].

Careful surveillance for the development of complications of sickle cell pain events is needed, which can become rapidly life threatening. These complications most commonly include the acute chest syndrome, which has been reported in 7% to 20% of pregnancies [13,14,18,20,23]. Acute sequestration or infarction of the spleen may occur in women with milder forms of sickle cell disease when the spleen is still present in adulthood [18,24]. Acute multiorgan failure may also occur, with a rapid decline in pulmonary, hepatic, and renal function. Early recognition of these complications with supportive care and judicious use of transfusion therapy may potentially halt their progression and prevent significant morbidity and mortality.

Transfusion Therapy in Pregnancy

Empiric therapy with transfusion of red blood cells has been used to support women with sickle cell disease in pregnancy. Both simple transfusion and erythrocytapheresis are well tolerated [20,33]. A single randomized trial was conducted to determine the maternal and fetal benefits of an aggressive transfusion regimen [24]. Pregnant women with HbSS were randomized between a program of "emergent" transfusion, given for acute severe anemia (Hb <6 g/dL) or complications during pregnancy, and a program of routine transfusion to suppress levels of HbS. Women in the emergent group had hemoglobin values throughout pregnancy as low as 6.0 g/dL, whereas women in the prophylactic group were maintained at a hemoglobin level of 10 g/dL. Despite aggressive prophylactic transfusion therapy, there was no significant reduction in obstetric complications or improvement in the fetal birth weight or incidence of intrauterine growth retardation (Table 4). This result is not surprising given the lack of correlation between maternal hemoglobin values and these complications, as previously noted. There was a significant reduction in the number of pain episodes but not in the complications (eg, acute chest syndrome) of these pain episodes, depicted in Table 4. These results were confirmed in a retrospective

Table 4
Effects of prophylactic transfusion compared with emergent transfusion on pregnancy outcomes in women with sickle cell anemia

| | Percentage of affected pregnancies | | | | | |
| | Randomized trial [24] | | Nonrandomized series [23] | | Prophylactic erythrocytapheresis program [20] | |
Outcome	Prophylactic (n = 36)	Emergent (n = 36)	Prophylactic (n = 22)	Emergent (n = 12)	Prophylactic (n = 103)	Emergent (n = 28)
Pain episodes	14	50*	55	50	3	75*
ACS	5	8	15	25	5	32*
Splenic sequestration	0	3	NR	NR	NR	NR
Preterm labor	17	17	32	42	8	31*
Birth weight (g)	2495	2654	NR	NR	NR	NR
Low birth weight	NR	NR	18	10	6	17*

Abbreviations: ACS, acute chest syndrome; NR, not reported.
* $P < 0.05$.

review of 81 pregnancies in women with HbSS and HbSC disease from 1991 to 1993 [23]. In that study, women who received transfusion as a prophylactic ally were compared with those who did not and with controls. There was no difference in the maternal or fetal outcomes, but a reduction was seen in the number of pregnancies complicated by pain events from 42% to 9% and a decrease in acute chest syndrome from 25% to 5%. In a nonrandomized trial, pregnancy outcomes with the use of chronic erythrocytapheresis instituted at an average of 19 weeks' gestation for 103 women with HbSS and HbSC were compared with the outcomes for 28 women who did not receive prophylactic transfusion [20]. There was a significant reduction in pain events and acute chest syndrome, as well as a reduction in low birth weight infants and perinatal death. Two patients sustained hepatitis, 5 had transfusion reactions, and 11 (10%) developed alloantibodies during prophylactic transfusion support. A recent Cochrane review [34] based on the single randomized trial of transfusion therapy [24] noted that there was not enough evidence to draw conclusions about prophylactic transfusion therapy for women with sickle cell disease. In the absence of consistent data supporting a reduction in obstetric or fetal outcomes, the use of transfusion therapy is generally limited to patients who experience a significant increase in sickle cell disease activity with severe complications, including acute chest syndrome and acute severe anemia (Hb <5.0–6.0 g/dL), and in anticipation of surgery [19].

Minor antigen matching of red blood cell units should be considered whenever possible for at least the full Rh blood group (C/c/D/E/e) and Kell antigens. As is true for anti-D, alloantibodies may result in hemolytic disease of the newborn. In a study of 30 pregnant women with sickle cell disease with a history of prior transfusion or transfusion during pregnancy, 20% developed alloantibodies during pregnancy, and one newborn was affected by mild hemolytic disease owing to an anti-c antibody [35]. In another series of pregnancies complicated by anti-c, 26% of infants developed hemolytic disease of the newborn [36]. In addition to avoidance of alloimmunization by the use of minor antigen matched blood whenever possible, awareness of previous transfusion history and associated alloantibodies should be recognized and monitored appropriately.

Other Sickle Cell Disease Comorbidities

Some patients with sickle cell disease sustain chronic complications before their pregnancy, including stroke, pulmonary hypertension with chronic restrictive lung disease, hepatic dysfunction associated with viral hepatitis or iron overload owing to transfusion therapy, and chronic renal failure. Pregnancies in these patients may be complicated or even contraindicated based on their end-organ damage. In some patients, these complications are well controlled using chronic transfusion therapy. Transfusion therapy should be continued in these patients throughout their pregnancy.

Sickle cell patients maintained on chronic transfusion therapy require chelation therapy with deferoxamine to treat or prevent secondary hemosiderosis.

This drug is considered a category C risk for pregnant women and should be withheld during pregnancy. Prenatal vitamins without iron should be prescribed to avoid further iron overload.

Chronic hydroxyurea therapy is used for severely affected patients with HbSS and HbSβ°-thalassemia to reduce the frequency of sickle cell pain crises. Hydroxyurea, even when used throughout pregnancy, has not been associated with birth defects in a small number of pregnancies [37]. Nevertheless, it is a teratogen in animals and should be stopped once pregnancy is recognized.

SICKLE CELL TRAIT

In general, women with the sickle cell trait tolerate pregnancy well without an increased risk of significant obstetric or fetal complications. During pregnancy, an increased rate of bacteriuria has been noted in women with the sickle cell trait when compared with those without it. This bacteriuria may be associated with the development of urinary tract infections or pyelonephritis [38], warranting monitoring of urinalysis and treatment of significant bacteriuria. A study of 126 women with the sickle cell trait suggested there was an increased risk of pre-eclampsia in a comparison with nontrait controls [39]. This finding was not confirmed in a subsequent study [40], which found that the relative risk of pre-eclampsia was actually somewhat lower in women with the sickle cell trait (relative risk, 0.5; 95% CI, 0.2–1.6). A small group of infants born to women with the sickle cell trait were noted to have increased nucleated red blood cells in cord blood, interpreted by the investigators as a potential indication of subtle fetal hypoxia [41]. Outcomes, including Apgar scores and birth weight, were not different in a comparison with controls, and the significance of this observation is unclear.

If a history of sickle cell trait is obtained, laboratory confirmation is recommended. Some women may report that they have been told they have the "sickle trait" plus "hemoglobin C trait" or "thalassemia trait," which may actually represent HbSC disease or HbSβ$^+$-thalassemia. In contrast to the sickle cell trait, the latter two conditions warrant careful pregnancy management, as for women with HbSS.

SUMMARY

Careful management of pregnancy in women with sickle cell disease, including access to prenatal care and to expertise in sickle cell disease and high-risk obstetrics, provides an opportunity for successful outcomes. The actual relative risk of obstetric complications has not been clearly defined. Based on observational data, there is likely some increased risk for miscarriage, preterm labor, and possibly placental abruption and hypertensive disorders in women with sickle cell anemia (HbSS). Infants born to women with HbSS generally have lower birth weight and are at risk for intrauterine growth retardation. Reduction of maternal anemia with transfusion support does not have an impact on these potential complications, suggesting that red blood cell adhesion and other factors leading to vaso-occlusion affect the uteroplacental unit. A prospective randomized trial demonstrated that transfusion therapy was successful in reducing the rate and potentially the severity of sickle cell manifestations, which are thought to be exacerbated during pregnancy.

Management recommendations focus on careful monitoring for obstetric and fetal complications and recognition of and early intervention for sickle cell–related complications. Labor and delivery should proceed as for other pregnant women. Transfusion support is indicated for acute severe events and during pregnancies complicated by persistent complications of sickle cell disease.

References

[1] Rappaport VJ, Valazquez M, Williams K. Hemoglobinopathies in pregnancy. Obstet Gynecol Clin North Am 2004;31:287–317.

[2] Veille JC, Hanson R. Left ventricular systolic and diastolic function in pregnant patients with sickle cell disease. Am J Obstet Gynecol 1994;170(1):107–10.

[3] Cines DB, Pollak ES, Buck CA, et al. Endothelial cells in physiology and in the pathophysiology of vascular disorders. Blood 1998;91(10):3527–61.

[4] Pantanowitz L, Schwartz R, Balogh K. The placenta in sickle cell disease. Arch Pathol Lab Med 2000;124:1565.

[5] Trampont P, Roudier M, Andrea AM, et al. The placental-umbilical unit in sickle cell disease pregnancy: a model for studying in vivo functional adjustments to hypoxia in humans. Hum Pathol 2004;35(11):1353–9.

[6] Brown AK, Sleeper LA, Pegelow CH, et al. The influence of infant and maternal sickle cell disease on birth outcome and neonatal course. Arch Pediatr Adolesc Med 1994;148: 1156–62.

[7] Billett HH, Langer O, Regan OT, et al. Doppler velocimetry in pregnant patients with sickle cell anemia. Am J Hematol 1993;42:305–8.

[8] Anyaegbunam A, Langer O, Brustman L, et al. Third-trimester prediction of small-for-gestational-age infants in pregnant women with sickle cell disease. J Reprod Med 1991; 36(8):577–80.

[9] Anyaegbunam A, Gauthier Morel M, Merkatz I. Antepartum fetal surveillance tests during sickle cell crisis. Am J Obstet Gynecol 1991;165(1):1081–3.

[10] Shaamash AH, Elsonosy ED, Zakhari MM, et al. Placental nitric oxide synthase (NOS) activity and nitric oxide (NO) production in normal pregnancy, pre-eclampsia and eclampsia. Int J Gynaecol Obstet 2001;72(2):127–33.

[11] Howard RJ, Tuck SM, Pearson TC. Blood transfusion in pregnancies complicated by maternal sickle cell disease: effects on blood rheology and uteroplacental Doppler velocimetry. Clin Lab Naematol 1994;16:253–9.

[12] Wilson WA, Alleyne GA. Total body water, extracellular and plasma volume compartments in sickle cell anemia. West Indian Med J 1976;25:241.

[13] Smith JA, Espeland M, Bellevue R, et al. Pregnancy in sickle cell disease: experience of the Cooperative Study of Sickle Cell Disease. Obstet Gynecol 1996;87(2):199–204.

[14] Serjeant GR, Look Loy L, Crowther M, et al. Outcome of pregnancy in homozygous sickle cell disease. Obstet Gynecol 2004;103(6):1278–85.

[15] Powars DR, Sandhu M, Niland-Weiss J, et al. Pregnancy in sickle cell disease. Obstet Gynecol 1986;67:217–28.

[16] Morris JS, Dunn DT, Serjeant GR. Haematological risk factors for pregnancy outcome in Jamaican women with homozygous sickle cell disease. Br J Obstet Gynaecol 1994;101: 770–3.

[17] Rust OA, Perry KG. Pregnancy complicated by sickle hemoglobinopathy. Clin Obstet Gynecol 1995;38:472–84.

[18] Koshy M, Burd L. Management of pregnancy in sickle cell syndromes. Hematol Oncol Clin North Am 1991;5(3):585–96.

[19] Koshy M, Chisum D, Burd L, et al. Management of sickle cell anemia and pregnancy. J Clin Apheresis 1991;6:230–3.

[20] Morrison J, Morrison F, Floyd R, et al. Use of continuous flow erythrocytapheresis in pregnant patients with sickle cell disease. J Clin Apheresis 1991;6:224–9.

[21] Seoud MAF, Cantwell C, Nobles G, et al. Outcome of pregnancies complicated by sickle cell and sickle C hemoglobinopathies. Am J Perinatol 1994;11(3):187–91.

[22] Sun PM, Wilburn W, Raynor BD, et al. Sickle cell disease in pregnancy: twenty years of experience at Grady Memorial Hospital, Atlanta, Georgia. Am J Obstet Gynecol 2001; 184(6):1127–30.

[23] Howard RJ, Tuck SM, Pearson TC. Pregnancy in sickle cell disease in the UK: results of a multicentre survey of the effect of prophylactic blood transfusion on maternal and fetal outcome. Br J Obstet Gynaecol 1995;102:947–51.

[24] Koshy M, Burd L, Wallace D, et al. Prophylactic red-cell transfusions in pregnant patients with sickle cell disease: a randomized cooperative study. N Engl J Med 1988;319: 1447–52.

[25] Wang X, Seaman C, Paik M, et al. Experience with 500 prenatal diagnoses of sickle cell diseases: the effect of gestational age on affected pregnancy outcome. Prenat Diagn 1994;14:851–7.

[26] Rementeria J, Nuang N. Narcotic withdrawal in pregnancy: stillbirth incidence with a case report. Am J Obstet Gynecol 1973;116:1152–6.

[27] Kaltenbach K, Berghella V, Finnegan L. Opioid dependence during pregnancy: effects and management. Obstet Gynecol Clin North Am 1998;25(1):139–51.

[28] Rathmell J, Viscomi C, Ashburn M. Management of nonobstetric pain during pregnancy and lactation. Anesth Analg 1997;85:1074–87.

[29] Finer P, Blair J, Rowe P. Epidural analgesia in the management of labor pain and sickle cell crisis—a case report. Anesthesiology 1988;68(5):799–800.

[30] Chiron B, Laffon M, Ferrandiere M, et al. Postdural puncture headache in a parturient with sickle cell disease: use of an epidural colloid patch. Can J Anest 2003;50:812–4.

[31] Sharpe C, Kuschel C. Outcomes of infants born to mothers receiving methadone for pain management in pregnancy. Arch Dis Child Fetal Neonatal Ed 2004;89(1):F33–6.

[32] Berghalla V, Lim PJ, Hill MK, et al. Maternal methadone dose and neonatal withdrawal. Am J Obstet Gynecol 2003;189(2):312–7.

[33] Lee W, Werch R, Rokey J, et al. Physiologic observations of pregnant women undergoing prophylactic erythrocytapheresis for sickle cell disease. Transfusion 1991;31:59–62.

[34] Mohomed K. Prophylactic versus selective blood transfusion for sickle cell anaemia during pregnancy. Cochrane Database Syst Rev 1996;2:CD000040.

[35] Narchi H, Ekuma-Nkama E. Maternal sickle cell anemia and neonatal isoimmunization. Int J Gynaecol Obstet 1998;62:129–34.

[36] Hackney DN, Knudtson EJ, Rossi KQ, et al. Management of pregnancies complicated by anti-c isoimmunization. Obstet Gynecol 2004;103(1):24–30.

[37] Diav-Citrin O, Hunnisett L, Sher G, et al. Hydroxyurea use during pregnancy: a case report in sickle cell disease and review of the literature. Am J Hematol 1999;60:148–50.

[38] Blank A, Freedman W. Sickle cell trait and pregnancy. Clin Obstet Gynecol 1969;12(1): 123–33.

[39] Larrabee K, Monga M. Women with sickle cell trait are at increased risk for pre-eclampsia. Am J Obstet Gynecol 1997;177:425–8.

[40] Stamilio D, Sehdev H, Macones G. Pregnant women with the sickle cell trait are not at increased risk for developing preeclampsia. Am J Perinatol 2003;20:41–8.

[41] Manzar S. Maternal sickle cell trait and fetal hypoxia. Am J Perinatol 2000;17(7):367–70.

Hematol Oncol Clin N Am 19 (2005) 917–928

HEMATOLOGY/ONCOLOGY CLINICS
OF NORTH AMERICA

Priapism in Sickle Cell Disease

Zora R. Rogers, MD[a,b,*]

[a]Division of Pediatric Hematology/Oncology, The University of Texas Southwestern Medical Center at Dallas, 5323 Harry Hines Boulevard, Dallas, TX 75390-9063, USA
[b]Southwestern Comprehensive Sickle Cell Center, Dallas, TX, USA

Priapism is an unwanted, painful erection of the penis. It has been recognized as a complication of sickle cell disease since 1934 [1]. Sickle cell disease is the single most common cause of priapism in adults and almost the only recognized specific cause in pediatric patients [2]. It occurs in two general patterns: (1) prolonged—an episode lasting 4 hours or more that carries with it a risk for permanent vascular damage and eventual impotence and (2) stuttering—brief episodes that resolve spontaneously, often occur in clusters, and may herald a prolonged event [3]. The relationship between stuttering and prolonged priapism is not clear, but both appear to be linked to the same pathophysiology.

Patients are reluctant to mention this problem to physicians, and when priapism does come to medical attention it may be inadequately managed. Treatment tends to be anecdotal, inconsistent, and at the discretion of individual practitioners who may only infrequently confront this problem and have no ongoing care relationship with the patient. Impotence is frequently the outcome. As yet there are scant data on the frequency of priapism, no good clinical trial data on the efficacy of different management approaches, and, essentially, no longitudinal data on the late effects of this little discussed but common major complication of sickle cell disease [4].

PHYSIOLOGY

The penis contains three vascular chambers: the paired lateral corpora cavernosa and a corpus spongiosum surrounding the urethra. Erection occurs when increased blood volume in the cavernosa and spongiosum is constrained by the tunica albuginea, leading to mechanical elongation of the penis. An erection is normally maintained by the partial obstruction of venous drainage [5]. Priapism occurs when there is either unregulated arterial inflow or persistent obstruction of venous outflow [2].

* Division of Pediatric Hematology/Oncology, The University of Texas Southwestern Medical Center at Dallas, 5323 Harry Hines Boulevard, Dallas, TX 75390-9063. E-mail address: zora.rogers@utsouthwestern.edu

0889-8588/05/$ – see front matter
doi:10.1016/j.hoc.2005.08.003

Priapism typically presents with involvement of the corpora cavernosa but spares the corpora spongiosum and glans. Tricorporal priapism has been reported in sickle cell disease [6] and may herald corporal infarction [6–8]. Multiple imaging modalities, including Doppler flow analysis of arteries [9], cavernosal pressure measurement, and Tc^{99m} scintigraphy [7], have been investigated without clarification of the pathophysiology or optimum management approach.

Priapism is often divided into low-flow and high-flow states, with each entailing a different prognosis, therapy, and urgency of management [2]. High-flow, or arterial, priapism is commonly due to cavernosal arterial injury, usually from external trauma, and is rarely associated with ischemia. Although it is often recurrent, high-flow priapism is seldom painful and does not require urgent intervention [3]. Cure is often surgical, with significant complications. Although arterial priapism has been reported in men who have sickle cell disease, priapism, whether prolonged or stuttering, is far more commonly a low-flow state related to venous stasis. It requires prompt resolution of prolonged episodes to prevent ischemia and minimize the risk for development of fibrosis and impotence [2,3].

The proposed pathophysiologic mechanism for development of low-flow priapism in patients who have sickle cell disease is sickling and sludging of erythrocytes in the corpora cavernosa, a process similar to sequestration of sickled erythrocytes in the spleen [5]. After prolonged erections, blood trapped in the corpora cavernosa becomes deoxygenated, resulting in local acidosis, further sludging, and an increase in intercavernosal pressure. When the intercavernosal pressure is increased to 80 to 120 mm Hg for 4 hours or more, the corpora cavernosa become ischemic, eliciting an inflammatory response that may result in fibrosis and impotence [2,5]. Histologic examination of tissue obtained during surgical procedures shows that irreversible fibrosis of the corpora cavernosa, but not usually of the glans or corpus spongiosum, may indeed be the outcome of prolonged episodes of priapism [10]. Retrospective reviews and small case series validate the notion that impotence is common after priapism in patients who have sickle cell anemia and that it appears to correlate with a longer duration of erection [2,11].

EPIDEMIOLOGY AND NATURAL HISTORY

Historically, only 5% to 10% of male patients of any age with sickle cell disease were said to have had priapism [6,12–14]. A retrospective review of adult patients now indicates that at least 30% to 45% of patients have a history of this complication [15,16]. An interview survey of sequential male patients aged 5 to 20 years from Dallas who had sickle cell anemia demonstrated a prevalence of 27.5% by 15 years of age. The calculated actuarial probability of experiencing priapism was 12.9% by 10 years of age, 50.3% by 15 years of age, and 89.3% by 20 years of age [17]. Episodes have been reported to occur as young as 3 years of age, and one series found that 16% of patients had their first episode of priapism before 5 years of age [18,19]. In a mail survey of 130 patients aged 4 to 66 years in the United Kingdom and Nigeria, 35% reported an episode of priapism. The mean age at first episode was 15 years, and 75% had their first episode before age 20 [20]. A large review of published cases concluded that approximately half of all reported sickle cell patients with priapism had their first episode before they were 18 years old [21]. Thus, priapism is a common problem even in young children.

Priapism is most common in patients who have sickle cell anemia, who account for 80% to 90% of reported cases [6,8,15,20,21]. However, it does occur in males with all forms of sickle cell disease (sickle hemoglobin C disease and both sickle beta^0 and beta$^+$ thalassemias) and is even reportedly increased in individuals who have sickle cell trait [20–22]. A single episode of priapism was reported by 31% to 64% of patients, a pattern that appears to be more common in childhood [6,16,17,19]. However, approximately half of all patients have recurrent episodes, from 2 to 50 times or more [15,17]. In one survey, the estimated mean duration of an episode of priapism was 125 minutes (range 30 to 480 minutes) [17]. The pattern of recurrent episodes is also variable and unpredictable. Stuttering spells may occur every few days for months before stopping abruptly or heralding a prolonged episode [16,19]. Other authors note no clustering of episodes and report patients with years of unpredictable recurrent events [15,17].

Although retrospective surveys are inconsistent [6,21], priapism in childhood appears to be associated with impotence [11]. A survey of 15 patients who had sickle cell disease and priapism in childhood and were later evaluated by questionnaire and objective RigiScan testing (a widely used objective monitor for the development of nocturnal penile tumescence, or erection during sleep) demonstrated that loss of potency was directly related to the duration of priapism and younger age at first episode. Only 4 of the 15 patients maintained normal erections at 10 to 46 years of age [23]. In the United Kingdom–Nigeria survey, 21% of respondents who had a history of priapism reported erectile dysfunction [20]. Not surprisingly, patients had trouble admitting loss of potency and overestimated the quality of erection compared with results of objective testing [20,23]. Overall, 10% to 50% of adults in published cases who have sickle cell disease and a history of priapism are impotent by self-report [6,15,16].

Most priapism episodes begin during sleep [17,21,24]. In the Dallas survey, episodes typically began around 4 am, and 75% of patients recalled at least one episode that started during or on awakening from sleep [17]. This finding may be due to the association of rapid eye movement sleep, which preferentially occurs during this time, with normal erections and to the relative nocturnal acidosis and dehydration that favor sickling of erythrocytes [21]. In a survey of adults, 17% of episodes were related to sexual activity and 3% each were related to excessive ethanol intake or were called spontaneous [21]. Today, cocaine or other drug use, a known risk factor in non–sickle cell–related priapism, would probably be a more significant factor [2].

The occurrence of priapism has been associated with higher levels of hemoglobin S [25] and inversely correlated with levels of fetal hemoglobin [26] in specific populations. This relationship is also suggested by the 42% prevalence reported in Jamaican patients who have sickle cell disease [16], compared with 2% of patients from Saudi Arabia, a population with higher fetal hemoglobin levels [26]. Other authors have observed no relationship to fetal hemoglobin levels [6].

Priapism has been suggested by some authors to be more common in patients who are or will be experiencing a severe course of their sickle cell disease [6,8,14]; other authors believe it occurs independently of overall severity [15]. In the Dallas review, no significant difference was found in the baseline hematologic data or number of hospital admissions for painful events between patients with and without a history of priapism [17,19]. One third of the boys described the pain of priapism as the worst complication of their sickle cell disease [17].

A National Institutes of Health–National Heart Lung and Blood Institute (NHLBI)–sponsored interview survey of 1650 male patients who have sickle cell disease is just beginning in the Clinical Trials Consortium of the Comprehensive Sickle Cell Centers Program. The survey is designed to provide solid epidemiologic data about how often and under what circumstances priapism occurs.

MANAGEMENT OF ACUTE EPISODES

Physical examination revealing a tumescent phallus with a history of the unwanted painful erection lasting 30 minutes or more is adequate for diagnosis of priapism. When priapism lasts 4 hours or more, the potential for permanent ischemic injury is present, and intervention is warranted [3]. A suggested approach to the patient presenting for medical attention during an episode of priapism is presented in Box 1.

Numerous therapeutic modalities have been used for treatment of priapism associated with sickle cell disease. Patients report that voiding, opioid and nonsteroidal analgesics, gentle exercise, ejaculation, or taking a warm bath or shower may terminate some events [15,17]. Physicians have offered intravenous hydration, opioid analgesia, erythrocyte transfusions, vasodilators, adrenergic agents, hormones, and surgical shunt procedures to treat acute events [19,21,27]. Hydration and opioid analgesia are the mainstays of management of all forms of sickle cell pain. Heat (hot water bottles, hot packs, sitz baths) is probably more beneficial than ice packs for comfort and does not precipitate painful crises in adjacent regions [8]. Anxiolysis with midazolam or benzodiazepines and alkalinization has never been demonstrated to be effective in inducing detumescence, but such maneuvers should not harm the patient so long as they do not delay other therapies. Oxygen is indicated when the patient is hypoxic but has no proven role when he is not. Indeed, routine use of supplemental oxygen could suppress erythropoiesis. However, none of these approaches is predictably effective in relieving priapism, and they may delay procedures that have been shown to result in rapid detumescence and reperfusion of the corpora cavernosa.

Box 1: Management of an acute episode of priapism in a patient who has sickle cell disease

I. Obtain brief history, with attention to

   1. Time since onset of priapism

   2. Precipitating events, if any [2]:

      • Excess or illicit drug use (alcohol, marijuana, cocaine)

      • Intracavernosal injection for impotence: aprostadil, papaverine, prostaglandin E1, phentolamine

      • Psychoactive medications: antihypertensives (prazosin), antidepressants (bupropion, trazdone, fluoxetine, sertraline, lithium), antipsychotics (clozapine), and tranquillizers (mesoridazine, perphenazine, chlorpromazine)

      • Perineal or pelvic trauma (more common in arterial priapism)

   3. Prior episodes of priapism and outcome

   4. Maneuvers taken to end this episode

II. Perform physical examination to confirm fully rigid painful penis

III. Consider an oral dose of a vasoactive agent, such as pseudoephedrine (see text)

IV. If episode duration has been or will soon be longer than 4 hours, obtain urologic consultation stat to perform aspiration and irrigation

V. While awaiting urologic consultant,

   1. Keep patient NPO for conscious sedation, if desired

   2. Provide pain relief with parenteral opioids

   3. Provide intravenous hydration

   4. Provide supplemental oxygen, if patient is hypoxic or if desired by patient

VI. If detumescence does not occur, aspiration and irrigation should be performed; Note that penis may remain edematous or semirigid after a prolonged episode, but pain should be diminished

---

Vasoactive Agents

Erection results from relaxation of smooth muscles of arterioles and trabeculae in the corpora, and detumescence is the result of smooth muscle contraction, opening emissary veins and increasing venous drainage [2,28]. Therefore, detumescence should be facilitated by α-adrenergic agonists, such as phenylephrine, a pure α-adrenergic agent, and epinephrine, which has mixed α, β-1, and β-2 activity [29]. These agents induce contraction of the smooth muscle of the trabecular arteries of the cavernosa, forcing blood out of the cavernosa and promoting detumescence [8]. Vasodilators, such as hydralazine, or β-agonists, such as terbutaline, activate β-adrenergic receptors. This effect leads to relaxation of the smooth muscles of the cavernosal vasculature, allowing arterial blood to "wash out" the sickled cells and permit detumescence [8,30].

Terbutaline, a β-agonist, in either subcutaneous and oral forms is effective in the management of pharmacologically induced priapism in some trials [31–33], but it has not been studied in sickle cell disease. Oral phenylephrine [34] and pseudoephedrine [32] have been reported to be equivalent to terbutaline in producing detumescence in patients who have pharmacologically induced priapism. Thus, a dose of one of these agents, or etilefrine where available (see later discussion), should be considered when evaluating a patient who presents during an episode of priapism.

Aspiration and Irrigation

Prolonged priapism is a urologic emergency requiring urgent intervention as the best chance of avoiding irreversible ischemic penile injury, which may terminate in corporal fibrosis and impotence [3]. Most traditional medical treatments yield a slow resolution of the problem and require hospitalization [21]. Aspiration and irrigation of the corpora with saline or dilute adrenergic agents (intracavernosal injection) has been shown to be effective in the treatment of priapism resulting from intrapenile injection of vasoactive drugs for the treatment of impotence [2,35]. This procedure induces rapid detumescence and thus allows oxygenated blood to re-enter the cavernosa.

The Dallas program reported rapid complete detumescence in 35 of 37 consecutive episodes of prolonged priapism in 15 pediatric patients treated with aspiration and irrigation with a dilute (1:1,000,000) epinephrine solution [27]. Two patients presenting after 27 and 36 hours of priapism did not respond [27], supporting the expert opinion that aspiration and irrigation may be unsuccessful after 12 hours [2]. This experience has been updated with immediate detumescence during 72 of 74 procedures (97%) performed in 20 patients. Three patients required repeat aspiration and irrigation within 24 hours and responded completely [19]. Although the majority of patients in this case series underwent the procedure only once, others have undergone aspiration and irrigation during as many as 40 episodes. The only complications were small, self-resolving penile hematomas. All boys who responded to aspiration and irrigation with detumescence self-reported normal erectile function a median of 40 months later [27]. The author's center's current protocol for emergency department aspiration and irrigation for prolonged priapism in pediatric patients who have sickle cell disease is detailed in Box 2.

Although aspiration and irrigation with dilute epinephrine is the only intervention published in a large United States series for relief of priapism in patients who have sickle cell disease, dilute phenylephrine may be a better agent. Epinephrine is theoretically more likely to increase the heart rate in already anemic patients and elevate blood pressure, with potentially more severe consequences in patients who have neurovascular compromise [8]. The practice guidelines of the American Urological Association endorse aspiration and irrigation with dilute phenylephrine as the treatment of choice, even in children, for relief of prolonged episodes of priapism regardless of hemoglobinopathy [35]. Methylene blue, a guanylate cyclase inhibitor, has been reported to relieve

Box 2: Aspiration and irrigation

This procedure should only be performed by a staff urologist or an experienced urology resident.

1. Conscious sedation may be administered at the discretion of the emergency department staff or attending urologist but is not, in general, required for an older patient or one who has undergone the procedure previously.

2. The lateral side of the penis is prepared with povidone-iodine, and approximately 0.5 mL of 1% lidocaine is infiltrated subcutaneously into the lateral surface of the penis, then more deeply into the tunica albuginea.

3. A 23-gauge needle is inserted into the corpora cavernosa, and as much blood as possible is aspirated into a dry 10-mL syringe through a three-way stopcock. This specimen is sent to the blood gas laboratory for analysis of pO_2, pCO_2, and pH (unless this analysis has been performed previously on the patient).

4. Another 10-mL syringe containing a dilute solution of an -adrenergic agent is attached to the three-way stopcock. The corpora cavernosa are irrigated with as much as 10 mL of the adrenergic solution, with additional blood aspirated by means of dry syringes until detumescence has occurred.

   The adrenergic solution is prepared with either phenylephrine or epinephrine (see text) as follows [2,29]:

   a. Phenylephrine (recommended in American Urological Association guidelines [35]), 1 mL of the stock vial (10 mg/mL), is diluted in 1000 mL of normal saline, making a 10 mcg/mL solution.

   b. Epinephrine (has published efficacy in patients with sickle cell disease [19,27,29]), 1 mL of 1:1,000 epinephrine, is diluted in 1 L of normal saline, making a 1:1,000,000 solution.

5. The needle is withdrawn, and 5 minutes (timed by the clock) of firm pressure are administered *by the physician* to prevent hematoma formation.

6. A cycle of aspiration and irrigation may be required every 5 minutes for as long as 1 hour before one may declare the treatment unsuccessful. Remember that the penis may be very edematous but that the endpoint of the procedure is a decrease in rigidity and less than 50% tumescence.

prolonged priapism but may be associated with the risk for cutaneous necrosis and penile fibrosis [36].

Outside the United States, investigators have used the adrenergic agent etilefrine in a similar fashion [22,24,37,38]. Etilefrine is a direct-acting sympathomimetic drug with both α- and β-agonist properties that is available only in Europe, Africa, and Asia [39]. It has been shown to cause detumescence in adults and children when used as an intracavernous injection alone or following aspiration [38]. Some investigators have even advocated teaching home self–intracavernosal injection with this agent to patients who have sickle cell anemia and recurrent episodes of prolonged priapism [22,24].

Transfusion

Red cell transfusion has been widely advocated as treatment of priapism, but the literature does not support its usefulness in the acute setting [8]. The original report advocated simple transfusion to a doubling of the baseline hematocrit and reported "relief" in 24 hours. Detumescence occurred 2 to 3 days later and in some patients took as long as 1 week. Although the report claims that potency was maintained [40], current understanding of the need to relieve ischemia within 4 to 12 hours suggests that this was unlikely. Simple transfusion to a hemoglobin concentration of approximately 10 g/dL has never been rigorously evaluated for benefits in mitigating priapism. Theoretically, once venous stasis and obstruction of outflow from spasm of the smooth muscles have occurred during priapism, it is unlikely that transfused cells can reach the area of involvement [8].

Exchange transfusion, although still widely employed, has been complicated by reports of the ASPEN Syndrome. This syndrome of acute, severe neurologic abnormalities, including severe headache, occurs 1 to 11 days after transfusion for priapism in patients who have sickle cell disease; it is thought to be related to the interaction of hyperviscosity and vasoactive substances released during penile tumescence following transfusion [14,41,42]. However, all these transfusion strategies require at least 4 hours to initiate and 8 hours or more to complete, after a patient reaches medical attention. Hence, transfusion may consume excessive time when the goal is to achieve detumescence before ischemia develops.

Surgical Shunts

Surgical management of priapism, including cavernospongiosum or cavernosaphenous vein shunts, should be reserved for use when conservative management fails to produce detumescence. In addition to the risk inherent in placing a patient who has sickle cell disease under anesthesia, these shunt procedures have been reported to result in skin sloughing and the formation of chordee or urethrocutaneous fistulas [43]. These procedures do not result in complete detumescence, and impotence is a common side effect [44]. However, one review found that shunts performed within 48 hours, particularly in postpubertal children, appeared more likely to preserve potency than supportive care alone [23].

STRATEGIES FOR THE SECONDARY PREVENTION OF PRIAPISM

For patients who have frequently recurrent stuttering spells or several prolonged episodes requiring repeated aspiration and irrigation, alternative strategies to prevent episodes should be considered. Treatment with hydroxyurea has been suggested by some authors to prevent priapism [45,46], although others found it ineffective [47]. A controlled trial of the efficacy of hydroxyurea treatment in the prevention of priapism has never been reported. However, this agent, which increases total and fetal hemoglobin levels, among other effects, may not be optimum for prevention of priapism. In patients with corporal bodies injured from prior episodes of priapism, a higher hemoglobin concentration with sickle hemoglobin present could make the episodes more frequent. Similarly, although a program of chronic transfusion therapy with the goal of maintaining the patient's hemoglobin S percentage below 30% is widely used for secondary prevention of stroke, acute chest syndrome, and painful events, there is no convincing evidence that this approach prevents recurrence of priapism.

Vasoactive agents, found to be useful in the urgent treatment of prolonged episodes, may also have a role in the prevention of recurrent priapism. A group from Togo has reported that oral etilefrine taken daily for 1 to 7 months hastened the "resolution" of stuttering priapism or prevented recurrent prolonged priapism in 11 pediatric patients treated for as long as 7 months [38]. Prophylactic bedtime administration of etilephrine, sometimes in combination with hydroxyurea or stilbestrol, resulted in a decrease of 69% to 72% in the frequency of both stuttering and prolonged episodes in adults [22,24] and a decrease of 100% in children [22,38]. With a mean treatment period of 14.7 months, none of the 18 patients developed hypertension or acknowledged sexual dysfunction [22].

It has been routine practice in the author's center to recommend 30 to 60 mg of oral pseudoephedrine at bedtime for patients who have previously required aspiration and irrigation. Patients are further advised to take an additional 30-mg dose when an episode of priapism occurs, in addition to other measures recommended to end the episode. This regimen is well tolerated, but some older patients receiving 60-mg or long-acting 120-mg doses initially report difficulty sleeping, which resolves with continued use. Review of medical records and self-reporting by patients and their families suggest that oral pseudoephedrine decreases recurrences of both stuttering and major episodes [19,27]. However, this effect has not been studied in a controlled fashion.

A number of other agents have been reported to decrease recurrent episodes of priapism in vivo and in vitro. Interestingly, a single oral dose of sildenafil citrate, taken at the onset of priapism in patients with recurrent severe episodes, has been reported to abort the episode with no ill effects [48]. Sildenafil may generate NO, which is known to relax the corpus cavernosum and allow egress of hypoxic sickled cells, thus relieving the episode. A small randomized trial with the estrogen diethylstilbestrol [49] showed efficacy, but this approach has not been widely adopted because of the feminizing side effect of this agent. Pentoxifylline enhances the rheologic properties of erythrocytes and has been of anecdotal benefit in priapism [21]. However, use of all these agents may be associated with unacceptable side effects, and none has been tried in large numbers of patients.

Levine and Guss [50] reported the successful use of leuprolide, an injectable synthetic analogue of gonadotropin-releasing hormone (GnRH or LH-RH), to prevent recurrent priapism in an 18-year-old who had sickle cell disease. Leuprolide acts to inhibit gonadotropin secretion and decrease serum testosterone levels. Leuprolide therapy may initially induce a testosterone flare that might precipitate an episode of priapism. Treatment with leuprolide is therefore initiated with a concomitant 1- to 2-week course of ketoconazole or casodex to block the effect of testosterone [19,50,51]. The author has reported similar success in preventing frequently recurrent stuttering and prolonged priapism in five (now seven) pediatric patients treated with a planned 6-month course of decreasing doses of depot leuprolide (2 months each of 3.88 mg, 1.94 mg, and 0.97 mg) [19,51]. Only one breakthrough episode of priapism occurred during 203 subsequent months of treatment [19]. Unfortunately, four of the seven patients again experienced recurrent episodes of priapism after the leuprolide was discontinued; they have chosen to receive repeat courses. A risk for decreased bone mineral density may exist during prolonged treatment (longer than 1 year) with gonadotropin-releasing hormone analogues [52]. However, the magnitude of this effect and whether it reverses after cessation of treatment are unknown. There are also case reports of successful prevention of recurrent priapism in patients who do not have sickle cell disease with the antiandrogen flutamide [53]. Thus, leuprolide and similar compounds may represent an alternative approach to the management of recurrent priapism requiring repeated aspiration and irrigation.

SUMMARY

Priapism is, for most patients, an unpredictable, recurrent event associated with devastating consequences for erectile function and quality of life. It occurs in a significant number of males who have all forms of sickle cell disease. Patients should be educated about priapism and currently available treatment options; this education should focus on the need to report recurrent events and to present for care within 4 hours of onset during a prolonged episode. Hematologists, as the physicians invested in the longitudinal care of such patients, must actively oversee the management of episodes, particularly of prolonged priapism, to ensure access to interventions such as aspiration and irrigation when these are required. Given such interest, it should be possible to design and conduct large-scale clinical trials of available intervention strategies to reach consensus about optimum strategies to terminate and prevent severe, frequently recurrent episodes of priapism in patients who have sickle cell disease.

References

[1] Diggs LW, Ching RE. Pathology of sickle cell anemia. South Med J 1934;27:839–45.
[2] Lue TF. Physiology of penile erection and pathophysiology of erectile dysfunction and priapism. In: Walsh PC, Retik AB, Vaughan Jr ED, et al, editors. Campbell's urology. 8th edition. Philadelphia: WB Saunders; 2002. p. 1591–613.
[3] American Foundation for Urologic Disease. Thought Leader Panel on Evaluation and Treatment of Priapism. Report of the American Foundation for Urologic Disease (AFUD) thought leader panel for evaluation and treatment of priapism. Int J Impot Res 2001; 13(Suppl 15):S39–43.
[4] Chinegwundoh F, Anie KA. Treatments for priapism in boys and men with sickle cell disease. Cochrane Database Syst Rev 2004;4:CD004198.
[5] Aboseif SR, Lue TF. Hemodynamics of penile erection. Urol Clin North Am 1988;15(1):1–7.
[6] Sharpsteen Jr JR, Powars D, Johnson C, et al. Multisystem damage associated with tricorporal priapism in sickle cell disease. Am J Med 1993;94(3):289–95.

[7] Hashmat AI, Raju S, Singh I, et al. 99mTc penile scan: an investigative modality in priapism. Urol Radiol 1989;11(1):58–60.

[8] Powars DR, Johnson CS. Priapism. Hematol Oncol Clin North Am 1996;10(6):1363–72.

[9] Lue TF, Hricak H, Marich KW, et al. Vasculogenic impotence evaluated by high-resolution ultrasonography and pulsed Doppler spectrum analysis. Radiology 1985;155(3):777–81.

[10] Yang Y-M, Donnell CA, Farrer JH, et al. Case report: corporectomy for intractable sickle-associated priapism. Am J Med Sci 1990;300(4):231–3.

[11] Mykulak DJ, Glassberg KI. Impotence following childhood priapism. J Urol 1990;144: 134–5.

[12] Kinney TR, Harris MB, Russell MO, et al. Priapism in association with sickle hemoglobin-opathies in children. J Pediatr 1975;86:241–2.

[13] Tarry WF, Duckett Jr JW, Snyder III HM. Urological complications of sickle cell disease in a pediatric population. J Urol 1987;138:592–4.

[14] Miller ST, Rao SP, Dunn EK, et al. Priapism in children with sickle cell disease, part 2. J Urol 1995;154:844–7.

[15] Fowler Jr JE, Koshy M, Strub M, et al. Priapism associated with the sickle cell hemo-globinopathies: prevalence, natural history and sequelae. J Urol 1991;145:65–8.

[16] Emond AM, Holman R, Hayes RJ, et al. Priapism and impotence in homozygous sickle cell disease. Arch Intern Med 1980;140:1434–7.

[17] Mantadakis E, Cavender JD, Rogers ZR, et al. Prevalence of priapism in boys with sickle cell anemia. J Pediatr Hematol Oncol 1999;21:518–22.

[18] Adeyokunnu AA, Lawani JO, Nkposong EO. Priapism complicating sickle cell disease in Nigerian children. Ann Trop Paediatr 1981;1(3):143–7.

[19] Rogers ZR, Ayoola F, Quinn CT, et al. The natural history of priapism in pediatric patients with sickle cell disease [abstract 2813]. Blood 2003;102:762s.

[20] Adeyoju AB, Olujohungbe ABK, Morris J, et al. Priapism in sickle-cell disease: inci-dence, risk factors and complications—an international multicentre study. BJU Int 2002; 90:898–902.

[21] Hamre MR, Harmon EP, Kirkpatrick DV, et al. Priapism as a complication of sickle cell disease. J Urol 1991;145:1–5.

[22] Okpala I, Westerdale N, Jegede T, et al. Etilefrine for the prevention of priapism in adult sickle cell disease. Br J Haematol 2002;118(3):918–21.

[23] Chakrabarty A, Upadhyay J, Dhabuwala CB, et al. Priapism associated with sickle cell hemoglobinopathy in children: long-term effects on potency. J Urol 1996;155:1419–23.

[24] Virag R, Bachir D, Lee K, et al. Preventive treatment of priapism in sickle cell disease with oral and self-administered intracavernous injection of etilefrine. Urology 1996;47(5): 777–81.

[25] Adedeji MO, Onuora VC, Ukoli FA. Hematological parameters associated with pria-pism in Nigerian patients with homozygous sickle cell disease. J Trop Med Hyg 1988; 91:157–9.

[26] Al-Awamy B, Taha SA, Naeem MA. Priapism in association with sickle cell anemia in Saudi Arabia. Acta Haematol 1985;73(3):181–2.

[27] Mantadakis E, Ewalt DH, Cavender JD, et al. Outpatient penile aspiration and epinephrine irrigation for young patients with sickle cell anemia and prolonged priapism. Blood 2000;95:78–82.

[28] Bosch RJ, Bernard F, Aboseif SR. Penile detumescence: characterization of three phases. J Urol 1991;146:867–71.

[29] Lee M, Cannon B, Sharifi R. Chart for preparation of dilutions of α-adrenergic agonists for intracavernous use in treatment of priapism. J Urol 1995;153:1182–3.

[30] Shantha TR, Finnerty DP, Rodriquez AP. Treatment of persistent penile erection and pria-pism using terbutaline. J Urol 1989;141:1427–9.

[31] Priyadarshi S. Oral terbutaline in the management of pharmacologically induced pro-longed erection. Int J Impot Res 2004;16(5):424–6.

[32] Lowe FC, Jarow JP. Placebo-controlled study of oral terbutaline and pseudoephedrine

in management of prostaglandin E1-induced prolonged erections. Urology 1993;42(1): 51–3.

[33] Govier FE, Jonsson E, Kramer-Levien D. Oral terbutaline for the treatment of priapism. J Urol 1994;151:878–9.

[34] Dittrich A, Albrecht K, Bar-Moshe O, et al. Treatment of pharmacologic priapism with phenylephrine. J Urol 1991;146:323–4.

[35] Priapism AUA. Guideline on the management of priapism. American Urological Association education and research. Available at: http://www.auanet.org/guidelines/priapism.cfm. Accessed April 1, 2005.

[36] Martínez Portillo FJ, Hoang-Boehm J, Weiss J, et al. Methylene blue as a successful alternative for pharmacologically induced priapism. Eur Urol 2001;39:20–3.

[37] Bachir D, Virag R, Lee K, et al. Prevention and treatment of erectile disorders in sickle cell disease. Rev Med Interne 1997;18(Suppl 1):46s–51s.

[38] Gbadoe AD, Atakouma Y, Kusiaku K, et al. Management of sickle cell priapism with etilefrine. Arch Dis Child 2001;85:52–3.

[39] DRUGDEX System (Etilefrine), Vol. 122. Greenwood Village (CO): Thompson MICRO-MEDEX; 2004.

[40] Seeler RA. Intensive transfusion therapy for priapism in boys with sickle cell anemia. J Urol 1973;110:360–1.

[41] Rackoff WR, Ohene-Frempong K, Month S, et al. Neurologic events after partial exchange transfusion for priapism in sickle cell disease. J Pediatr 1992;120:882–5.

[42] Siegel JF, Rich MA, Brock WA. Association of sickle cell disease, priapism, exchange transfusion and neurological events: ASPEN syndrome. J Urol 1993;150:1480–2.

[43] Snyder GB, Wilson CA. Surgical management of priapism and its sequelae in sickle cell disease. South Med J 1966;59:1393–6.

[44] Winter CC, McDowell G. Experience with 105 patients with priapism: update review of all aspects. J Urol 1988;140:980–3.

[45] Saad STO, Lajolo C, Gilli S, et al. Follow-up of sickle cell disease patients with priapism treated by hydroxyurea. Am J Hematol 2004;77(1):45–9.

[46] Al Jam'a AH, Al Dabbous IA. Hydroxyurea in the treatment of sickle cell associated priapism. J Urol 1998;159:1642.

[47] Rogers ZR. Hydroxyurea therapy for diverse pediatric populations with sickle cell disease. Semin Hematol 1997;34(3 Suppl 3):42–7.

[48] Bialecki ES, Bridges KR. Slidenafil relieves priapism in patients with sickle cell disease. Am J Med 2002;113(3):252.

[49] Serjeant GR, deCeulaer K, Maude GH. Stilboestrol and stuttering priapism in homozygous sickle-cell disease. Lancet 1985;2(8467):1274–6.

[50] Levine LA, Guss SP. Gonadotropin-releasing hormone analogues in the treatment of sickle cell anemia–associated priapism. J Urol 1993;150:475–7.

[51] Nguyen MT, Ewalt DH, Cavender JD, et al. Leuprolide therapy in the treatment of sickle cell anemia–associated priapism in adolescents [abstract 13a]. Blood 2000;96:41.

[52] Stoch SA, Parker RA, Chen L, et al. Bone loss in men with prostate cancer treated with gonadotropin-releasing hormone agonists. J Clin Endocrinol Metab 2001;86:2787–91.

[53] Dahm P, Rao DS, Donatucci CF. Antiandrogens in the treatment of priapism. Urology 2002;59(1):138.

Hematol Oncol Clin N Am 19 (2005) 929–941

HEMATOLOGY/ONCOLOGY CLINICS
OF NORTH AMERICA

Bone and Joint Disease in Sickle Cell Disease

Christine Aguilar, MD*, Elliott Vichinsky, MD,
Lynne Neumayr, MD

Children's Hospital & Research Center, 747 52nd Street, Oakland, CA 94609, USA

I n sickle cell disease, various disturbances commonly affect the bones and joints. Vaso-occlusive events in blood vessels that traverse the bones cause acute and chronic morbidity. Damage of the vessels may result in metabolic and structural changes. Limited joint mobility, along with acute and chronic pain can be severely disabling. Bone and joint disorders are the most common cause of chronic pain in people who have sickle cell disease. This article highlights aspects of sickle cell disease that affect healthy bone and joint function.

FEMORAL INFARCTS

The femoral head is the most common area of bone destruction in patients who have sickle cell disease [1]. The initial infarcts often occur in the subchondrial regions where the collateral circulation is minimal. These subchondral infarcts usually involve necrosis of a triangular or wedge-shaped segment of tissue that has the subchondral bone plate as its base and the center of the epiphysis as its apex. The overlying articular cartilage often remains viable in the early stages of the disease because it receives nutrition from the synovial fluid. In the healing response, osteoclasts resorb the necrotic trabeculae; however, the trabeculae that remain act as scaffolding for the new living bone that is deposited in a process known as "creeping substitution." If within the subchondral infarct, the pace of "creeping substitution" is too slow to be effective, then microfractures develop that eventually lead to collapse of the necrotic cancellous bone and ultimately to joint destruction [2]. Joint destruction almost always includes the anterior superior portion of the proximal femur, where the weight bearing forces are the greatest [3]. Radiographs frequently show collapse or flattening of this area.

PATHOPHYSIOLOGY AND RISK FACTORS

The exact pathophysiology of sickle osteonecrosis is unknown. It appears to be a progressive occlusion of microcirculation within the femoral head, which leads

---

* Corresponding author. *E-mail address:* caguilar@mail.cho.org (C. Aguilar).

0889-8588/05/$ – see front matter
doi:10.1016/j.hoc.2005.07.001

to increased intraosseous pressure and subsequent cell death. This process is followed by bone resorption and variable structural collapse of the head of the femur. There are several potential clinical, laboratory, and genetic risk factors for sickle bone disease, including steady state hematocrit, coagulation levels, β-globin mutations, and, recently, genes associated with bone metabolism. Clinically, increased painful crises are associated with bone disease. Higher hematocrit levels are also a risk factor for osteonecrosis. Other laboratory findings, including hypofibrinolysis, have been implicated as etiologic factors but have not been proven [4]. Early reports found a higher rate of osteonecrosis in hemoglobin sickle cell disease compared with other sickle mutations. Recent studies have found no significant difference between the SS or SC genotype [5,6]. The only consistent globin mutation associated with an increased risk of osteonecrosis is in patients who have the HbSS genotype and α-thalassemia [6]. Recent studies have found several mutations, unrelated to the hemoglobin disorder, influence the severity of the disease by altering genes involved in its pathophysiology [7]. Single nucleotide polymorphisms affecting genes important to bone metabolism appear to influence the natural history of sickle bone disease. These genes include *KL*, a gene that participates in vitamin D regulation; BMP6, a bone morphogenic protein important in bone formation and inflammation; and ANXA2, a calcium-dependent phospholipid-protein, which regulates cell growth and osteoblast mineralization.

PREVALENCE AND INCIDENCE

The prevalence rate of avascular necrosis in the femoral head increases with age. A 3% prevalence rate has been reported in those less than 15 years old [3]. Milner [6] reports a 10% overall prevalence rate, and a rise to 50% in those over 35 years old.

CLINICAL IDENTIFICATION

Pain is likely to be the first symptom of an acute infarct of the femur. If the infarct takes place at the proximal portion of the femoral head, then pain may be experienced in the groin, anterior or medial thigh, buttocks, knee, or as low back pain. Acute pain is constant and increases with weight bearing of the limb. Activities that increase forces across the hip joint, such as running or stair climbing, are avoided. Even walking is minimized. With time the pain may abate but limitation of movement, such as a hip flexion contracture or pain only with end range of motion, often remains.

GROWTH DISTURBANCES

Growth disturbances have been reported in sickle cell disease. Leg-length discrepancy and abnormalities of hip development are common sequelae [8]. If the growth disturbances occur asymmetrically in the lower extremities, a significant leg-length disturbance may arise. A leg-length discrepancy >2 cm results in an obvious limp. The limp may enhance forces on the hip and lower back causing muscular pain and spasm. In general, gait disturbances are frequent and not always secondary to growth problems; it is important to determine the cause by evaluating physical changes. If a leg-length discrepancy is found, then treatment with an appropriate shoe lift or insert should be prescribed early to prevent further complications. Usually, the initial lift is half the distance of total discrepancy.

RADIOGRAPHY

There are a number of radiographic ways to identify avascular necrosis of the femoral head. Plain film changes are seen late, only after there is healing of the infarct. The standard technique should include antero–posterior (AP) radiographs of the pelvis and frog leg lateral views of both hips.

CT scans can be helpful for surgical planning if two-dimensional reconstruction in the coronal and sagittal planes is used, but three-dimensional reconstruction is not helpful since it loses too much resolution [9].

MRI on the other hand, is the most accurate imaging modality for the diagnosis of avascular necrosis of the femoral head. An accuracy rate >90% was found with routine MRI techniques and it has become the mainstay in diagnosis and staging of the disease process [9–11].

Bone scintigraphy can visualize the blood flow throughout the bones, but it is not able to measure the efficiency of the vascular supply or repair mechanism. The interruption of the blood supply is detected as a cold spot and is unspecific in its pattern; thus, can be found in several other bone marrow processes [9].

STAGING

There have been many attempts to effectively classify and stage avascular necrosis of the hip [12]. They are primarily based on radiography, either by plain radiographs, bone scans, MRIs, or a combination of these. More invasive diagnostic procedures such as scintigraphy are generally not used. Ficat and Arlet [13] were among the first to describe a classification system of five stages (O through IV), where stages I through IV are based on standard radiographs. Stage I consists of a symptomatic patient who has no visible defect on plain radiographs. Stage II consists of a normal femoral head contour but the radiograph reveals evidence of bone-remodeling, cystic, or sclerotic areas. Stage III involves subchondral collapse or flattening of the proximal femoral head. In stage IV, there is narrowing of the joint space with secondary degenerative changes in the acetabulum. Steinberg and colleagues [14] modified and expanded the staging system of Ficat and Arlet when magnetic resonance imaging became available. The expansion included six stages (0 through VI) that integrated subdivisions to quantify the percent of necrosis. This quantification provides a more accurate evaluation of the progression or resolution of treatments.

NON-SURGICAL TREATMENT

Although there are many methods for treating avascular necrosis, none have been completely satisfactory. Moreover, it is extremely difficult to compare the effectiveness since most of these methods have not been prospective

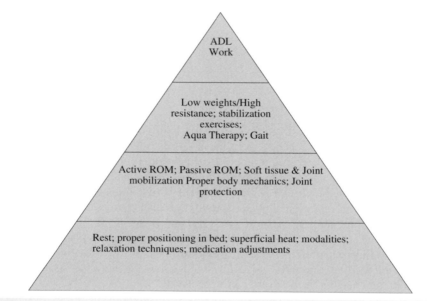

Fig. 1. A therapeutic treatment pyramid.

controlled studies. Nevertheless, general guidelines for treatment have been developed that include pharmacological and non-pharmacological measures. Pain relief is the primary indication for pharmacological measures. Currently there are no drugs available that reverse the structural abnormalities or improve the healing process of infarctions. Medications, as discussed in other chapters, should include the consideration of nonsteroidal antiinflammatory agents unless the patient has an allergy or other common contraindication. Non pharmacological therapies include modalities to relieve or control pain, stretching programs to improve range of motion, strengthening curriculums for stabilization and ultimately a route to restore normal function or minimizing disability. This type of therapy needs to be implemented by a multidisciplinary team. The team should at least include a hematologist, physiatrist, physical therapist, occupational therapist, and psychologist. Initial goals are to educate the patient and caregivers about the goal oriented therapeutic plan. Fig. 1 shows an example of a therapeutic treatment pyramid.

SURGICAL TREATMENT

There are no standardized surgical treatments for early avascular necrosis of the femoral head in sickle cell disease [15]. The treatments are drawn from people who have other diseases, which may not always be successful in those who have sickle cell disease. For example, hemiresurfacing of the femoral head for the treatment of avascular necrosis in the general population who are younger than 30 years may be a promising alternative to total hip arthroplasty [16]. For those who have sickle cell disease, the failure rate has been reported to be 100% [17]. Attempting to minimize the invasiveness of procedures is ideal since perioperative complications occur in 67% of people who have sickle cell disease and higher risk procedures are more likely to be associated with these complications [18].

CORE DECOMPRESSION

Core decompression of the femoral head is the most common procedure used to treat early stages of avascular necrosis [13]. Although the procedure has been used for more than 25 years [19], it remains controversial as to the indications and success. Core decompression requires further investigation because preliminary reports indicate beneficial results, not only in the general population [20,21] but also in those who have sickle cell disease [1]. Unfortunately, none of the existing studies have had the statistical power to make a definitive conclusion. Preliminary results from the national hip sickle cell study are encouraging [22]. The goal of this prospective randomized trial is to evaluate hip coring decompression and aggressive physical therapy. Patients enrolled in the study include (Ficat) stage I, II, and III patients. The study noted two-thirds of all patients have bilateral disease. Preliminary results suggest both arms improve outcome in stages I–III. Therefore, until the study is completed, both options should be considered in early avascular necrosis of the hip.

Core decompression has been combined with various interventions such as introducing non-vascularized bone grafts, vascular bone grafts, and electrical stimulation into the core procedure. The purpose is to promote osteogenesis and improve bone repair. The procedure of the core decompression with vascularized fibular transplant appears to be very promising in the general population. But it has not been evaluated in those who have sickle cell disease. Unfortunately, it does not completely alleviate pain and is associated with a longer rehabilitation period [23], both of which are disturbing to those who have sickle cell disease.

OSTEOTOMIES

Femoral osteotomies may be an alternative to partial or total hip arthroplasty. The purpose of a femoral osteotomy is to move the necrotic tissue away from the weight-bearing forces of the hip and avoid prosthetic hardware. This procedure remains controversial because it has a significant surgical risk and does not have the success of total hip arthroplasty [24].

TOTAL HIP ARTHROPLASTY

Avascular necrosis of the femoral head frequently progresses to total collapse and end stage destruction of the hip [25]. This total collapse leads to chronic pain that necessitates hip replacement [25]. Overall, patients who have sickle cell disease are younger than the general population at the time of needing total hip arthroplasty (THA) [6]. Milner and colleagues reported in a large, cooperative sickle cell study, that 80% of those who underwent THA were younger than 35 years [6]. Studies have shown that THA in those younger than 45 years have a greater failure rate than those who are older [26,27]. In the general population, using cementless bipolar arthroplasty in the young allows for a more successful future replacement of a THA without compromising the life of the first THA [24,28]. By and large, of all the treatment options, THA provides the best opportunity for clinical improvements but the early and late complication rates are high [1,29–31]. Technical difficulties related to marrow hyperplasia and the presence of sclerotic intramedullary bone, vaso-occlusive crises, major transfusion reactions, blood loss, acute chest syndrome, congestive heart failure, intraoperative femoral fractures, femoral perforations, greater than usual infection rates, and late aseptic loosening are some of the added complications to performing a THA in a patient who has sickle cell disease. Failure rates > 10% in fewer than 6 years are reported [32]. The risk-to-benefit ratio of this procedure needs to be assessed for each patient. Overall, further studies are needed to determine the best course of action when dealing with avascular necrosis of the femoral head.

HUMERAL INFARCTS

Avascular necrosis of the humeral head has been described as a problem related to sickle cell disease for over 50 years [33–35]. It usually occurs in the quadrants supplied by the anterior circumflex humeral artery—possibly because of the longer course of this artery and the susceptibility for impingement underneath the subscapularis during abduction and rotation of the shoulders—as opposed to the posterior circumflex artery which lies mainly posterior and inferiorly [36].

The same pathological chain of events that occurs in the femoral head appears likely to occur in the humeral head [37]. But unlike the femoral head, the destructive secondary changes are less likely to be seen at the shoulder, primarily because there is less stress on the humeral head compared with the femoral head. Only rarely is the gleno-humeral joint used in a weight-bearing manner. Also when infarcts develop, it is easier to rest and to splint the shoulder than the hip. If collapse does occur in the humeral head, it usually happens at the superior medial quadrant, where most of the pressure arises with shoulder abduction [38]. Pain can occur acutely with or without shoulder range of motion. In time, many affected shoulders become asymptomatic. They frequently remain asymptomatic unless there are structural failures [39]. But some are asymptomatic only because major stresses or maximum ranges of motion are not applied to the joint. On physical examination, the range of motion maneuvers that characteristically cause pain are shoulder abduction and internal rotation. Performing these movements passively or actively may elicit pain in an otherwise asymptomatic patient.

The incidence of avascular necrosis of the humeral head is best attained from the Cooperative Study of the Clinical Course of Sickle Cell Disease (CSSCD), organized in 1978 by the Sickle Cell Branch of the National Heart, Lung, and Blood Institute and reported by Milner and colleagues [40]. Avascular necrosis of the humeral head was found in 5.6% of the patients at entry to the study. The prevalence increased with age: 2.7% in patients younger than 25 years of age; 9.7% in patients 25–34 years of age; and 19.8% in patients 35 years of age and older [40]. According to the CSSCD, avascular necrosis of the humeral head was most common in those with HbSS (6%), followed by HbS/β°-thalassemia (5.7%), HbSC (4.6%), and HbS/β$^+$-thalassemia (3.6%) patients [40]. Coexistence of femoral head infarction, when humeral head necrosis was present, ranges between 60% and 75% [37,40]. When a humeral head infarct is suspected, it is important to examine the patient's hips, and with any suspicion of an abnormality, perform radiographic studies. Bilateral disease of the shoulder is seen in approximately 44% to 67% [39,41] and often one side is asymptomatic; therefore, when performing radiographic studies, consider evaluating both shoulders, even if only one is symptomatic.

Plain radiographs of the gleno-humeral joint should include an AP view and an axillary–lateral view. Staging of the avascular necrosis can be performed similarly to the staging of the femoral head [42]. If plain radiographs in a symptomatic shoulder do not detect lesions, then MRI of the shoulder is warranted to rule out early stages of the disease process.

TREATMENT

In addition to appropriate pain medications, rest with part-time splinting should be considered. Full-time splinting should be avoided after the first few days from the onset of acute pain, to avoid a "frozen shoulder syndrome." If adjacent muscle spasms are a cause of pain, then heat in the form of whirlpool or heating pads can be beneficial. In general, ice may initiate a vaso-occlusive crisis and should be avoided [43]. In a very few cases, chronic pain develops and can be functionally limiting. In these circumstances, arthroscopic debridement, core decompression, or an arthroplasty need to be performed.

VERTEBRAL INFARCTS

Changes in the thoracic and lumbar spine are frequently seen in those who have sickle cell disease. The findings of the vertebra are very distinct and have been named for their radiographic appearances such as "fish vertebrae" or "tower vertebra" [44–46]. The vertebral changes consist of central deterioration with preserved peripheral areas of the vertebral end-plates. This central destruction is a result of the anatomic blood supply to the end-plates. The central portion of the vertebral end-plate derives its blood supply from the long branches of the vertebral nutrient artery, while the peripheral portion of the end-plate is supplied by short perforating branches of the periosteal vessels. The longer end arterial vessels are more likely than the shorter vessels to exhibit vaso-occlusion and destructive events (Fig. 2) [47]. The back pain caused by this vertebral destruction is difficult to treat. Pain medications, particularly muscle relaxants, may be useful but chronic use may bring their own functional limitations. Regardless of which muscle relaxer is chosen, the most significant side effect is sedation and medication should be taken at bedtime. Cyclobenzaprine, despite being particularly effective, has anticholinergic uncomfortable side effects such as dry mouth and constipation. Rest or physical therapy is often only minimally

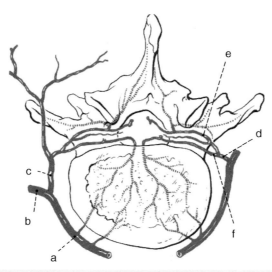

Fig. 2. Diagram of the blood supply of a vertebra seen from below. (*a*) is a segmental (lumbar) artery, (*b*) its ventral continuation, (*c*) its dorsal branch; (*d*) is the spinal branch, (*e*) and (*f*) are dorsal and ventral twigs of the spinal branch to tissue of the epidural space and vertebral column. The unlabeled twig between (*e*) and (*f*) (a radicular artery) is to the nerve roots, and at some levels, to the spinal cord. (*Modified from* Hollinshead W. Textbook of anatomy. 3rd edition. Hagerstown [MD]: Medical Department, Harper & Row Publishers, Inc.; 1974. p. 313 [Fig. 14-13]; with permission.)

helpful, but a proper thoracic or lumbar orthosis can be beneficial and diminish the need for medications.

DACTYLITIS

Symptomatic microinfarcts in the phalanges and metatarsal bones—known as dactylitis—usually occur before 5 years of age [48–50], although there is a report of dactylitis developing in a 26-year-old who has HbS/β-thalassemia [51]. Symptoms of dactylitis consist of unilateral or bilateral painful swelling of the distal extremities. This painful swelling of the hands and feet is often associated with leukocytosis and fever. The symptoms mimic osteomyelitis or cellulitis, but unlike these, the symptoms of dactylitis are self-limiting and usually resolve within a month [52]. The occurrence appears to be equal between boys and girls [49]. Initial radiographs may reveal only soft tissue enlargement; but after 7 to 14 days of symptoms, radiographs can reveal evidence of irregular density, subperiosteal new-bone formation, and cortical thinning [48]. These radiographic changes are completely reversible but it may take 2 to 8 months before complete normalization transpires [48,52]. Having dactylitis in infancy is a strong predictor of the possibility of severe sickle cell disease later in life [41]. Milner and colleagues [40] report that patients who had dactylitis before their first birthday were 2.67 times more likely to have severe disease than those who did not have dactylitis before one year of age. Treatment consists of symptomatic relief with pain medication, rest, and elevation. Mild heat is acceptable but avoidance of ice or cold is necessary to avoid a vaso-occlusive crisis [53].

OSTEOMYELITIS

Hematologic dissemination is a common cause of infections in the bone and joints [54]. Sickle cell patients have functional asplenia, diminished opsonic activity of the serum, and poor antibody response to the polysaccharide component of the bacterial capsule. All these factors predispose patients who have sickle cell disease to infection with encapsulated organisms. *Salmonella* and *staphylococcal aureus* are the most common organisms [55]. Salmonella is a well-known cause of osteomyelitis in those who have sickle cell disease [56,57]. Worldwide, it may be twice as common in causing osteomyelitis than staphylococcus [55,58], despite the fact that it is relatively uncommon in those without sickle cell disease. Symptoms of osteomyelitis, including fever, tenderness, swelling, and limitation of movement, can mimic those of acute infarction, making osteomyelitis clinically indistinguishable from infarcts [59].

Infarction can be 50 times more common than bacterial osteomyelitis in those who have sickle cell disease [60]. Many have tried to distinguish the two using numerous radiographic methods [61–64], but despite improvements in nuclear and magnetic resonance imaging, biopsy for histopathology and culture remain the gold standard for diagnosis. Determining which patients to treat can be challenging. Many algorithms have been devised [65] and sequential bone scans seem to be the most successful but are repeatedly invasive [66].

Treatment for osteomyelitis requires surgical debridement and prolonged parental antibiotics [67]. Depending on the site of the osteomyelitis, orthotics or non-weight bearing may be indicated.

BONE MARROW DISTURBANCES

Infarcts and hyperplasia affect the bone marrow in sickle cell disease. Both can cause growth and structural abnormalities. Bone marrow infarcts are extremely common in those who have sickle cell disease [68–70]. Pain and swelling are the frequent symptoms; limitation of movement is less problematic. In general, marrow necrosis predominates in fatty marrow. However, in sickle cell disease, the marrow infarctions occur in areas of active hematopoiesis as well as fatty marrow [71].

Imaging bone marrow infarcts with scintigraphy (Technetium 99m-sulfphur colloid) can reveal stages of marrow necrosis within 24 hours [72]. The interruption of the blood supply is detected as a cold spot. Unfortunately, this finding is nonspecific and can be seen in other bone marrow disorders. But the repair process that occurs in the revascularization of the area of infarction is detected as a hot spot. Thus, the combination of a cold and hot spot represents a diagnostic pattern for a necrotic area that is undergoing the healing process of new vessels.

Chronic hemolytic anemia of sickle cell disease results in erythroid hyperplasia. In the skull, marrow hyperplasia causes widening of the diploic space and a "hair on end " pattern can be seen [73]. The widening of the diploic space is bilaterally symmetrical and involves the frontal or parietal bones [70]. If the hyperplasia occurs in the maxilla, overgrowth of the anterior maxilla can occur, and result in an overbite. Maxillary sinuses have been reported to cause severe calvarial and mandibular changes [74]. Other sites of marrow hyperplasia are in the pelvis and ribs, although more commonly these areas are affected by infarcts.

OTHER BONY EFFECTS

Dental effects go well beyond the overgrowth of the anterior maxilla. Dental concerns can also result from enamel hypomineralization, calcified canals, and increased overjet [75]. If marrow infarcts occur in the mandibular condyle, then fibrous ankylosis of the temporomandibular joint may be a painful and limit outcome [76].

Osteopenia results from bone marrow hyperplasia in the long bones and can eventually lead to osteoporosis and fractures. Bisphosphonates have been shown to increase bone mineral density and decrease the risk for new fractures [77]; however, there have not been any randomized controlled studies to evaluate them in sickle cell disease. Determining their effects on infarcts and hyperplasia could be beneficial.

SUMMARY

Sickle cell disease has many bone and joint effects. Most are a result of infarctions, hyperplasia, or infections. These complications can occur at any location: epiphyseal, metaphyseal, or diaphyseal. The location and the extensiveness of any of these problems determine the pain and structural damage. The hip joint is particularly vulnerable and unfortunately, is frequently affected in sickle cell disease. The treatments for the pain and functional problems that are caused by any of the bone and joint disorders need to be systematically implemented and further studied to determine the best course of action.

Acknowledgments

The authors acknowledge Owen F. Hurley for his acquisition of references and Erica Dolor for editorial support.

References

[1] Styles LA, Vichinsky EP. Core decompression in avascular necrosis of the hip in sickle-cell disease. Am J Hematol 1996;52(2):103–7.

[2] Chung SM, Alavi A, Russell MO. Management of osteonecrosis in sickle-cell anemia and its genetic variants. Clin Orthop Relat Res 1978;130:158–74.

[3] Gupta R, Adekile AD. MRI follow-up and natural history of avascular necrosis of the femoral head in Kuwaiti children with sickle cell disease. J Pediatr Hematol Oncol 2004;26(6):351–3.

[4] Glueck CJ, Freiberg R, Glueck HI, et al. Idiopathic osteonecrosis, hypofibrinolysis, high

plasminogen activator inhibitor, high lipoprotein(a), and therapy with Stanozolol. Am J Hematol 1995;48(4):213–20.

[5] Mukisi-Mukaza M, Elbaz A, Samuel-Leborgne Y, et al. Prevalence, clinical features, and risk factors of osteonecrosis of the femoral head among adults with sickle cell disease. Orthopedics 2000;23(4):357–63.

[6] Milner PF, Kraus AP, Sebes JI, et al. Sickle cell disease as a cause of osteonecrosis of the femoral head. N Engl J Med 1991;325(21):1476–81.

[7] Baldwin C, Nolan VG, Wyszynski DF, et al. Association of klotho, bone morphogenic protein 6, and annexin A2 polymorphisms with sickle cell osteonecrosis. Blood 2005; 106:372–5.

[8] Hernigou P, Galacteros F, Bachir D, et al. Deformities of the hip in adults who have sickle-cell disease and had avascular necrosis in childhood. A natural history of fifty-two patients. J Bone Joint Surg Am 1991;73(1):81–92.

[9] Hofmann S, Kramer J, Plenk Jr H, et al. Imaging of osteonecrosis. In: Urbaniak J, Jones Jr J, editors. Osteonecrosis: etiology, diagnosis, and treatment. Rosemont (IL): American Academy of Orthopaedic Surgeons; 1997. p. 213–23.

[10] Mitchell DG, Steinberg ME, Dalinka MK, et al. Magnetic resonance imaging of the ischemic hip. Alterations within the osteonecrotic, viable, and reactive zones. Clin Orthop Relat Res 1989;244:60–77.

[11] Kramer J, Breitenseher M, Imhof H, et al. [Diagnostic imaging in femur head necrosis]. Orthopade 2000;29(5):380–8 [in German].

[12] Steinberg ME, Steinberg DR. Classification systems for osteonecrosis: an overview. Orthop Clin North Am 2004;35(3):273–83 [vii–viii].

[13] Ficat RP. Idiopathic bone necrosis of the femoral head. Early diagnosis and treatment. J Bone Joint Surg Br 1985;67(1):3–9.

[14] Steinberg ME, Hayken GD, Steinberg DR. A quantitative system for staging avascular necrosis. J Bone Joint Surg Br 1995;77(1):34–41.

[15] Marti-Carvajal A, Dunlop R, Agreda-Perez L. Treatment for avascular necrosis of bone in people with sickle cell disease. Cochrane Database Syst Rev 2004;4:CD004344.

[16] Cuckler JM, Moore KD, Estrada L. Outcome of hemiresurfacing in osteonecrosis of the femoral head. Clin Orthop Relat Res 2004;429:146–50.

[17] Nelson CL, Walz BH, Gruenwald JM. Resurfacing of only the femoral head for osteonecrosis. Long-term follow-up study. J Arthroplasty 1997;12(7):736–40.

[18] Vichinsky EP, Neumayr LD, Haberkern C, et al. The perioperative complication rate of orthopedic surgery in sickle cell disease: report of the National Sickle Cell Surgery Study Group. Am J Hematol 1999;62(3):129–38.

[19] Hungerford DS, Zizic TM. Alcoholism associated ischemic necrosis of the femoral head. Early diagnosis and treatment. Clin Orthop Relat Res 1978;130:144–53.

[20] Stulberg BN, Davis AW, Bauer TW, et al. Osteonecrosis of the femoral head. A prospective randomized treatment protocol. Clin Orthop Relat Res 1991;268:140–51.

[21] Koo KH, Kim R, Ko GH, et al. Preventing collapse in early osteonecrosis of the femoral head. A randomised clinical trial of core decompression. J Bone Joint Surg Br 1995; 77(6):870–4.

[22] Vichinsky EP, Neumayr LD, Earles AN, et al. Progression of avascular necrosis of the hip in sickle cell disease: 2 year follow-up of randomized trial of aggressive physical therapy and hip coring decompression. Blood 2004;104(11):468a.

[23] Soucacos PN, Beris AE, Malizos K, et al. Treatment of avascular necrosis of the femoral head with vascularized fibular transplant. Clin Orthop Relat Res 2001;386:120–30.

[24] Launay F, Jouve JL, Guillaume JM, et al. Total hip arthroplasty without cement in children and adolescents: 17 cases. Rev Chir Orthop Reparatrice Appar Mot 2002;88(5):460–6.

[25] Hernigou P, Bachir D, Galacteros F. The natural history of symptomatic osteonecrosis in adults with sickle-cell disease. J Bone Joint Surg Am 2003;85-A(3):500–4.

[26] NIH Consensus Development Panel on total hip replacement. NIH consensus conference: total hip replacement. JAMA 1995;273(24):1950–6.

[27] Dorr LD, Takei GK, Conaty JP. Total hip arthroplasties in patients less than forty-five years old. J Bone Joint Surg Am 1983;65(4):474–9.
[28] Alonge TO, Shokunbi WA. The choice of arthroplasty for secondary osteoarthritis of the hip joint following avascular necrosis of the femoral head in sicklers. J Natl Med Assoc 2004;96(5):678–81.
[29] Bishop AR, Roberson JR, Eckman JR, et al. Total hip arthroplasty in patients who have sickle-cell hemoglobinopathy. J Bone Joint Surg Am 1988;70(6):853–5.
[30] Moran MC. Osteonecrosis of the hip in sickle cell hemoglobinopathy. Am J Orthop 1995;24(1):18–24.
[31] Fink B, Ruther W. [Partial and total joint replacement in femur head necrosis]. Orthopade 2000;29(5):449–56 [in German].
[32] Clarke HJ, Jinnah RH, Brooker AF, et al. Total replacement of the hip for avascular necrosis in sickle cell disease. J Bone Joint Surg Br 1989;71(3):465–70.
[33] Carrington HT, Ferguson AD, Scott RB. Studies in sickle-cell anemia. XI. Bone involvement simulating aseptic necrosis. AMA J Dis Child 1958;95(2):157–63.
[34] Ehrenpreis B, Schwinger HN. Sickle cell anemia. Am J Roentgenol Radium Ther Nucl Med 1952;68(1):28–36.
[35] Golding JS, Maciver JE, Went LN. The bone changes in sickle cell anaemia and its genetic variants. J Bone Joint Surg Br 1959;41-B:711–8.
[36] Clemente CD, editor. Gray's anatomy. 30th American edition. Philadelphia: Lea & Febiger; 1985.
[37] Chung SM, Ralston EL. Necrosis of the humeral head associated with sickle cell anemia and its genetic variants. Clin Orthop Relat Res 1971;80:105–17.
[38] Beck JS, Nordin BE. Histological assessment of osteoporosis by iliac crest biopsy. J Pathol Bacteriol 1960;80:391–7.
[39] David HG, Bridgman SA, Davies SC, et al. The shoulder in sickle-cell disease. J Bone Joint Surg Br 1993;75(4):538–45.
[40] Milner PF, Kraus AP, Sebes JI, et al. Osteonecrosis of the humeral head in sickle cell disease. Clin Orthop Relat Res 1993;289:136–43.
[41] Miller ST, Sleeper LA, Pegelow CH, et al. Prediction of adverse outcomes in children with sickle cell disease. N Engl J Med 2000;342(2):83–9.
[42] Cruess RL. Osteonecrosis of bone. Current concepts as to etiology and pathogenesis. Clin Orthop Relat Res 1986;(208):30–9.
[43] Resar LM, Oski FA. Cold water exposure and vaso-occlusive crises in sickle cell anemia. J Pediatr 1991;118(3):407–9.
[44] Reynolds J. A re-evaluation of the "fish vertebra" sign in sickle cell hemoglobinopathy. Am J Roentgenol Radium Ther Nucl Med 1966;97(3):693–707.
[45] Marlow TJ, Brunson CY, Jackson S, et al. "Tower vertebra": a new observation in sickle cell disease. Skeletal Radiol 1998;27(4):195–8.
[46] Westerman MP, Greenfield GB, Wong PW. "Fish vertebrae," homocystinuria, and sickle cell anemia. JAMA 1974;230(2):261–2.
[47] Hollinshead W. Textbook of anatomy. 3rd edition. Hagerstown (MD): Medical Department, Harper & Row Publishers, Inc.; 1974.
[48] Worrall VT, Butera V. Sickle-cell dactylitis. J Bone Joint Surg Am 1976;58(8):1161–3.
[49] Stevens MC, Padwick M, Serjeant GR. Observations on the natural history of dactylitis in homozygous sickle cell disease. Clin Pediatr (Phila) 1981;20(5):311–7.
[50] Serjeant GR. Sickle-cell disease. Lancet 1997;350(9079):725–30.
[51] Rao KR, Patel AR, Shah PC, et al. Sickle cell dactylitis. Arch Intern Med 1980;140(3):439.
[52] Watson RJ, Burko H, Megas H, et al. The handfoot syndrome in sickle-cell disease in young children. Pediatrics 1963;31:975–82.
[53] Michaels LA, Maraventano MF, Drachtman RA. Thrombosis and gangrene in a patient with sickle cell disease and dactylitis. J Pediatr 2003;142(4):449.
[54] Ebong WW. Septic arthritis in patients with sickle-cell disease. Br J Rheumatol 1987;26(2):99–102.

[55] Burnett MW, Bass JW, Cook BA. Etiology of osteomyelitis complicating sickle cell disease. Pediatrics 1998;101(2):296–7.

[56] Bennett OM, Namnyak SS. Bone and joint manifestations of sickle cell anaemia. J Bone Joint Surg Br 1990;72(3):494–9.

[57] Webb DK, Serjeant GR. Systemic salmonella infections in sickle cell anaemia. Ann Trop Paediatr 1989;9(3):169–72.

[58] Piehl FC, Davis RJ, Prugh SI. Osteomyelitis in sickle cell disease. J Pediatr Orthop 1993;13(2):225–7.

[59] Chambers JB, Forsythe DA, Bertrand SL, et al. Retrospective review of osteoarticular infections in a pediatric sickle cell age group. J Pediatr Orthop 2000;20(5):682–5.

[60] Keeley K, Buchanan GR. Acute infarction of long bones in children with sickle cell anemia. J Pediatr 1982;101(2):170–5.

[61] Rao S, Solomon N, Miller S, et al. Scintigraphic differentiation of bone infarction from osteomyelitis in children with sickle cell disease. J Pediatr 1985;107(5):685–8.

[62] Kim HC, Alavi A, Russell MO, et al. Differentiation of bone and bone marrow infarcts from osteomyelitis in sickle cell disorders. Clin Nucl Med 1989;14(4):249–54.

[63] Rifai A, Nyman R. Scintigraphy and ultrasonography in differentiating osteomyelitis from bone infarction in sickle cell disease. Acta Radiol 1997;38(1):139–43.

[64] Umans H, Haramati N, Flusser G. The diagnostic role of gadolinium enhanced MRI in distinguishing between acute medullary bone infarct and osteomyelitis. Magn Reson Imaging 2000;18(3):255–62.

[65] Wong AL, Sakamoto KM, Johnson EE. Differentiating osteomyelitis from bone infarction in sickle cell disease. Pediatr Emerg Care 2001;17(1):60–3 [quiz 64].

[66] Skaggs DL, Kim SK, Greene NW, et al. Differentiation between bone infarction and acute osteomyelitis in children with sickle-cell disease with use of sequential radionuclide bone-marrow and bone scans. J Bone Joint Surg Am 2001;83-A(12):1810–3.

[67] Mallouh A, Talab Y. Bone and joint infection in patients with sickle cell disease. J Pediatr Orthop 1985;5(2):158–62.

[68] Alavi A, Bond JP, Kuhl D, et al. Scan detection of bone marrow infarcts in sickle cell disorders. J Nucl Med 1974;15(11):1003–7.

[69] Charache S, Page DL. Infarction of bone marrow in the sickle cell disorders. Ann Intern Med 1967;67(6):1195–200.

[70] Diggs LW. Bone and joint lesions in sickle-cell disease. Clin Orthop Relat Res 1967; 52:119–43.

[71] Rao VM, Mitchell DG, Rifkin MD, et al. Marrow infarction in sickle cell anemia: correlation with marrow type and distribution by MRI. Magn Reson Imaging 1989;7(1):39–44.

[72] Meyers MH, Telfer N, Moore TM. Determination of the vascularity of the femoral head with technetium 99m-sulphur-colloid. J Bone Joint Surg Am 1977;59(5):658–64.

[73] Sebes JI, Diggs LW. Radiographic changes of the skull in sickle cell anemia. AJR Am J Roentgenol 1979;132(3):373–7.

[74] Fernandez M, Slovis TL, Whitten-Shurney W. Maxillary sinus marrow hyperplasia in sickle cell anemia. Pediatr Radiol 1995;25(Suppl 1):S209–11.

[75] Taylor LB, Nowak AJ, Giller RH, et al. Sickle cell anemia: a review of the dental concerns and a retrospective study of dental and bony changes. Spec Care Dentist 1995; 15(1):38–42.

[76] Baykul T, Aydin MA, Nasir S. Avascular necrosis of the mandibular condyle causing fibrous ankylosis of the temporomandibular joint in sickle cell anemia. J Craniofac Surg 2004;15(6):1052–6.

[77] Brenckmann C, Papaioannou A. Bisphosphonates for osteoporosis in people with cystic fibrosis. Cochrane Database Syst Rev 2001;4:CD002010.

Hematol Oncol Clin N Am 19 (2005) 943–956

HEMATOLOGY/ONCOLOGY CLINICS
OF NORTH AMERICA

Leg Ulceration in Sickle Cell Disease: Medieval Medicine in a Modern World

Graham R. Serjeant, MD, FRCP[a,b,*], Beryl E. Serjeant, FIMLS[a,b], Junette S. Mohan, PhD[a], Andrea Clare, MD[a]

[a]*former MRC Laboratories—Jamaica, University of the West Indies, Kingston, Jamaica, West Indies*
[b]*Sickle Cell Trust—Jamaica, 14 Milverton Crescent, Kingston 6, Jamaica, West Indies*

L eg ulceration is now recognized as an important complication of sickle cell disease, especially of the SS genotype. Since there is no convincing evidence of delayed healing of operation scars or of wounds elsewhere in the body, it must be concluded that factors specific to the lower leg render patients prone to delayed healing at this site. Many lesions are traumatic in origin and since there is considerable variation in healing rates among the normal population, it is useful to define chronic leg ulceration on the basis of a minimal duration, which in Jamaican studies has required at least 3 months and sometimes 6 months before healing. This minimal duration avoids the difficulties of interpreting the significance of briefer lesions since the moment of final healing may be poorly defined (patients may conclude that a scab represents healing whereas small lesions persist beneath) and often goes undocumented as patients may not report and medical attendants may not enquire, the date of final healing.

HISTORY

Leg ulcers occurred in the first four reports of sickle cell disease but were not recognized as a specific complication. Cases were reported in the dermatological literature [1–5] but the etiology was confused by positive syphilis serology and it was not until Cummer and LaRocco [6] that a causal role of sickle cell disease was suspected. Even before this recognition, several reviews of clinical features reported active ulcers or healed scars in approximately 75% of adult patients [7–9].

INCIDENCE AND PREVALENCE
Age and Genotype
Jamaican data indicate that leg ulcers are rare before 10 years, occur most frequently for the first time between 10 and 25 years, and become increasingly

---

* Corresponding author. Sickle Cell Trust—Jamaica, 14 Milverton Crescent, Kingston 6, Jamaica, West Indies. *E-mail address:* grserjeant@cwjamaica.com (G.R. Serjeant).

0889-8588/05/$ – see front matter
doi:10.1016/j.hoc.2005.08.005
hemonc.theclinics.com

uncommon after 30 years. A similar pattern occurred in the Cooperative Study of Sickle Cell Disease (CSSCD) in the United States, although the maximum incidence occurred slightly later: between 20 and 50 years [10]. Ulceration is most common in SS disease and much less frequent in other genotypes [10].

Geographic Region

There are striking regional differences in leg ulcer prevalence, some of which may be attributable to differing age structures of the studied population, but there are also real differences within the same age group. Among patients of West African origin, Jamaica has a very high (70%–80%) prevalence of leg ulcers (Fig. 1), whereas comparable ages in the CSSCD suggest a much lower (5%–10%) prevalence. A lower prevalence has been reported from Ghana and Nigeria [11–13], but in these populations, relatively few people reach the high-risk age groups. Among patients who have the Asian haplotype, leg ulceration is rare among adults in both the eastern province of Saudi Arabia [14,15] and central India [16].

RISK FACTORS

Gender

A male preponderance has been reported from Ghana [17] and in the CSSCD, where the relative incidence rates were 15 per 100 patient-years for males and 5 per 100 patient-years for females [10]. No gender difference occurred in a study from Nigeria [18] or in the Jamaican Cohort Study.

Hematology

α-thalassemia is commonly associated with SS disease and patients who have homozygous α^+-thalassemia are less prone to leg ulceration [10,19], although such protection has not been documented in connection with the more common

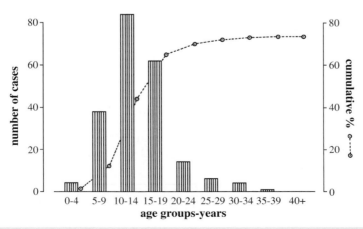

Fig. 1. Incidence of leg ulcers in Jamaican patients with SS disease. Columns represent occurrence of leg ulcers for the first time and the line shows the cumulative incidence.

heterozygous α^+- thalassemia. The CSSCD yielded data which showed that low hemoglobin may be a risk factor: an incidence of 43.2 per 100 patient-years in subjects who have steady state levels <6 g/dL, compared with 2.6 per 100 patient-years in subjects who have levels >10 g/dL. This study also showed that a high fetal hemoglobin (HbF) level may protect: an incidence of 0.7 per 100 patient-years in those who have levels >10%, compared with 13.0 per 100 patient-years in subjects who have HbF levels <5%. These effects were confined to subjects without α^+ thalassemia. The complex interactions between hematological indices, such as the association between high hemoglobin and high HbF levels, may complicate interpretation of univariate analyses. A clearer picture may emerge with datasets that are sufficiently large to allow a multivariate approach.

Autonomic Vascular Control

The cardiac output is increased in patients who have SS disease and this may affect the distribution of peripheral blood flow and reflex vascular responses [20,21]. Cutaneous vasoconstriction occurs when the leg is lowered from the horizontal to the dependent position; this reflex was reported absent in two female SS patients and was postulated to be an adaptation rendering leg ulceration less likely [22]. Later studies with the leg horizontal showed that red cell flux (an indicator of skin blood flow) in normal lower leg skin was significantly higher in SS subjects than in healthy HbAA controls. When compared in SS subjects with and without ulceration, skin blood flow at the abnormal skin site (active ulcers or a history of ulcers, Fig. 2) was higher than in normal skin of the same individual [23]. With the leg dependent, skin blood flow fell to a similar degree in both genotypes, but in SS subjects who have abnormal skin, the fall was greater at the abnormal skin site than in normal skin. This more pronounced vasoconstriction in abnormal skin could be a factor contributing to the recurrence of ulcers at these sites.

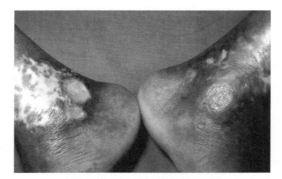

Fig. 2. Skin appearance of bilateral leg ulcers. Note the depigmented skin of the healed ulcer on the right medial malleolus and the small satellite ulcers around the lesion on the left medial malleolus, as well as the irregular pigmentation, atrophic areas, and healed scars.

Role of Venous Incompetence

Until recently, data on venous incompetence were limited and conflicting. A comparison of SS subjects with and without leg ulcers showed delayed clearance of ^{99m}Tc [24] and differences in magnetic resonance spectroscopy [25], both consistent with venous stasis in calf muscle of the ulcer group. Studies of 16 SS subjects who had leg ulcers found rapid venous refilling times and attributed these to high cardiac output rather than venous incompetence, because invasive venous pressure measurements were normal in 4 subjects, and an additional 4 subjects failed to show venous incompetence on angiography [26]. The change in leg volume induced during a period of venous occlusion or exercise can provide simple non-invasive methods for the assessment of venous function that correlate well with direct measurements of venous pressure [27,28]. The change in leg volume induced by venous occlusion allows indices of venous capacitance, venous outflow, and venous emptying time to be derived. These indices were similar in SS subjects (with or without ulcers), and in HbAA controls, inconsistent with deep venous obstruction. The abnormal venous function in SS subjects, was, therefore, more likely to result from failure of the calf muscle pump, either primary or secondary to venous incompetence. Further studies of the change in leg volume during ankle exercise showed shorter venous refilling times at the ankle in SS subjects compared with HbAA controls, and these were further reduced in SS subjects who had ulcers compared with those who did not. In addition, after ankle exercise, the time taken for skin blood flow to return to pre-exercise levels was shorter in SS subjects than HbAA controls and further shortened in SS subjects with ulcers compared with those without [29]. In the normal leg after exercise, the veins fill from the arteries in about 15 seconds, but in venous insufficiency, they fill faster by retrograde flow or venous reflux [30]. The shorter venous refilling times and skin flow recovery times in SS ulcer subjects were consistent with abnormal venous function and the following hypothesis: incompetence of venous valves, which drain the ankle region, and the resulting raised venous pressure, contribute to the slow healing and possibly to the onset of leg ulceration in SS disease. The concept of abnormal venous function in SS patients who have leg ulcers is supported by Doppler ultrasound imaging, which confirmed venous reflux in 21% of SS patients who have leg ulcers [31]. Subsequent studies of venous incompetence by hand-held Doppler in the Jamaican Cohort Study showed venous incompetence in 75% of 183 SS subjects compared with 39% of 137 non-pregnant HbAA controls and a highly significant association ($P<.001$) between leg ulceration and venous incompetence in the same leg of SS subjects [32]. The association between venous incompetence and the SS genotype should come as no surprise because of the low oxygen tension in the venous system, the turbulence inevitable around venous valves, and the high white blood cell and platelet counts that promote endothelial adhesion. This adds another potential pathology to the morbidity of SS disease. Although the mechanism of these changes may not be fully understood, both the pronounced vasoconstriction on standing and the high prevalence of venous incompetence may contribute to ulcer formation or retard healing.

Other Clinical Events and Potential Risk Factors
Data on the association between leg ulceration and other clinical features are conflicting. In the CSSCD, acute or chronic complications of the disease did not differ between patients with and without leg ulcers. Conversely, Ballas [33] noted that patients with leg ulcers were less likely to experience painful crises. This observation was confirmed and extended in the Jamaican Cohort Study [34], in which 78% of 311 SS subjects could be classified into either leg ulcer or painful crisis phenotypes with 95% confidence. The leg ulcer group had lower frequencies of dactylitis, meningitis/septicemia and acute chest syndrome compared with the painful crisis group. It is unknown whether such phenotypes are genetically determined or reflect dynamic changes in which the presence of a leg ulcer renders a patient less prone to painful crises.

A significant association with HLA-B35 and HLA-Cw4 antigens was reported in nine patients who had leg ulceration [35], but this study requires confirmation in larger populations before the link can be considered established.

CHARACTERISTICS OF ULCERATION
Mode of Onset
Two principal modes of onset are seen in Jamaican patients: traumatic or spontaneous. Trauma accounts for approximately half the cases which present with physical damage to the skin around the ankles from scratching insect bites, dog bites, or scraping the skin. Initially small lesions may cease to heal, and may develop into large ulcers, which characteristically have a healing–relapsing course over many years. In spontaneous ulcers, there is no history of trauma, but a lesion develops within the dermis often with surrounding induration and hyperpigmentation (Fig. 3). Initially, lesions may be covered by an intact epidermis, which then breaks down forming small, deep, and painful

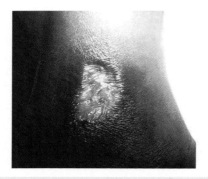

Fig. 3. Spontaneous ulceration believed to result from skin infarction. Note the hyperpigmentation around the ulcer, and the ulcer in the subcutaneous tissues covered by an almost intact epidermis.

lesions which heal relatively quickly. The lack of trauma in these lesions is consistent with an etiology from skin infarction, which is supported by an association with low HbF levels [36]. The relative rarity of ulcers before 10 years suggests that repeated vaso-occlusion is necessary before skin blood flow is sufficiently compromised for skin infarction to occur. Once this stage is reached, the healing capacity of the affected skin is reduced allowing persistence of ulcers from either traumatic or spontaneous origin.

Site
Leg ulcers typically affect the skin around the medial or lateral malleoli (see Fig. 2), but also occur less frequently on the anterior shin or the dorsum of the foot. The malleolar distribution is characteristic of ulceration in other hematological conditions (hereditary spherocytosis, β—thalassemia, Felty's syndrome) which suggests that the blood flow in this area is barely adequate. Blood flow is further restricted by high venous pressure (see earlier section) and lymphedema consistent with observations that ulcers tend to heal on complete bed rest and deteriorate on prolonged standing. Medial involvement was more common in two studies [36,37], but the CSSCD found no predilection for medial, lateral, right or left legs [10].

Size
Ulcers 0.5 cm, 5–10cm, and 10–15cm diameter occurred with equal frequencies in the CSSCD. In Jamaica, most ulcers are less than 10 cm diameter, although occasionally they may involve most of the skin between the ankle and knee. Circumferential ulcers have a particularly poor prognosis because of the inevitable damage to superficial veins and lymphatics.

Appearance
Most established ulcers have a punched out appearance with well defined margins and a slightly raised edge (see Fig. 3). The base consists of granulation tissue, which is often covered with a yellow slough. Sometimes, multiple small ulcers develop simultaneously and merge to form a larger lesion. Histological examination of an early leg ulcer reveals atrophic epithelial margins, cellular infiltration, debris, and dilated capillaries filled with sickled cells. Arterioles in the ulcer base show marked intimal proliferation, neovascularization around occluded arterioles, and perivascular cellular infiltrates. It is unknown whether this arteriolar occlusion is a cause or consequence of leg ulceration, but it seems likely that this pathology would retard healing.

Healing and Recurrence
Healing of ulcers is typically slow, proceeding over months or years (Fig. 4). The ulcer fills in with granulation tissue and in a clean ulcer bluish epithelium may be seen growing in from the ulcer margin. Healing rates of 3.3–8.1 mm^2/d have been reported in SS disease [38,39] compared with rates of 400 mm^2/d in other types of leg ulcer [40]. Even after satisfactory healing, 25%–52% recurred in the CSSCD.

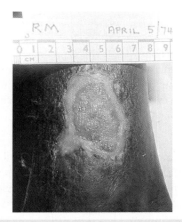

Fig. 4. Rapid healing in a leg ulcer of traumatic origin. Note the new bluish epithelium around the ulcer margin.

Bacteriology

Secondary bacterial infection is usually regarded as inevitable and of limited importance in the persistence of these lesions [12,41]. *Staphylococcus aureus, Pseudomonas,* β-hemolytic streptococci, and salmonellae were common in African reports [12,17,42–44], and anaerobes accounted for over half the isolations in one series [44]. In Jamaica, the bacterial flora is predominantly aerobic and polymicrobial; *Staphylococcus aureus* (51%), *Pseudomonas aeruginosa* (51%), and β-hemolytic streptococci (40%) occur in 80 unilateral ulcers [45]. Repeat sampling over a period of 6 months showed persistence of these three organisms either singly or in combination in over 80% of lesions. *Corynebacterium diphtheriae* occurred in eight ulcers and four strains were toxigenic [46], but no clinical diphtheria was observed.

Whether these organisms are harmless colonizers or delay healing of ulcers is important in the debate about the role of antibiotics in their therapy.

TREATMENT

The treatment of leg ulceration is unsatisfactory and information from controlled trials is sparse. Prevention of trauma is important, and active treatment of early lesions may prevent the development of extensive fibrosis as well as the healing–relapsing course of large lesions. The cornerstones of therapy are keeping the lesions clean and providing firm supporting bandages to reduce hemostasis and lymphedema if the patient is ambulant.

Debridement and Dressings

Debridement may be necessary if ulcer healing is inhibited by a dirty fibrous ulcer base and this may be achieved with the use of papaya, enzyme preparations, or by surgical excision. Many hydrocolloid based dressings have been proposed [47], but the only one subjected to randomized, placebo-controlled trial has been an RGD peptide matrix, which healed ulcers nearly three times faster than control saline treatment over a 10-week study [48]. Randomized, controlled trials of Solcoseryl or Duoderm [49] or of propionyl-L-carnitine [50] failed to show beneficial effect. Amnion dressings may induce a striking neovascularisation [51] and might possibly induce healing or render ulcers more suitable for grafting, but their use has not been explored in sickle cell ulcers.

Antimicrobial Agents

The ulcer surface always yields bacteria but in most cases, these are colonizers and are rarely invasive enough to justify systemic antibiotics. Systemic antibiotics may be indicated if there is other evidence of infection (cellulitis, inguinal lymphadenopathy) but may simply change the sensitivity of colonizing organisms. Local antiseptic agents are commonly used to clean ulcers but do not appear to affect the bacteriology [45]. The role of local antibiotics is unclear; however, a topical antibiotic spray, containing neomycin, polymyxin B, and bacitracin, improved leg ulcers in one study [52] but repeated use may induce skin sensitivity.

Other Interventions

Zinc

Patients who have SS disease have lower serum zinc levels, and oral zinc sulfate, 220 mg 3 times daily, tripled the healing rate from 2.8 mm^2/d to 8.1 mm^2/d [38], but the rate remained slow compared with rates in patients with non-sickle ulcers.

Vasodilating agents

Methylxanthine pentoxifylline has several effects likely to improve blood flow, and improved healing has been reported in a single case [53], but the vasodilating agent, isoxsuprine HCl (Vasodilan) had no effect in a controlled trial [54].

Granulocyte-macrophage colony-stimulating factor

Observations that intradermal injections of granulocyte-macrophage colony-stimulating factor improved wound healing [55,56], led to its use in sickle cell ulcers where injection [57,58] or dripping onto the ulcer surface [59,60] produced some striking improvement. However, these are anecdotal reports, there has been no proper randomized trial, the induced leucocytosis may precipitate severe painful crises [57], and the high cost is likely to limit its application.

Blood transfusion

Blood transfusion has become widely advocated in the management of sickle cell ulcers [61] despite no data to support its effect. Transfusion to normal hemoglobin levels for 1–3 months appeared to improve healing of leg ulcers in 3 patients [62], although much of this effect may have been because of in-patient management and bed rest. Transfusion use appears to be entirely theoretical, and assumes that increasing the hemoglobin level will improve oxygen delivery and that reducing the HbS level will improve small vessel blood flow. These assumptions may not recognize the low oxygen affinity of HbS or the lack of data supporting a direct role of vaso-occlusion. Transfusion carries the potential for serious risks especially in multiple transfused populations, and there is an urgent need for data from a controlled trial.

Hydroxyurea

Hydroxyurea is widely used in the management of sickle cell disease because of its effect in reducing painful crises, acute chest syndrome, and transfusion requirements. Sickle cell ulcers have either failed to improve [63–65] or have developed during therapy [66] and hydroxyurea may actually precipitate leg ulcers in other conditions [67].

Other agents

Other therapies that may have improved healing in individuals or small groups include recombinant human erythropoietin [63], arginine butyrate [64,68], and antithrombin III concentrate [69].

Bed rest, although never subjected to controlled trial, almost always results in a dramatic healing of chronic leg ulcers but cessation of bed rest may result in an equally dramatic deterioration if the ulcer is not completely healed. The data supporting a role of venous incompetence in the delayed healing of leg ulcers suggests that supporting elastic bandages may be beneficial. Although only anecdotal information is available, their use in Jamaica has been attended by rapid improvement in many chronic ulcers.

Pain relief

Chronic ulcers may be extremely distressing, painful, and require ingestion of large amounts of analgesia. Topical opioids have been successful in controlling pain in some patients [70].

Surgery

Surgical approaches to leg ulceration have included full thickness grafts, myocutaneous grafts [71], latissimus dorsi flaps [72], use of omentum [73], microsurgical free flaps [74,75], split skin grafts, and pinch grafts. Some dramatic improvements in indolent ulcers have been reported, but observations remain anecdotal and larger groups of patients, preferably randomized trials, and longer follow-up are needed to assess the value of these methods. Comparison of the skin grafting techniques [76] recommended pinch grafting, which had the advantages of a minor procedure done under local anesthesia and could be repeated if necessary. Experience in Jamaica suggests that ulcers must be completely healed before discharge from hospital and recurrence rates of 80%–97% within 2 years occur, even in successfully grafted and healed ulcers [76,77].

COMPLICATIONS

Social and Educational Effects

Social and educational effects are the most important contributors to the overall morbidity of leg ulceration in Jamaica. Leg ulceration causes a child to leave school and there is a direct relationship between age at onset of leg ulceration and educational attainment [78]. This educational deprivation places patients who have sickle cell disease, who are less suited to physical activity, at a special disadvantage and is reflected in their difficulty obtaining and retaining employment compared with sickle cell patients without ulcers [78].

Depression and Social Withdrawal

Sickle cell patients who have leg ulcers find it less easy to form stable family and social relationships. In the Jamaican experience, depression may complicate leg ulcers and impair a patient's capacity to dress the ulcer properly, which contributes to its chronicity. Anti-depressive agents may have remarkable effects in improving morale and ulcer management.

Subcutaneous Fibrosis

Local complications related to leg ulceration include the effect of chronic subcutaneous fibrosis impairing venous and lymphatic drainage. Occasionally fibrosis may be so marked as to cause an equinus deformity with fixed flexion of the ankle joint [79].

Bone and Synovial Effects

In leg ulceration, direct involvement of the periosteum is rare, but periosteal reaction to the overlying inflammation is common, and affected the tibia or fibula in 61% of Jamaican patients [80]. Malignant epithelial change, which may complicate chronic leg ulceration in other conditions, has never been described in sickle cell disease. Osteomyelitis, secondary to chronic ulceration, has not occurred in the Jamaican experience, although sometimes patients present with an apparent small deep 'ulcer' which represents a draining sinus from an underlying chronic osteomyelitis. Acute ankle arthritis complicates some cases of spontaneous leg ulceration, possibly as a result of associated ischemic synovial damage [81]. It resolves spontaneously with improvement of the leg ulcer.

Other Associations

The association of proteinuria and leg ulceration (GD Nicholson, MD thesis, 1977) led to the suggestion that β-hemolytic streptococci also gain access through these lesions, causing an increased prevalence of acute glomerulonephritis, but subsequent observations suggest that both proteinuria and leg ulceration are independently age related and not directly associated [82]. Further studies on the effect of leg ulceration on immunity [83] indicated that patients who have leg ulcers had significant increases in IgG, IgA, factor B, serum cryoprecipitates and anticomplementary activity, and decreased complement C3.

Leg ulcers also act as a portal of entry for other organisms or toxins, and tetanus is sufficiently common [36,84,85] to justify vaccine prophylaxis in sickle cell disease.

SUMMARY

The unsatisfactory treatment of leg ulceration is apparent from the variety of proposed therapies. Avoidance of trauma, which may initiate chronic ulceration, is essential and minor traumatic lesions must be taken seriously. Ambulatory care can reduce the dangers of loss of schooling and employment, but carries the risk of increasing venous stasis. The apparent high frequency of venous incompetence suggests that firm supportive dressings (elastic or compression bandaging) would help healing and the use of hydrocolloid dressings, which can be changed every 3–6 days, reduces the dangers of damage to the new epithelium. Bed rest is recommended but is rarely as effective in the home as in hospital, and patients are advised to keep the affected leg elevated whenever possible. Pinch grafting is confined to clean, vascular ulcers and is only used after failure of conservative measures. Physiotherapy may be necessary to prevent fixation of the ankle. Once healed, support stockings should be worn to reduce the risks of breakdown and every effort should be made to prevent trauma, which may cause a recurrence.

Finally, there is an urgent need to increase understanding of the mechanisms giving rise to leg ulceration. Proposed therapies must be submitted to randomized, controlled trials to produce data on which rational therapies can be based.

References

[1] King AD. Sickle cell anemia. Arch Dermatol Syphilol 1936;33:756.
[2] Netherton EW. Sickle cell anemia with ulcer of the leg. Arch Dermatol Syphilol 1936;34: 158–9.
[3] Schwartz WF. Sickle cell anemia associated with ulcer on the legs. Arch Dermatol Syphilol 1938;37:866–7.
[4] Cummer CL, LaRocco CG. Ulcers on the legs in sickle cell anemia. Arch Dermatol Syphilol 1939;40:459–60.
[5] Krugh FJ. Sickle cell anemia. Ulcer on the leg. Arch Dermatol Syphilol 1939;40:656.
[6] Cummer CL, LaRocco CG. Ulcers on the legs in sickle cell anemia. Arch Dermatol Syphilol 1940;42:1015–39.
[7] Hein GE, McCalla RL, Thorne GW. Sickle cell anemia. With report of a case with autopsy. Am J Med Sci 1927;173:763–72.
[8] Anderson WW, Ware RL. Sickle cell anemia. Am J Dis Child 1932;44:1055–70.
[9] Diggs LW, Ching RE. Pathology of sickle cell anemia. South Med J 1934;27:839–45.
[10] Koshy M, Entsuah R, Koranda A, et al. Leg ulcers in patients with sickle cell disease. Blood 1989;74:1403–8.
[11] Konotey-Ahulu FID. The sickle cell diseases. Arch Intern Med 1974;133:611–9.
[12] Akinyanju O, Akinsete I. Leg ulceration in sickle cell disease in Nigeria. Trop Geogr Med 1979;31:87–91.
[13] Durosinmi MA, Gevao SM, Esan GJF. Chronic leg ulcers in sickle cell disease: experience in Ibadan, Nigeria. Afr J Med Sci 1991;20:11–4.
[14] Perrine RP, Pembrey ME, John P, et al. Natural history of sickle cell anemia in Saudi Arabs. A study of 270 subjects. Ann Intern Med 1978;88:1–6.
[15] Padmos MA, Roberts GT, Sackey K, et al. Two different forms of homozygous sickle cell disease occur in Saudi Arabia. Br J Haematol 1991;79:93–8.
[16] Kar BC, Satapathy RK, Kulozik AE, et al. Sickle cell disease in Orissa State, India. Lancet 1986;ii:1198–201.
[17] Ankra-Badu GA. Sickle cell leg ulcers in Ghana. E Afr Med J 1992;69:366–9.
[18] Adedeji MO, Ukoli FAM. Haematologic factors associated with leg ulcer in sickle cell disease. Trop Geogr Med 1987;39:354–6.
[19] Higgs DR, Aldridge BE, Lamb J, et al. The interaction of alpha-thalassemia and homozygous sickle-cell disease. N Engl J Med 1982;306:1441–6.
[20] Mohan JS, Marshall JMM, Reid HL, et al. Daily variability in resting levels of cardiovascular variables in normal subjects and those with homozygous sickle cell disease. Clin Auton Res 1995;5:1–6.

[21] Mohan JS, Marshall JM, Reid HL, et al. Comparison of responses evoked by mild indirect cooling and by sound in the forearm vasculature in patients with homozygous sickle cell (SS) disease and in normal subjects. Clin Auton Res 1998;8:25–30.

[22] Gniadecka M, Gniadecka R, Serup J, et al. Microvascular reactions to postural changes in patients with sickle cell anaemia. Acta Derm Venereol 1994;74:191–3.

[23] Mohan JS, Marshall JM, Reid HL, et al. Postural vasoconstriction and leg ulceration in homozygous sickle cell disease. Clin Sci 1997;92:153–8.

[24] Saad STO, Zago MA. Leg ulceration and abnormalities of calf blood flow in sickle-cell anemia. Eur J Haematol 1992;46:188–90.

[25] Norris SL, Gober JR, Haywood J, et al. Altered muscle metabolism shown by magnetic resonance spectroscopy in sickle cell disease with leg ulcers. Magn Reson Imaging 1993; 11:119–23.

[26] Billett HH, Patel Y, Rivers SP. Venous insufficiency is not the cause of leg ulcers in sickle cell disease. Am J Hematol 1991;37:133–4.

[27] Yao ST, Hobbs JT, Irvine WT. Ankle systolic pressure measurements in arterial disease affecting the lower extremities. Br J Surg 1969;56:676–9.

[28] Mason R, Giron F. Noninvasive evaluation of venous function in chronic venous disease. Surgery 1982;91:312–7.

[29] Mohan JS, Vigilance JE, Marshall JM, et al. Abnormal venous function in patients with homozygous sickle cell (SS) disease and chronic leg ulcers. Clin Sci 2000;98:667–72.

[30] Fernandes J, Fernandes E, Horner J, et al. Ambulatory calf volume plethysmography in the assessment of venous insufficiency. Br J Surg 1979;66:327–30.

[31] Chalchal H, Rodino W, Hussain S, et al. Impaired venous hemodynamics in a minority of patients with chronic leg ulcers due to sickle cell anemia. Vasa 2001;30:277–9.

[32] Clare A, FitzHenley M, Harris J. Chronic leg ulceration in homozygous sickle cell disease: a role of venous incompetence. Br J Haematol 2002;119:567–71.

[33] Ballas SK. Sickle cell anemia with few painful crises is characterized by decreased red cell deformability and increased number of dense cells. Am J Hematol 1991;36: 122–30.

[34] Alexander N, Higgs D, Dover G, et al. Are there clinical phenotypes of homozygous sickle cell disease? Br J Haematol 2004;126:606–11.

[35] Ofosu MD, Castro O, Alarif L. Sickle cell ulcers are associated with HLA-B35 and Cw4. Arch Dermatol 1987;123:482–4.

[36] Serjeant GR. Leg ulceration in sickle cell anemia. Arch Intern Med 1974;133:690–4.

[37] Sawhney H, Weedon J, Gillette P, et al. Predilection of haemolytic anemia-associated leg ulcers for the medial malleolus. Vasa 2002;31:191–3.

[38] Serjeant GR, Galloway RE, Gueri M. Oral zinc sulphate in sickle-cell ulcers. Lancet 1970; 2:891–3.

[39] Margraf HW, Covey TH. A trial of silver-zinc-allantoinate in the treatment of leg ulcers. Arch Surg 1977;112:699–704.

[40] Husain SL. Oral zinc sulphate in leg ulcers. Lancet 1969;i:1069–71.

[41] Charache S. Treatment of sickle cell anemia. Annu Rev Med 1981;32:195–206.

[42] Oluwasanmi JO, Ofodile FA, Akinyemi OO. Leg ulcers in haemoglobinopathies. E Afr Med J 1980;57:60–4.

[43] Adedeji MO, Emokpare CI. Bacteriology of sickle-cell ulcers in the equatorial forest belt of South West Nigeria. J Trop Med Hyg 1987;90:297–300.

[44] Ademiluyi SA, Rotimi VO, Coker AO, et al. The anaerobic and aerobic bacterial flora of leg ulcers in patients with sickle-cell disease. J Infect 1988;17:115–20.

[45] MacFarlane DE, Baum KF, Serjeant GR. Bacteriology of sickle cell leg ulcers. Trans R Soc Trop Med Hyg 1986;80:553–6.

[46] Baum KF, MacFarlane DE, Cupidore L, et al. Corynebacterium diphtheriae in sickle cell leg ulcers in Jamaica. West Ind Med J 1985;34:24–8.

[47] Reindorf CA, Walker-Jones D, Adekile AD, et al. Rapid healing of sickle cell ulcers treated with collagen dressing. J Natl Med Assoc 1989;81:866–8.

[48] Wethers DL, Ramirez GM, Koshy M, et al. Accelerated healing of chronic sickle-cell leg ulcers treated with RGD peptide matrix. Blood 1994;84:1775–9.

[49] La Grenade L, Thomas PW, Serjeant GR. A randomized controlled trial of Solcoseryl and Duoderm in chronic sickle cell leg ulcers. West Ind Med J 1993;42:121–3.

[50] Serjeant BE, Harris J, Thomas P, et al. Propionyl-L-carnitine in chronic leg ulcers of homozygous sickle cell disease; a pilot study. J Am Acad Dermatol 1997;37:491–3.

[51] Bennett JP, Matthews R, Faulk WP. Treatment of chronic ulceration of the legs with human amnion. Lancet 1980;i:1153–6.

[52] Baum KF, MacFarlane DE, Maude GH, et al. Topical antibiotics in chronic sickle leg ulcers. Trans R Soc Trop Med Hyg 1987;81:847–9.

[53] Frost ML, Treadwell P. Treatment of sickle cell leg ulcers with pentoxifylline. Int J Dermat 1990;29:375–6.

[54] Serjeant GR, Howard C. Isoxsuprine hydrochloride in the therapy of sickle cell ulceration. West Ind Med J 1977;26:164–6.

[55] Kaplan G, Walsh G, Guido LS, et al. Novel responses of human skin to intradermal recombinant granulocyte/macrophage-colony-stimulating factor: Langerhans cell recruitment, keratinocyte growth, and enhanced wound healing. J Exp Med 1992;175:1717–28.

[56] Da Costa RM, Jesus FM, Aniceto C, et al. Double-blind, randomized placebo-controlled trial of the use of granulocyte-macrophage colony stimulating factor in chronic ulcers. Am J Surg 1997;173:165–8.

[57] Pieters RC, Rojer RA, Saleh AW, et al. Molgramostim to treat SS-sickle cell leg ulcers [letter]. Lancet 1995;345:528.

[58] Voskaridou E, Kyrtsonis M-C, Loutradi-Anagnostou A, et al. Healing of chronic leg ulcers in the hemoglobinopathies with perilesional injections of granulocyte-macrophage colony-stimulating factor. Blood 1999;93:3568–9.

[59] Alikhan MA, Carter G, Mehta P. Topical GM-CSF hastens healing of leg ulcers in sickle cell disease. Am J Hematol 2004;76:192.

[60] Mery L, Girot R, Aractingi S. Topical effectiveness of molgramostim (GM-CSF) in sickle cell leg ulcers. Dermatol 2004;208:135–7.

[61] Trent JT, Kirsner RS. Leg ulcers in sickle cell disease. Adv Skin Wound Care 2004;17:410–6.

[62] Chernoff AI, Shapleigh JB, Moore CV. Therapy of chronic ulceration of the legs associated with sickle cell anemia. JAMA 1954;155:1487–91.

[63] Al-Momen AM. Recombinant human erythropoietin induced rapid healing of a chronic leg ulcer in a patient with sickle cell disease. Acta Haematol 1991;86:46–8.

[64] Cackovic M, Chung C, Bolton LL, et al. Leg ulceration in the sickle cell patient. J Am Coll Surg 1998;187:307–9.

[65] Kersgard C, Osswald MB. Hydroxyurea and sickle cell leg ulcers. Am J Hematol 2001;68: 215–6.

[66] Loukopoulos D, Voskaridou E, Kalotychou V, et al. Reduction of the clinical severity of sickle cell/b-thalassemia with hydroxyurea: the experience of a single center in Greece. Blood Cells Mol Dis 2000;26:453–66.

[67] Best PJ, Daoud MS, Pittelkow MR, et al. Hydroxyurea-induced leg ulceration in 14 patients. Ann Intern Med 1998;128:29–32.

[68] Sher GD, Olivieri NF. Rapid healing of chronic leg ulcers during arginine butyrate therapy in patients with sickle cell disease and thalassemia [letter]. Blood 1994;84:7.

[69] Cacciola E, Musso R, Giustolisi R, et al. Blood hypercoagulability as a risk factor for leg ulcers in sickle cell disease. Blood 1990;75:2467–8.

[70] Ballas SK. Treatment of painful sickle cell ulcers with topical opioids. Blood 2002; 99:1096.

[71] Heckler FR, Dibbell DG, McGraw JB. Successful use of muscle flaps or myocutaneous flaps in patients with sickle cell disease. Plast Reconstr Surg 1977;59:902–8.

[72] Khouri RK, Upton J. Bilateral lower limb salvage with free flaps in a patient with sickle cell ulcers. Ann Plast Surg 1991;27:574–6.

[73] Weinweig N, Schuler J, Marschall M, et al. Lower limb salvage by microvascular free-

tissue transfer in patients with homozygous sickle cell disease. Plast Reconstr Surg 1995; 96:1154–61.

[74] Spence RJ. The use of a free flap in homozygous sickle cell disease. Plast Reconstr Surg 1985;76:616–9.

[75] Richards RS, Bowen CVA, Glynn MFX. Microsurgical free flap transfer in sickle cell disease. Ann Plast Surg 1992;29:278–81.

[76] Gueri M, Serjeant GR. Leg ulcers in sickle cell anaemia. Trop Geogr Med 1970;22: 155–60.

[77] Wolfort FG, Krizek TJ. Skin ulceration in sickle cell anemia. Plast Reconstr Surg 1969;43: 71–7.

[78] Alleyne SI, Wint E, Serjeant GR. Social effects of leg ulceration in sickle cell anemia. South Med J 1977;70:213–4.

[79] Brown JS, Middlemiss JH. Bone changes in tropical ulcer. Br J Radiol 1956;29:213–7.

[80] Ennis JT, Gueri MC, Serjeant GR. Radiological changes associated with leg ulcers in the tropics. Br J Radiol 1972;45:8–14.

[81] De Ceulaer K, Forbes M, Roper D, et al. Non-gouty arthritis in sickle cell disease: report of 37 consecutive cases. Ann Rheum Dis 1984;43:599–603.

[82] Morgan AG. Proteinuria and leg ulcers in homozygous sickle cell disease. J Trop Med Hyg 1982;85:205–8.

[83] Morgan AG, Venner AM. Immunity and leg ulcers in homozygous sickle cell disease. J Lab Clin Immunol 1981;6:51–5.

[84] Montgomery RD. Tetanus as a complication of sickle cell disease. Trans R Soc Trop Med Hyg 1960;54:385–8.

[85] Greco JB, Sacramento E, Tavares-Neto J. Chronic ulcers and myasis as ports of entry for Clostridium tetani. Braz J Infect Dis 2001;5:319–23.

Hematol Oncol Clin N Am 19 (2005) 957–973

HEMATOLOGY/ONCOLOGY CLINICS
OF NORTH AMERICA

Effects of Sickle Cell Disease on the Eye: Clinical Features and Treatment

Geoffrey G. Emerson, MD[a], Gerard A. Lutty, PhD[b],*

[a]Casey Eye Institute, 3375 SW Terwilliger Boulevard, Portland, OR 97239, USA
[b]Wilmer Ophthalmological Institute, 170 Woods Research Building, Johns Hopkins Hospital,
600 North Wolfe Street, Baltimore, MD 21287-9115, USA

The eyes provide a unique opportunity for direct observation of the sickle cell vaso-occlusive phenomenon. Vaso-occlusion can affect all of the vascular beds in the eye, including the conjunctiva, anterior segment, retina, or choroid, with a risk of devastating visual consequences. Because the early stages of sickle cell eye disease are not always accompanied by symptoms, evolving disease can remain undetected unless a careful eye examination is performed by an ophthalmologist. This examination should include an assessment of visual acuity and intraocular pressure, an evaluation of the anterior structures with slit-lamp biomicroscopy, and an examination of the posterior and peripheral retina including fluorescein angiography. Examination of patients with sickling hemoglobinopathies should begin in childhood and continue throughout life at annual intervals.

CLINICAL FEATURES

The clinical manifestations of sickle hemoglobinopathies in the eye can be grouped according to the presence or absence of vasoproliferative changes. Nonproliferative ocular manifestations of the sickle hemoglobinopathies have been well described and include altered conjunctival vasculature, hyphema, retinal "salmon patch" hemorrhages, retinal "iridescent spots," retinal "black sunbursts," and various abnormalities of the retinal vasculature, macula, choroid, and optic disk.

Conjunctival Vasculature

Clinical evidence of vaso-occlusion may be seen in the conjunctival vasculature in the form of dark red, comma-shaped or corkscrew-shaped vascular fragments that appear to be isolated from other neighboring vessels [1]. The anomalous vascular segments are most obvious in the inferior bulbar conjunctiva (Fig. 1).

Dr. Lutty's studies on sickle disease were supported by National Institutes of Health grant HL45922 and the Reginald Lewis Foundation.
* Corresponding author. E-mail address: galutty@jhmi.edu (G.A. Lutty).

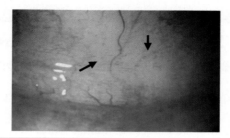

Fig. 1. Sickle conjunctival sign. Note the comma-shaped capillary segments, some of which appear to be isolated from the remaining circulation (*arrows*).

HbSS patients show more prominent conjunctival changes than do HbSC patients, and patients possessing the sickle cell trait (AS) almost never have conjunctival findings. Nagpal and coworkers [2] reported a positive correlation between the severity of conjunctival sickling and the number of irreversibly sickled cells in HbAS, HbSC, and HbSS patients. The radiant heat of the examining light may induce vasodilatation, reversing the anomalous vascular changes [3,4]. The characteristic comma-shaped pattern may also disappear after oxygen inhalation or blood transfusion [1]. In contrast, pharmacologic agents inducing vasoconstriction, such as phenylephrine, may enhance the conjunctival sign [5]. Histopathologic examination of the aberrant conjunctival vessels reveals endothelial proliferation, aggregation of red blood cells in distal portions of capillaries, and dilatation and thinning of the proximal segments of the vessels [6].

Hyphema

The anterior chamber of the eye (between the cornea and the iris) is ordinarily filled with a transparent and noncellular fluid, the aqueous humor. With its relatively low oxygen tension, low pH, and high ascorbate concentration, the aqueous humor serves to enhance sickling. Aqueous humor ascorbate may be as much as 15 times greater than the concentration found in circulating blood. When blood cells abnormally enter the anterior chamber as a result of trauma or intraocular surgery, a condition called hyphema (blood in the anterior chamber) occurs. In this sequestered environment, metabolizing erythrocytes and leukocytes use oxygen and liberate CO_2 and lactic acid, with resultant hypoxia, hypercarbia, and acidosis in the local microenvironment. The aggregate effect of this unusual chemical milieu is to induce and maintain sickling of predisposed erythrocytes in the anterior chamber. Even sickle trait cells become sickled in this particularly noxious medium. As a result, the elongated rigid sickled erythrocytes become trapped in the anterior chamber because they can no longer pass with ease out of the eye via Schlemm's canal and the trabecular meshwork that ordinarily provides outflow for normal pliable red cells. Log jamming of the sickled erythrocytes within the outflow apparatus provides sufficient mechanical obstruction that even aqueous humor cannot escape easily.

Because the production of new aqueous humor continues unabated, the pressure in the entire eye increases, with a resultant reduction of vascular perfusion pressure (vascular perfusion pressure equals the intravascular pressure minus the intraocular pressure). The net result is a slowing and sometimes a cessation of blood flow in all portions of the eye. Only a moderate increase in intraocular pressure may cause a reduction in perfusion of the optic nerve head and retina, placing the eye at risk for optic atrophy and artery occlusion [7]. If the blood flow is substantially compromised in the retina or optic nerve at the back of the eye (as a result of the events in the front of the eye), irreversible loss of vision or blindness may occur quickly and without warning [8].

A hyphema can usually be detected by simple inspection of the anterior chamber through the transparent cornea. A very bright focal beam of light from a high-quality penlight is usually sufficient for its visualization by an examiner. The presence of blood in the anterior chamber should prompt a measurement of visual acuity and intraocular pressure. The intraocular pressure should be around 25 mm Hg or less [9–11].

Salmon Patch Hemorrhage

Salmon patch hemorrhage is a round to oval area of hemorrhage located within the superficial retina. The lesion may be up to 2 mm in diameter, with well-defined boundaries and a flattened or dome-shaped configuration. Such hemorrhages, which usually occur in the midperipheral retina adjacent to an intermediate arteriole, are thought to result from a blowout of vascular walls weakened by prior episodes of occlusion and ischemia. Although the hemorrhage is initially red, it may turn salmon-colored over time because of progressive hemolysis [12,13].

Iridescent Spots

After resorption of a salmon patch hemorrhage, the retina may appear entirely normal without any evidence of residual blood; however, a faint indentation or depression representing thinning of the inner retina may be present in the location of the hemorrhage. This area appears on ophthalmoscopy as a dimple that may contain multiple glistening, refractile, yellowish granules, which are hemosiderin-laden macrophages. Histopathologic study discloses the presence of intracellular and extracellular iron in the area [12]. The finding of iridescent spots has been observed in 33% of HbSC patients, 18% of HbSThal patients, and 13% of HbSS patients [14–16].

Black Sunburst

The black sunburst lesion [17] appears as a flat round to oval black patch about 0.5 to 2 mm in size (Fig. 2). Glistening refractile granules, similar to those observed in iridescent spots, may be present. The black sunburst represents intraretinal migration of hyperplastic retinal pigment epithelium (RPE) in response to blood that has dissected between the RPE and neurosensory retina [12]. Histopathologic study discloses focal hypertrophy of the RPE along with areas of RPE hyperplasia and migration (Fig. 3D–E). Also present are diffuse

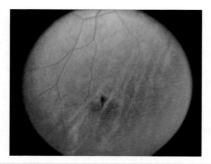

Fig. 2. Fundus photograph of a black sunburst surrounded by iridescent spots.

iron deposits, hemosiderin-laden macrophages, and pigment deposition. Black sunbursts are found in 41% of HbSC patients [14], 35% of HbSS patients [15], and 20% of HbSThal patients [16].

Retinal Vasculature

The major vessels of the posterior pole usually appear normal, although non-specific increased tortuosity may be observed in as many as 47% of HbSS patients and 32% of HbSC patients [17]. Posterior pole vascular tortuosity is rare in HbAS and HbSThal patients. Although the cause of the tortuosity is not known, some researchers hypothesize that it is due to peripheral arteriovenous shunting. Other posterior pole changes range from subtle perifoveal capillary dropout to occluded arterioles that appear as silver wires (Fig. 4) and central retinal artery occlusion [18,19].

Retinal occlusive events occur first and most often in the peripheral retina. Occlusions of the peripheral retinal microvasculature have been documented in HbSS patients at as early as 20 months of age (Fig. 5) [20]. Although retinal capillaries seem to be the initial site of occlusion early in life, larger-caliber vessels eventually become nonperfused with age (see Fig. 3). Where vessels end abruptly, hairpin-shaped loops may form. These loops are short at sites of capillary occlusion (see Fig. 5) and longer where major vessels end (see Fig. 3). One channel of the loop is the original blood vessel that became occluded; the second channel is a recanalization of the wall of the occluded segment (see Fig. 5C). With repeated vaso-occlusive events in the peripheral retina over a prolonged time, centripetal recession of the most peripheral vascular arcades occurs, away from the ora serrata and toward the equator. The result is a totally ischemic peripheral retina (see Fig. 3) [19].

Macula

Fluorescein angiographic studies of HbSS patients have demonstrated perifoveal capillary dropout resulting from arteriolar occlusion in the macula [18]. This nonperfusion causes degeneration and thinning of the inner retina, producing a concave dimple or depression in the macula known as the macular depression sign (Fig. 6). The depression is highlighted on ophthalmoscopy by

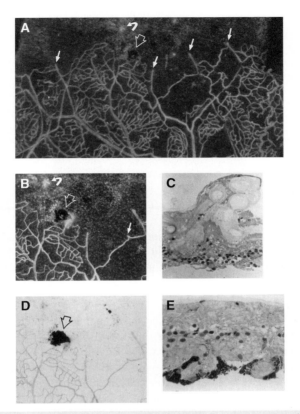

Fig. 3. Peripheral retinal specimen from a 54-year-old HbSC patient incubated for adenosine diphosphatase (ADPase) and embedded in glycol methacrylate. (A) The entire peripheral retina lacks viable blood vessels (no ADPase activity), and there are small areas of capillary loss. There are many characteristics of sickle cell retinopathy at the border of perfused and avascular peripheral retina, including hairpin loops (*thin arrows*) at the tips of perfused large vessels and arteriovenous anastomoses. A black sunburst lesion is present at the edge of the vasculature (*open arrow*). (B) At higher magnification, a hairpin loop (*thin arrow*) is appearant with the arteriovenous anastomosis. (C) When the avascular periphery was sectioned, the atrophic stalk of an auto-infarcted sea fan was found in (A) and (B) (*curved arrow*). The apparent feeder or draining blood vessel had a large lumen, and the retina is atrophic in this area. (D) The black sunburst lesion (*open arrow*) is apparent when the same area in the glycol methacrylate block is viewed with brightfield illumination. (E) A section through the sunburst lesion demonstrates that the retina is atrophic and the RPE cells have migrated into the retina and assembled around a core of basement membranelike material in the posterior retina (*bottom*) (A and B, darkfield illumination; D, brightfield illumination).

the surrounding light reflex at the border between healthy and atrophic retina. The depression stands out darkly from the normal internal light reflexes. The macular depression may or may not be accompanied by diminution of visual acuity [21].

Vascular irregularities may also occur in the macula. They include micro-aneurysmal dots, dilated precapillary arterioles and capillary segments, nerve

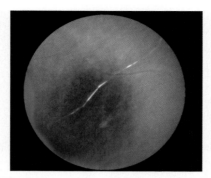

Fig. 4. Arteriolar silver wire.

fiber layer infarcts, and hairpin-shaped venous loops with adjacent capillary dropout [5,18,22]. Approximately 32% of HbSS patients, 36% of HbSC patients, and 20% of HbSThal patients have one or more of these findings [18,22,23].

Choroidal Occlusions
Described numerous times in patients with sickling hemoglobinopathies [20,24–26], choroidal nonperfusion is thought to result from occlusive events in the posterior ciliary arterial circulation. Some investigators have suggested that vaso-occlusive events in the choroidal vasculature may be involved in the formation of the black sunburst lesion [27,28]. Histopathologic features associated with choroidal vaso-occlusion include impacted erythrocytes, increased fibrin, and platelet-fibrin thrombi [20,29].

Occlusions of the choroidal vasculature may also contribute to the orange-red or brown streaks that emanate radially in the fundus from the optic nerve called angioid streaks. These streaks appear as crack lines in the choroid and are thought to be due to calcification and brittleness of Bruch's membrane, the limiting membrane between the retina and choroid.

Vascular Changes at the Optic Nerve Head
Vascular changes at the optic disk are transient and consist of dilated, dark capillary vessels that demonstrate occlusion on fluorescein angiography [5,15,30]. These vessels, which appear as small red dots with a linear or Y-shaped configuration on highly magnified ophthalmoscopy, are essentially precapillary arterioles plugged with sickled erythrocytes. The involved vessels intermittently open and close, and the ischemic insult is apparently not severe enough to have an impact on visual function. Neovascularization of the optic disk is rare but has been reported in four HbSC patients [31–34] and one HbSS patient [15].

Proliferative Sickle Retinopathy
Peripheral retinal arteriolar occlusion is the initiating event in the pathogenesis of proliferative sickle retinopathy. Arteriolar closure preferentially occurs at or

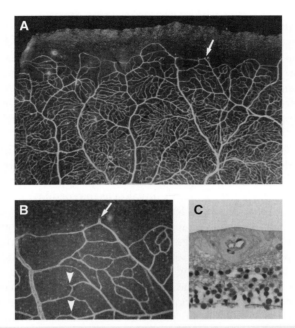

Fig. 5. Postmortem peripheral retinal specimen from a 20-month-old HbSS patient incubated for ADPase activity and embedded flat in glycol methacrylate polymer. (A) Retinal vasculature (white ADPase activity) at ora seratta (*top*) appears normal at low magnification, but some capillaries have reduced ADPase activity, and a small hairpin loop is already present (*arrow*). (B) The hairpin loop (*arrow*) is more obvious at higher magnification, and capillaries that end abruptly (*arrowheads*) suggest that capillary occlusions (loss of ADPase activity) have already occurred. (C) Cross-section of the hairpin loop in (A) and (B) shows that both lumens share a common basement membrane (A and B, darkfield illumination).

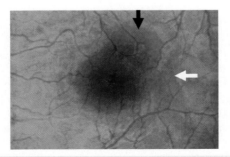

Fig. 6. Macular depression sign. Note the areas of macular thinning superotemporal to the fovea (*black arrow*) and along the temporal raphe (*white arrow*).

near Y-shaped bifurcations [22]. Occlusions also often occur at arteriovenous crossings (Fig. 7) [35]. The occlusive process produces local ischemia, which stimulates the production of vascular growth factors. Vascular endothelial growth factor and basic fibroblast growth factor (FGF-2) are associated with neovascularization [36]. The end result is the emergence of sea fan–shaped neovascular fronds that are predisposed to vitreous hemorrhage, subsequent tractional vitreous membrane formation, and, ultimately, retinal detachment [19,37].

Goldberg and coworkers have developed a widely recognized classification scheme detailing the stages of proliferative sickle retinopathy (Goldberg stages I–V). The hallmark of stage I retinopathy is peripheral arteriolar occlusion [5]. Presumably, sickled erythrocytes function as microemboli in capillaries and precapillary arterioles, impeding flow and turning the arteriolar segment a dark red cyanotic color and resulting in peripheral retinal nonperfusion.

In stage II, vascular remodeling occurs at the boundary between perfused and nonperfused peripheral retina. Connections form between occluded arterioles and adjacent terminal venules by way of pre-existing capillaries, resulting in arteriovenous anastomoses at the border separating the vascularized and the ischemic peripheral retina (see Fig. 3B). The anastomoses do not show leakage on fluorescein angiography, confirming that they indeed represent enlargement of pre-existing vessels with intact blood-retinal barrier properties rather than true neovascularization [5,34,38].

In stage III, peripheral retinal neovascularization (Figs. 8, 9) often assumes a frondlike configuration, resembling the marine invertebrate *Gorgonia flabelum* (sea fan). Most neovascular sea fan formations are found at the interface between perfused and nonperfused peripheral retina, growing toward the ischemic pre-equatorial retina (see Fig. 7) [19,34]. Sea fans may have multiple feeding arterioles and draining venules, probably owing to their origin from multiple buds

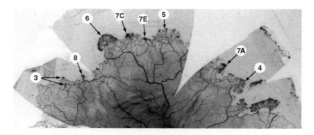

Fig. 7. Specimen from the superior peripheral retina in a 40-year-old woman with HbSS that was incubated for ADPase activity. The entire peripheral retina is nonperfused (vessels lack ADPase activity). There is a neovascular formation at every numbered arrow, ranging from sea fan–shaped viable structures (*arrow 6*) to autoinfarcted neovascular structures (*arrow 8*) (bright-field illumination of wet retinal flatmount). (*From* McLeod DS, Merges C, Fukushima A, et al. Histopathologic features of neovascularization in sickle cell retinopathy. Am J Ophthalmol 1997;124(4):458; with permission.)

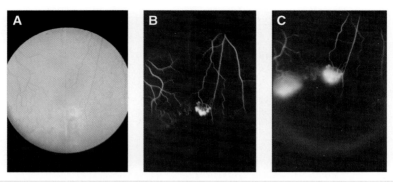

Fig. 8. Proliferative sickle retinopathy (sea fan). (A) Note the neovascular sea fan (white tissue) growing anterior to the retina at the interface of vascularized and ischemic retina. (B) An early image from a fluorescein angiogram highlights the sea fan. (C) Later, the sea fan is clearly leaking, demonstrating breakdown of the blood-retinal barrier. Additional neovascular tissue superior to the sea fan also leaks.

of angiogenesis that break through the internal limiting membrane of retina and grow along the surface of the retina at the vitreoretinal interface [35]. The sea fan is a dynamic neovascular formation in that the same formation may have actively growing blood vessels, established lumens ensheathed with pericytes, and autoinfarcted segments (see Fig. 9). Statistically, sea fans are most commonly found in the superotemporal quadrant, followed in order by the inferotemporal, superonasal, and inferonasal quadrants. They usually are limited to the equatorial retina, rarely extending to the posterior pole. Sea fans represent true neovascular tissue and show profuse leakage of intravascular fluorescein dye, indicating loss of the blood-retinal barrier (see Fig. 8). The clinician can take advantage of this property by using intravenous fluorescein angiography or angioscopy to detect subtle patches of neovascularization not evident during standard ophthalmoscopy [19].

Stage IV is defined by the presence of vitreous hemorrhage. As sea fans grow into the vitreous cavity, traction on their delicate vascular channels results in bleeding at irregular intervals for years. Traction-induced hemorrhage may occur in the setting of minor ocular trauma, normal vitreous movement, or contraction of vitreous bands induced by previous hemorrhage. Vitreous hemorrhage may be asymptomatic if it remains localized to the region adjacent to the sea fan. Stage IV retinopathy occurs more commonly in HbSC patients (21% to 23%) and is less common in HbSS patients (2% to 3%) [15,17,39] and other sickle hemoglobinopathies [17,39].

Vitreous bands and condensed contractile membranes are common sequelae of chronic vitreous hemorrhage and plasma transudation from incompetent neovascular tissue. They serve as key mechanical players in the progression to stage V retinopathy, defined as the presence of tractional or rhegmatogenous retinal detachment. As one would expect, retinal detachment is found most frequently

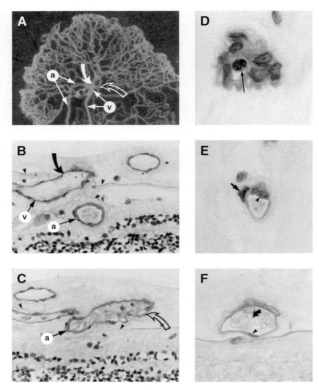

Fig. 9. Sea fan formation shown at arrow 6 in Fig. 7. (A) The sea fan has formed at the crossing of an artery (a) and vein (v). (B) The draining venule (v) (*solid curved arrow* here and in part A) breaches the internal limiting membrane (*arrowhead*) of retina at the arteriovenous crossing. (C) The feeding arteriole (*open arrow* here and in part A) breaching the internal limiting membrane (*arrowhead*). (D–F) This sea fan has forming capillaries that appear as undifferentiated angioblastic masses (D), mature capillaries that have endothelial cells (*arrowhead*) and pericytes (*arrow*) (E), and capillaries that have autoinfarcted (F) (A, darkfield illumination). (*From* McLeod DS, Merges C, Fukushima A, et al. Histopathologic features of neovascularization in sickle cell retinopathy. Am J Ophthalmol 1997;124(4):466; with permission.)

in HbSC patients [17] because these patients are most plagued by proliferative disease. Retinal detachment is rarely present in HbAS [40] or HbSS [15,41] patients.

Autoinfarction

Sea fan fronds may regress over time, with an eventual rate as high as 60% because of the process of autoinfarction [13,31,42–44]. Although not completely understood, the pathophysiology of autoinfarction is probably multifactorial. In a milieu of chronic hypoxia and ischemia, multiple recurrent episodes of thromboses and sickling within sea fans may eventually lead to permanent infarction of the lesion. The atrophic sea fans may slough off into vitreous, leaving a stalk containing the major feeding and draining blood vessels (see

Figs. 3B, C and 9B, C). Sea fans have elevated expression of leukocyte-endothelial cell adhesion molecules and greatly increased numbers of neutrophils, which undoubtedly contribute to autoinfarction [45].

Major nutrient vessels may also become kinked or even avulsed by vitreous traction, resulting in complete interruption of feeder flow [20]. Although sea fans may autoinfarct in one region of the eye, they may continue to flourish in other regions of the same eye (see Fig. 7). For this reason, most neovascular lesions are considered potentially dangerous and should be treated and obliterated.

TREATMENT

Given the high rate of spontaneous regression or the lack of progression of sea fan neovascularization in some eyes, indications for treatment of retinal neovascularization are not always clear. Nevertheless, therapeutic intervention is usually undertaken in cases of bilateral proliferative disease, spontaneous hemorrhage, large elevated sea fans, or rapid growth of neovascular tissue, or cases in which one eye has already been lost owing to proliferative retinopathy. On the other end of the spectrum, a single eye containing one small sea fan frond may be followed conservatively until expansion of the lesion or hemorrhage occurs.

The usual goal of management is the early treatment of stage III lesions before progression to substantial hemorrhage or retinal detachment occurs. If early treatment is successful, the need for pars plana vitrectomy or scleral buckling will be obviated, with avoidance of the concomitant surgical complications that often occur in sickle cell patients [37,43,46,47]. Techniques such as laser photocoagulation and cryotherapy have been employed to achieve involution of neovascular lesions. Of these techniques, laser photocoagulation has a lesser chance of damaging Bruch's membrane, which separates the retina and choroid, with a risk of choroidal neovascularization. Specific methods of laser application include direct coagulation of feeder vessels, local scatter photocoagulation with and without focal treatment of the sea fan, and 360-degree peripheral scatter delivery.

Feeder Vessel Photocoagulation

Direct heavy laser treatment of nutrient arterioles and subsequently draining venules has been shown to cause closure of sea fans in 88% of eyes studied in a controlled clinical trial [48]. With effective closure of sea fans comes a reduced likelihood of vitreous hemorrhage and concomitant secondary visual loss. Although xenon arc and argon lasers have been effective in achieving sea fan closure, the argon laser is currently most widely used for this purpose, because xenon has a greater chance of injuring Bruch's membrane, causing choroidal neovascularization. Once segmentation of the feeder arteriole has been accomplished, the same steps are used to treat the draining venule. This approach can prove difficult because sea fan formations may have multiple feeding and draining blood vessels. Because relatively high power settings are required to treat the sea fan in this manner, significant complications have been observed, including chorioretinal neovascularization, choriovitreal neovascularization, and retinal detachment [48–57]. One study documented complications in 32% of treated patients in the 6 months after treatment [48]. Most retinal specialists have abandoned feeder vessel treatment in favor of scatter photocoagulation, except in recalcitrant cases with repetitive bleeding.

Scatter Photocoagulation

Scatter photocoagulation has also been shown to reduce the chance of vitreous hemorrhage and secondary visual loss in patients with proliferative disease [42] and is preferred by many clinicians over feeder vessel photocoagulation because of the lower rate of complications. One important advantage of feeder vessel photocoagulation over local scatter is that direct feeder vessel treatment seems to be more successful in promoting closure if the sea fan is elevated [58].

In local scatter treatment, the spots are placed approximately one burn width apart in the local vicinity of proliferative sickle retinopathy [57]. In 360-degree scatter photocoagulation, a similar pattern of laser burns is placed around the entire peripheral retina. Scatter photocoagulation is thought to cause involution of sea fans by reducing the retinal production of angiogenic factors initially triggered in the milieu of ischemia created by prior vaso-occlusion. The laser scar enhances chorioretinal adhesion, theoretically preventing or minimizing the extent of subsequent retinal detachment. If the sea fan is not elevated, direct treatment may be performed in conjunction with local scatter applications. Failure to induce regression of the neovascular tissue, especially in the context of developing vitreous hemorrhage, may prompt the clinician to pursue aggressive feeder vessel photocoagulation.

In an eye with a lone sea fan or in any eye that contains 60 degrees or less of circumferential neovascularization, the risk of vitreous hemorrhage and secondary visual loss is relatively low [50]; therefore, the indications for treatment are less clear. Many clinicians believe that, because the risks of scatter treatment are also low, it probably should be performed whenever neovascularization is detected [42]. A possible exception may be the subset of HbSS patients over 40 years of age, 86% of who tend to remain stable or demonstrate regression of neovascular tissue [59].

Regular follow-up is necessary to monitor the regression or progression of neovascular disease; therefore, the reliable patient is the preferred candidate for local scatter photocoagulation. Despite previous scatter treatment, new fronds of neovascularization may develop in as many as 34% of eyes [42]. With regular follow-up, new sea fans may be detected early and receive proper treatment in a timely fashion.

Cryotherapy

If lenticular or vitreous opacities preclude an adequate view of the retina for laser photocoagulation, transconjunctival cryotherapy may be necessary to treat neovascularization. The single freeze-thaw technique has been successful in approximately 70% of treated sea fans [60]. During cryotherapy application, care should be taken to surround completely the neovascular tissue and to avoid overlap of neighboring applications. Re-treatment in the same area (eg, a triple freeze-thaw technique) may create retinal breaks and detachment and should be avoided [61].

Pars Plana Vitrectomy for Nonclearing Vitreous Hemorrhage

Vitrectomy surgery carries a significantly higher risk of intraoperative and postoperative complications in patients with sickle hemoglobinopathies when compared with patients with normal hemoglobin [46,62]. As a result, the indications for proceeding with vitrectomy are stringent [47,63]. Patients with new visually significant vitreous hemorrhages are usually followed up for at least 6 months to allow clearing of the media. If the view permits, cryotherapy or laser treatment is initiated. If no view of the fundus is possible, the patient is observed with approximately monthly ultrasound examinations to detect retinal detachments, for which early surgery is indicated. If visual acuity improves to a level permitting the patient to function to his or her satisfaction, vitrectomy is deferred. Pars plana vitrectomy in combination with endolaser photocoagulation may be considered in cases of long-standing vitreous hemorrhage (duration usually greater than 6 months) in which the view is inadequate for laser or cryotherapy.

After combined vitrectomy/lensectomy or vitrectomy in an aphakic patient, sickled erythrocytes may migrate forward from the vitreous cavity into the anterior chamber, clogging the trabecular meshwork and creating secondary glaucoma [7]. The intraocular pressure should be maintained at an average of less than 25 mm Hg [9–11]. Methazolamide, which produces less of a systemic acidosis and may even raise the pH somewhat, is the most appropriate of the systemic intraocular pressure–lowering agents to use in this setting. Most topical intraocular pressure–lowering agents can be used to treat glaucoma resulting from outflow obstruction by sickled erythrocytes. Anterior chamber paracentesis is indicated in cases in which topical and systemic therapies fail to achieve the desired target pressure (usually, 24 mm Hg or lower) [46].

Scleral Buckling Surgery for Retinal Detachment

As is true for pars plana vitrectomy, scleral buckling surgery in patients with sickle cell disease carries an increased risk of intraoperative and postoperative complications when compared with the risk in the general population [43]. Complications are similar to those seen in pars plana vitrectomy, including persistent intraocular hemorrhage, hyphema with secondary glaucoma, infarctions of the macula and optic nerve from elevated intraocular pressure, and the potential for intraoperative sickling crises [43,64]. Buckle placement also may cause anterior segment ischemia, as demonstrated by Ryan and Goldberg [65]. For these reasons, scleral buckling surgery usually is avoided unless it is absolutely necessary. Rhegmatogenous detachments usually require immediate buckling, but tractional detachments are buckled only when definite progression has been documented. In cases of extensive traction and vitreous hemorrhage, a combined buckle/vitrectomy may be performed.

To lower the risk of intraoperative vaso-occlusion and ischemia, an exchange blood transfusion may be considered before surgery to achieve a target hemoglobin A level of 50% to 60% (measured by electrophoresis) and a target hematocrit of 35% [66]. These goals may be accomplished by the withdrawal of 1 or 2 units of blood followed by repeated simple transfusions of packed cells over several days. Alternatively, erythrocytapheresis makes use of an automated blood cell separator to replace sickled red blood cells with donor erythrocytes within a few hours [64]. Preoperative consultation with an experienced hematologist is advised [64].

SUMMARY

Ocular complications of the sickling disorders are multiple and require continuing assessment to detect lesions early enough for effective prophylactic therapy to maximize visual functioning. The natural history of proliferative sickle retinopathy is incompletely understood; therefore, the risk factors for visual outcome are largely unknown. The disease requires close monitoring of the patient for progression or regression of lesions in determining the selection of therapeutic options.

Acknowledgments

The authors acknowledge Scott McLeod for his assistance with the figures and the histologic studies presented in this article.

References

[1] Paton D. The conjunctival sign of sickle-cell disease. Arch Ophthalmol 1961;66:90–4.

[2] Nagpal KC, Asdourian GK, Goldbaum MH, et al. The conjunctival sickling sign, hemoglobin S, and irreversibly sickled erythrocytes. Arch Ophthalmol 1977;95(5):808–11.

[3] Fink AI, Funahashi T, Robinson M, et al. Conjunctival blood flow in sickle-cell disease: preliminary report. Arch Ophthalmol 1961;66:824–9.

[4] Paton D. The conjunctival sign of sickle-cell disease: further observations. Arch Ophthalmol 1962;68:627–32.

[5] Nagpal KC, Goldberg MF, Rabb MF. Ocular manifestations of sickle hemoglobinopathies. Surv Ophthalmol 1977;21(5):391–411.

[6] Funahashi T, Fink A, Robinson M, et al. Pathology of conjunctival vessels in sickle-cell disease: a preliminary report. Am J Ophthalmol 1964;57:713–8.

[7] Al-Abdulla NA, Haddock TA, Kerrison JB, et al. Sickle cell disease presenting with extensive perimacular arteriolar occlusions in a nine-year-old boy. Am J Ophthalmol 2001; 131(2):275–6.

[8] Deutsch TA, Weinreb RN, Goldberg MF. Indications for surgical management of hyphema in patients with sickle cell trait. Arch Ophthalmol 1984;102(4):566–9.

[9] Goldberg MF. The diagnosis and treatment of secondary glaucoma after hyphema in sickle cell patients. Am J Ophthalmol 1979;87(1):43–9.

[10] Goldberg MF. The diagnosis and treatment of sickled erythrocytes in human hyphemas. Trans Am Ophthalmol Soc 1978;76:481–501.

[11] Serjeant G. Sickle cell disease. Oxford (UK): Oxford University Press; 1985.

[12] Romayanada N, Goldberg MF, Green WR. Histopathology of sickle cell retinopathy. Trans Am Acad Ophthalmol Otolaryngol 1973;77(5):642–76.

[13] Gagliano DA, Goldberg MF. The evolution of salmon-patch hemorrhages in sickle cell retinopathy. Arch Ophthalmol 1989;107(12):1814–5.

[14] Condon PI, Serjeant GR. Ocular findings in hemoglobin SC disease in Jamaica. Am J Ophthalmol 1972;74(5):921–31.
[15] Condon PI, Serjeant GR. Ocular findings in homozygous sickle cell anemia in Jamaica. Am J Ophthalmol 1972;73(4):533–43.
[16] Condon PI, Serjeant GR. Ocular findings in sickle cell thalassemia in Jamaica. Am J Ophthalmol 1972;74(6):1105–9.
[17] Welch RB, Goldberg MF. Sickle-cell hemoglobin and its relation to fundus abnormality. Arch Ophthalmol 1966;75(3):353–62.
[18] Asdourian GK, Nagpal KC, Busse B, et al. Macular and perimacular vascular remodeling sickling haemoglobinopathies. Br J Ophthalmol 1976;60(6):431–53.
[19] Goldberg MF. Retinal neovascularization in sickle cell retinopathy. Trans Am Acad Ophthalmol Otolaryngol 1977;83(3 Pt 1):409–31.
[20] McLeod DS, Goldberg MF, Lutty GA. Dual-perspective analysis of vascular formations in sickle cell retinopathy. Arch Ophthalmol 1993;111(9):1234–45.
[21] Goldbaum MH. Retinal depression sign indicating a small retinal infarct. Am J Ophthalmol 1978;86(1):45–55.
[22] Stevens TS, Busse B, Lee CB, et al. Sickling hemoglobinopathies; macular and perimacular vascular abnormalities. Arch Ophthalmol 1974;92(6):455–63.
[23] Marsh RJ, Ford SM, Rabb MF, et al. Macular vasculature, visual acuity, and irreversibly sickled cells in homozygous sickle cell disease. Br J Ophthalmol 1982;66(3):155–60.
[24] Condon PI, Serjeant GR, Ikeda H. Unusual chorioretinal degeneration in sickle cell disease: possible sequelae of posterior ciliary vessel occlusion. Br J Ophthalmol 1973;57(2):81–8.
[25] Dizon RV, Jampol LM, Goldberg MF, et al. Choroidal occlusive disease in sickle cell hemoglobinopathies. Surv Ophthalmol 1979;23(5):297–306.
[26] Stein MR, Gay AJ. Acute chorioretinal infarction in sickle cell trait: report of a case. Arch Ophthalmol 1970;84(4):485–90.
[27] Wise G, Dollery C, Henkind P. The retinal circulation. New York: Harper & Row; 1971.
[28] Cogan DG. Ophthalmic manifestations of systemic vascular disease. Major Probl Intern Med 1974;3:1–187.
[29] Lutty GA, Merges C, Crone S, et al. Immunohistochemical insights into sickle cell retinopathy. Curr Eye Res 1994;13(2):125–38.
[30] Goldberg MF. Retinal vaso-occlusion in sickling hemoglobinopathies. Birth Defects Orig Artic Ser 1976;12(3):475–515.
[31] Condon PI, Sergeant GR. Behaviour of untreated proliferative sickle retinopathy. Br J Ophthalmol 1980;64(6):404–11.
[32] Kimmel AS, Magargal LE, Tasman WS. Proliferative sickle retinopathy and neovascularization of the disc: regression following treatment with peripheral retinal scatter laser photocoagulation. Ophthalmic Surg 1986;17(1):20–2.
[33] Ober RR, Michels RG. Optic disk neovascularization in hemoglobin SC disease. Am J Ophthalmol 1978;85(5 Pt 1):711–4.
[34] Raichand M, Goldberg MF, Nagpal KC, et al. Evolution of neovascularization in sickle cell retinopathy: a prospective fluorescein angiographic study. Arch Ophthalmol 1977;95(9):1543–52.
[35] McLeod DS, Merges C, Fukushima A, et al. Histopathologic features of neovascularization in sickle cell retinopathy. Am J Ophthalmol 1997;124(4):455–72.
[36] Cao J, Mathews MK, McLeod DS, et al. Angiogenic factors in human proliferative sickle cell retinopathy. Br J Ophthalmol 1999;83(7):838–46.
[37] Jampol LM, Green Jr JL, Goldberg MF, et al. An update on vitrectomy surgery and retinal detachment repair in sickle cell disease. Arch Ophthalmol 1982;100(4):591–3.
[38] Goldberg MF. Classification and pathogenesis of proliferative sickle retinopathy. Am J Ophthalmol 1971;71(3):649–65.
[39] Clarkson JG. The ocular manifestations of sickle-cell disease: a prevalence and natural history study. Trans Am Ophthalmol Soc 1992;90:481–504.

[40] Isbey H, Clifford G, Tanaka K. Vitreous hemorrhage associated with sickle-cell trait and sickle-cell hemoglobin C disease. Am J Ophthalmol 1958;45:870–9.

[41] Kearney WF. Sickle cell ophthalmopathy. N Y State J Med 1965;65(21):2677–81.

[42] Farber MD, Jampol LM, Fox P, et al. A randomized clinical trial of scatter photocoagulation of proliferative sickle cell retinopathy. Arch Ophthalmol 1991;109(3):363–7.

[43] Goldberg MF, Jampol LM. Treatment of neovascularization, vitreous hemorrhage, and retinal detachment in sickle cell retinopathy. Trans New Orleans Acad Ophthalmol 1983; 31:53–81.

[44] Nagpal KC, Patrianakos D, Asdourian GK, et al. Spontaneous regression (autoinfarction) of proliferative sickle retinopathy. Am J Ophthalmol 1975;80(5):885–92.

[45] Kunz Mathews M, McLeod DS, Merges C, et al. Neutrophils and leukocyte adhesion molecules in sickle cell retinopathy. Br J Ophthalmol 2002;86(6):684–90.

[46] Cohen SB, Fletcher ME, Goldberg MF, et al. Diagnosis and management of ocular complications of sickle hemoglobinopathies: part IV. Ophthalmic Surg 1986;17(5): 312–5.

[47] Goldbaum MH, Peyman GA, Nagpal KC, et al. Vitrectomy in sickling retinopathy: report of five cases. Ophthalmic Surg 1976;7(4):92–102.

[48] Jacobson MS, Gagliano DA, Cohen SB, et al. A randomized clinical trial of feeder vessel photocoagulation of sickle cell retinopathy: a long-term follow-up. Ophthalmology 1991; 98(5):581–5.

[49] Carney MD, Paylor RR, Cunha-Vaz JG, et al. Iatrogenic choroidal neovascularization in sickle cell retinopathy. Ophthalmology 1986;93(9):1163–8.

[50] Condon P, Jampol LM, Farber MD, et al. A randomized clinical trial of feeder vessel photocoagulation of proliferative sickle cell retinopathy. II. Update and analysis of risk factors. Ophthalmology 1984;91(12):1496–8.

[51] Condon PI, Serjeant GR. Choroid neovascularization: an important complication of photocoagulation for proliferative sickle cell retinopathy. Trans Ophthalmol Soc U K 1981; 101(Pt 4):429.

[52] Condon PI, Jampol LM, Ford SM, et al. Choroidal neovascularisation induced by photocoagulation in sickle cell disease. Br J Ophthalmol 1981;65(3):192–7.

[53] Dizon-Moore RV, Jampol LM, Goldberg MF. Chorioretinal and choriovitreal neovascularization: their presence after photocoagulation of proliferative sickle cell retinopathy. Arch Ophthalmol 1981;99(5):842–9.

[54] Fox PD, Acheson RW, Serjeant GR. Outcome of iatrogenic choroidal neovascularisation in sickle cell disease. Br J Ophthalmol 1990;74(7):417–20.

[55] Galinos SO, Asdourian GK, Woolf MB, et al. Choroido-vitreal neovascularization after argon laser photocoagulation. Arch Ophthalmol 1975;93(7):524–30.

[56] Goldbaum MH, Galinos SO, Apple D, et al. Acute choroidal ischemia as a complication of photocoagulation. Arch Ophthalmol 1976;94(6):1025–35.

[57] Jampol LM, Farber M, Rabb MF, et al. An update on techniques of photocoagulation treatment of proliferative sickle cell retinopathy. Eye 1991;5(Pt 2):260–3.

[58] Rednam KR, Jampol LM, Goldberg MF. Scatter retinal photocoagulation for proliferative sickle cell retinopathy. Am J Ophthalmol 1982;93(5):594–9.

[59] Fox PD, Vessey SJ, Forshaw ML, et al. Influence of genotype on the natural history of untreated proliferative sickle retinopathy—an angiographic study. Br J Ophthalmol 1991; 75(4):229–31.

[60] Lee CB, Woolf MB, Galinos SO, et al. Cryotherapy of proliferative sickle retinopathy. Part I. Single freeze-thaw cycle. Ann Ophthalmol 1975;7(10):1299–308.

[61] Goldbaum MH, Fletcher RC, Jampol LM, et al. Cryotherapy of proliferative sickle retinopathy, II: triple freeze-thaw cycle. Br J Ophthalmol 1979;63(2):97–101.

[62] Leen JS, Ratnakaram R, Del Priore LV, et al. Anterior segment ischemia after vitrectomy in sickle cell disease. Retina 2002;22(2):216–9.

[63] Ryan SJ. Role of the vitreous in the haemoglobinopathies. Trans Ophthalmol Soc U K 1975;95(3):403–6.

[64] Cohen SB, Fletcher ME, Goldberg MF, et al. Diagnosis and management of ocular complications of sickle hemoglobinopathies. Part V. Ophthalmic Surg 1986;17(6):369–74.
[65] Ryan SJ, Goldberg MF. Anterior segment ischemia following scleral buckling in sickle cell hemoglobinopathy. Am J Ophthalmol 1971;72(1):35–50.
[66] Brazier DJ, Gregor ZJ, Blach RK, et al. Retinal detachment in patients with proliferative sickle cell retinopathy. Trans Ophthalmol Soc U K 1986;105(Pt 1):100–5.

Hematol Oncol Clin N Am 19 (2005) 975–987

HEMATOLOGY/ONCOLOGY CLINICS
OF NORTH AMERICA

New Therapies for Sickle Cell Disease

Iheanyi E. Okpala, MBBS (Hons), MSc, FRCPath, FWACP

Hematology Department, St. Thomas' Hospital, University of London, Lambeth Palace Road, London, SE1 7EH, England, UK

The various entities generally called sickle cell disease (SCD) share two characteristics: sickle erythrocytes in the blood and clinical illness as a result of having these abnormal red cells. They include the homozygous HbSS condition sickle cell anemia, and the compound heterozygous states HbSC disease and HbS/thalassaemia, but not sickle cell trait (HbAS). Oral history passed down through generations in Africa relays accounts of an inherited illness that manifests as recurrent episodes of sudden onset bone pain, and death during childhood [1]. In the medical literature, the earliest publication of the features of the disorder now called sickle cell disease was in 1874 by Africanus Horton [2]. Born of Igbo parents from Nigeria who lived in Sierra Leone, Horton graduated from the medical school of King's College London, and served as a colonel in the British army (Fig. 1). In his book *The Diseases of Tropical Climates and Their Treatment,* Horton [2] described the recurrent pain that is the hallmark of clinical manifestation of sickle cell disease, as well as the association of fever and cold weather. The characteristic hematological feature of sickle cell disease, "peculiar elongated and sickled red cells" was published in the 1910 issue of *Archives of Internal Medicine* by James Herrick, a Chicago cardiologist [3]. It was the first account of the pathology of SCD, and gave the condition the name it bears today.

Since 1910, there have been remarkable advances in understanding the pathological basis of SCD. Three disease mechanisms stand out: haemolysis, vaso-occlusion, and impaired defense against infections. Premature destruction of red blood cells is mostly the end effect of erythrocyte sickling and membrane damage induced by crystallization and polymerization of deoxy-HbS [4]. However, in the uncommon condition of hyperhaemolysis syndrome, immunological mechanisms appear to play a dominant role in destruction of both the patient's own and transfused red blood cells [5]. Blood vessel occlusion in SCD is a process fairly simple in conception. However, the cellular and molecular details are complex. Various gaps in knowledge notwithstanding, the current model of vaso-occlusion in SCD views the process as the result of interactions between sickled and unsickled erythrocytes, leukocytes, platelets,

E-mail address: iheanyi.okpala@gstt.sthames.nhs.uk

0889-8588/05/$ – see front matter
doi:10.1016/j.hoc.2005.08.004

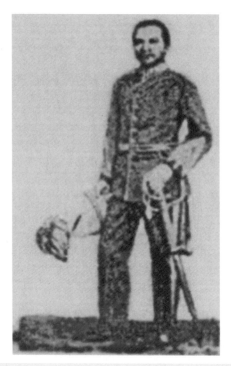

Fig. 1. Colonel James Africanus Horton (1835–83), MBBS (London), MD (Edinburgh). First to publish the clinical features of the condition now called sickle cell disease.

plasma proteins, and the blood vessel wall [6,7]. The causes of impaired defense against infections in SCD include splenic hypofunction [8], a defect in the alternative pathway of complement [9,10], and possible reduction in the microbicidal capacity of white blood cells [11,12]. Despite substantial developments in understanding the pathophysiology of SCD, application of this immense body of knowledge to medical treatment remains a major challenge. Interference with various disease mechanisms is the basis of many treatment modalities in SCD. This review will discuss new and developing therapies for SCD as a whole, and for specific manifestations of the hemoglobinopathy.

HYDROXYUREA THERAPY

Although it is licensed in the United States for administration to sickle cell patients who have ≥3 crises a year in steady state, hydroxyurea (HU) remains unlicensed in most countries where it is regarded as an experimental drug [13,14]. In the author's hospital in the United Kingdom, where HU is unlicensed for SCD, it is offered to patients who have ≥5 crises a year; or 3–4 crises a year with either neutrophil count $\geq 10 \times 10^9$/L or platelet count $\geq 500 \times 10^9$/L in steady state [7]; bearing in mind that the reference range for neutrophil count in black people is $1-3 \times 10^9/L$ [15,16], and is $100-300 \times 10^9/L$ for platelets [17]. Since high neutrophil count in steady state is a marker of severe SCD [12,18–22], these criteria usually identify individuals who have a clinical course sufficiently severe to ensure that the benefits of hydroxyurea therapy justify the potential risks. HU therapy is offered if the patient does not want to have (more) children, and is weighed against any severe impairment of liver or kidney function, or blood cytopenia. HU is unlicensed in most countries because the long-term adverse effects are unknown, not because the clinical efficacy is in doubt. In fact, after over 9 years of follow-up, HbSS subjects who received HU in the US placebo-controlled trial, had significantly less painful crises, acute chest syndrome, and mortality [23]. Potential long-term toxic effects that reduce enthusiasm for HU include teratogenicity, carcinogenesis and, for young children, impaired cognitive development.

How much of an issue have these potential adverse effects been in clinical practice? With respect to possible effects on unborn babies, about 15 women have taken HU all through pregnancy, and none of the children had a congenital anomaly [24,25]. Although these reports may reduce anxiety about the outcome of pregnancy in humans taking HU, it is a cytotoxic drug, teratogenic in mice [26]. Therefore, the manufacturers and most clinicians currently hold the view that HU is contra-indicated in pregnancy, and advise contraception in patients of child-bearing age who take the medication [27]. Sperm banking before starting HU therapy may be considered in males who plan to have children later. Neurocognitive deficits have not been observed in children who have sickle cell disease who are taking HU [28], who may indeed have better school performance than those not on the therapy. Twenty-nine children who have sickle cell disease (median age 14 months) treated for 2 years with HU at the initial dose of 20 mg/kg, then had the dose increased to 30 mg/kg. At a time when 19 of the 29 had completed a median treatment period of 2.8 years, growth and development remained normal [29]. A much longer median follow-up period of 5 years in 60 children taking HU for secondary erythrocytosis has resulted in no malignant disease in any of the cohort [30]. Acute leukemia has developed in 3 sickle cell patients on HU, in 2 of the 3 patients, after 6 and 8 years respectively of treatment [31–33]. However, the leukemogenic risk of HU therapy is difficult to quantify from these case reports because the total number of patients treated and the duration of therapy are not certain. The Medical College of Georgia (Augusta, GA) recently published their 15 years of experience with HU therapy in SCD. Leukemia was not reported among the 226 patients treated [34]. After 9 years of follow-up, the US multi-center trial observed 2 cases of cancer among 204 sickle cell subjects who actually took HU (irrespective of the original randomization to the drug or placebo), and 1 case among 96 subjects who never did [23]. The data do not suggest a significant increase in the risk of malignant disease caused by HU therapy. As a ribonucleotide reductase inhibitor that is mutagenic [35] and impairs DNA and protein synthesis with adverse effects on cell division, HU has a theoretical potential to be carcinogenic.

Whether this will translate into a practical problem in hematology clinics, remains to be seen.

The clinical benefits of HU are mediated by increased total HbF, mean cell HbF, number of erythrocytes with detectable amounts of HbF and possibly nitric oxide [36,37], as well as with reduction in reticulocyte, leukocyte, and platelet counts, and in the expression of adhesion molecules in blood and vascular endothelial cells [38,39]. The dose of HU used in SCD is 5–35 mg/kg/d. In the author's hospital, treatment of adults is started with 0.5 g/d, and increased by 5 mg/kg every 6 weeks, until clinical benefit is observed. Clinical experience shows that the maximum tolerable dose (as used during the initial trials) is not necessary to achieve the benefits of HU therapy in SCD. The short-term adverse effects of HU, such as blood cytopenias, are more likely to occur with higher doses and, though not yet proven, it is possible this may also apply to the long-term toxicities. Therefore, in the author's hospital, the minimum effective dose is used, where about 25 adult sickle cell patients are on HU 1–2 g/d, with good effect. The dose at which side effects or clinical benefits occur may vary between individuals. Therefore, it is important to monitor each patient for adverse effects, especially during the initial period of treatment. Blood cell counts and chemistry to assess liver and renal functions are done every 2 weeks in the first month, monthly for the next 3 months, and every 2–3 months thereafter. Treatment is suspended in black patients if the neutrophil count drops below 1×10^9/L, and the platelet or reticulocyte count below 80×10^9/L. HU therapy is restarted at a lower dose when neutrophil count rises to 2×10^9/L, platelet count to 100×10^9/L, and reticulocyte count to 100×10^9/L. For white patients who have higher reference ranges of blood cell counts, the criteria for suspending therapy are neutrophils $<2 \times 10^9$/L, platelets $<100 \times 10^9$/L, and retics $<80 \times 10^9$/L. Other therapeutic agents that increase HbF levels are used less extensively than HU in SCD. This is probably because, despite their effectiveness, these agents lack the convenience of oral administration. Arginine butyrate infused once or twice a month led to a remarkable rise in HbF sustained for 1–2 years [40]. Subcutaneous infusion of decitabine, an analog of azacytidine that is less cytotoxic than HU, significantly increased total Hb level and percentage HbF in HbSS patients who did not have such improvements in hematological parameters during previous treatment with hydroxyurea [41].

OMEGA-3 FATTY ACIDS

These food substances that occur naturally in fish oil are essential to humans because we do not have the biosynthetic machinery. They are important structural and functional components of the membranes of cells and various organelles. In a placebo-controlled pilot trial, oral supplements of two omega-3 polyunsaturated fatty acids (PUFA)– docosahexanoic acid (DHA) and eicosapentanoic acid (EPA)–reduced the mean number of sickle cell crises requiring hospital attendance from 7.8 per year to 3.8 per year in 5 HbSS individuals [42]. By contrast, 5 HbSS patients who received placebo (olive oil) had pre- and post-treatment crisis rates of 7.6 per year and 7.1 per year, respectively. In addition, the thrombogenicity of blood (as measured by various coagulation parameters) and expression of the adhesion molecule platelet selectin (CD62P) were significantly reduced. Omega-3 PUFA was given as 0.25 g/kg/d of menhaden fish oil containing 18% DHA and 12% EPA. The placebo was given at the same dose. If confirmed in a controlled trial involving a large number of sickle cell patients, the dramatic reduction in the number of crises would hold promise for the future. This is because, unlike hydroxyurea, DHA and EPA are not cytotoxic, they are naturally occurring nutrients, they are more widely available and affordable in developing countries where the majority of SCD patients live, and they will be more acceptable to both patients and physicians. Concerns about carcinogenicity, teratogenicity and impaired cognitive development are far less likely to arise. Fish oil is generally consumed as a food substance in many countries. Supplements of DHA and EPA have been safely given in previous studies to pregnant women, as well as term and pre-term babies [43,44]. In fact, there is evidence that DHA enhances development of the brain and nervous system [45,46].

Hongmei Ren and coworkers [47–49] have studied omega-3 fatty acids in steady state sickle cell disease, and observed a striking correlation between the proportions of DHA and EPA in the blood, and indices of disease severity. There was global reduction of DHA and EPA in erythrocytes, leukocytes, platelets, and plasma of sickle cell patients relative to healthy HbAA controls. In addition, steady state hemoglobin levels increased with the proportion of omega-3 PUFA in red cell membranes, and patients with complications of SCD had significantly less platelet DHA than those who have uncomplicated disease. Several factors may contribute to the biological basis of these findings. As stated previously, omega-3 fatty acids are vital to the structural integrity of erythrocyte membranes. So, increased proportions confer resistance against hemolyis, as demonstrated following dietary supplementation in animal models [50]. This improves hemoglobin levels in SCD because haemolysis is the dominant cause of anemia in this hemoglobinopathy. Also, increased proportions of DHA and EPA inhibit production of pro-inflammatory cytokines, activation of vascular endothelium, and adhesion of blood cells to the vessel wall [51–53]. In SCD, the end-effect is reduction in vaso-occlusive episodes, ischemic organ damage, and disease complications. Together with reduced blood coagulability and adhesion molecule expression reported in the pilot trial [42], the findings of Ren and colleagues [47–49] have shed some light on how omega-3 fatty acid therapy confers clinical benefit in SCD. Administration of these PUFA ameliorates various diseases of the cardiovascular, skeletal, and other organ systems [54–56]. Available data provide sufficient grounds for a large clinical trial of omega-3 fatty acids in the multi-system disorder that is SCD.

GARDOS CHANNEL BLOCKERS

A calcium-dependent mechanism for potassium transport across cell membranes, the Gardos channel, regulates K^+ ion and water loss from erythrocytes. In humans and animal models who have SCD, inhibition of this potassium flux system by the antifungal clotrimazole, prevented intra-cellular dehydration of erythrocytes and reduced the polymerization of HbS and sickling of red blood cells [57]. An analog of clotrimazole that is less toxic to the liver and urinary tract because it has no imidazole moiety, ICA-17043 is a more potent Gardos channel inhibitor and specifically blocks potassium efflux from red blood cells mediated by this transport mechanism [58]. In a phase II placebo-controlled clinical trial reported by Ataga and colleagues [59], oral ICA-17043 10 mg/d for 12 weeks raised the mean steady state Hb by 0.68 ± 0.11 g/dL; with significant reduction in reticulocyte count, bilirubin level, and lactate dehydrogenase ($P < .001$). The main side-effects of ICA-17043 were nausea and diarrhea. The beneficial effects of this Gardos channel inhibitor on hematological indices has prompted a phase III multi-center clinical trial designed to find out if it reduces the frequency of vaso-occlusive events in SCD.

PROSPECTS FOR ANTI-ADHESION THERAPY

Adhesion of blood cells to each other and the vascular endothelium contributes to vaso-occlusion in SCD [6,7]. Therefore, the molecules that mediate these cellular interactions are potential targets in the treatment of sickle hemoglo-binopathies. There are prospects for the use of chemical or biological agents to interfere with the intercellular adhesions that facilitate blood vessel obstruction. Such anti-adhesion therapy could reduce tissue ischaemia or infarction, and ameliorate the clinical manifestations of vaso-occlusion in SCD. Early investi-gators recognized that sickled erythrocytes are rigid, a property that facilitates mechanical obstruction of the micro-vasculature [60]. More recent studies demonstrate that both sickled and unsickled erythrocytes bind to blood vessel walls via adhesion molecules [61]. So, red blood cells also contribute to vaso-occlusion in SCD through an active process distinct from passive mechanical obstruction. $\alpha_5\beta_3$ integrin on vascular endothelium is the ligand for several adhesion molecules on erythrocytes (eg, phosphatidyl serine, sulfated gly-cans, CD47, and CD36) [6]. Administration of a monoclonal antibody to $\alpha_5\beta_3$ integrin led to remarkable inhibition of vaso-occlusion in a mouse model that had SCD [62]. Therefore, $\alpha_5\beta_3$ integrin is a candidate adhesion molecule for targeted blockade or reduction, with the hope of achieving clinical benefit in SCD. Since vascular obstruction in SCD also involves adhesion of leuko-cytes and platelets to other blood cells and the endothelium, these cellular inter-actions present opportunities for therapeutic intervention. Two molecules that mediate leukocyte adhesion to vascular endothelium—L-selectin (CD62L) and $\alpha_M\beta_2$ integrin (CD11b and CD18)—are highly expressed by individuals who have severe manifestations of SCD; such as vaso-occlusive crisis, stroke, ne-phropathy, and other organ complications [38]. Reducing the surface expression of these adhesion molecules or blocking their interactions with vascular endothe-lial ligands could reduce vaso-occlusion and yield clinical benefits in SCD.

There is evidence to suggest that two new therapies already tried in SCD work partly by reducing intercellular adhesion. An early clinical benefit of hydroxy-urea therapy, amelioration of mild 'niggling' pains experienced even during steady state, is reported by patients within a month of commencing treatment, at a time when leukocyte adhesion molecule expression has fallen significantly, without a significant rise in HbF level [38]. HU therapy also reduces the expression of adhesion molecules on erythrocytes, evidenced by decreased in vitro adherence of sickle erythrocytes to thrombospondin and laminin [39]. An emerging therapy for SCD that has shown clinical benefit in a pilot trial, oral supplementation with omega-3 fatty acids, reduces platelet expression of the adhesion molecule CD62P (platelet selectin) [42], the counterpart of leukocyte selectin (CD62L) that is down-regulated by HU therapy [38]. How do hydroxy-urea and omega-3 fatty acids reduce adhesion molecule expression on blood cells? A plausible explanation is that by inhibiting DNA synthesis, HU ulti-mately interferes with protein synthesis. This effect of HU appears to be non-specific because different adhesive proteins on leukocytes, erythrocytes, and possibly vascular endothelial cells, are reduced during therapy. With regard to omega-3 fatty acids, it is recognized that the lipid composition of the cell membrane affects not only its structure and function, but also membrane expression of adhesion molecules [51]. It has been demonstrated that adminis-tration of omega-3 fatty acids increases the proportion of these lipids in the membranes of blood cells [42]. This alteration of membrane lipid constitution is thought to modulate the expression of adhesion molecules. Anti-adhesion therapy has some prospects in SCD. Targeted inhibition, blockade, or down-regulation of specific adhesion molecules most relevant to intercellular bonding is preferable to global reduction. This strategy will minimize interference with normal body function dependent on physiological processes that require different adhesive proteins and their ligands.

TREATMENT OF SPECIFIC MANIFESTATIONS
Pulmonary Hypertension

Acute lung injury, manifesting as the chest syndrome, is the leading cause of death in adults who have sickle hemoglobinopathy [21,63]. The overall increase in survival of sickle cell patients means that chronic sickle lung disease, including pulmonary hypertension, is becoming increasingly important as a cause of poor health. That lung disease is a dominant cause of morbidity and mortality in SCD is hardly surprising considering the crucial role of the organ in oxygenation of the blood, and that it is hypoxaemia that causes sickling of erythrocytes. The normal blood pressure in the pulmonary artery is 25/15 mm Hg, with a mean pulmonary artery systolic pressure (PASP) of 18 mm Hg. Pulmonary hyper-tension (PHT) is defined as pulmonary artery systolic pressure >30 mm Hg, or mean PASP >25 mm Hg, or tricuspid valve regurgitant jet velocity (of blood flow) >2.5 m/s. The pathogenesis of PHT in SCD is probably multi-factorial. However, intravascular haemolysis with binding of free plasma hemoglobin to endogenous nitric oxide (NO, a natural vasodilator) is thought to play an important causative role. This concept is supported by the occurrence of PHT in other hemolytic conditions such as thalassaemia [64]. The development of PHT in SCD carries a poor prognosis [65], and there is no generally used effective therapy for this complication. The effects include reduced blood oxygen saturation in steady state (SaO_2 < 90%), fatigue, chronic chest pain, dyspnoea on exertion, a loud pulmonary component of the second heart sound, pansystolic murmur if there is tricuspid regurgitation, ECG changes of right ventricular hypertrophy, syncope, and sudden death [64] Several new therapies for PHT in SCD are coming into clinical practice. The rationale for these treatment modalities is to interfere with the pathogenesis of PHT. Regular exchange blood transfusion reduces the rate of haemolysis by replacing erythrocytes containing HbS with normal red blood cells. Inhalation of NO to replenish the endogenous gas consumed by free plasma Hb corrects the relative NO deficiency that occurs in sickle cell patients including the pulmonary vasculature, stimulates vasodilation, and reduces the pulmonary blood pressure [66]. Oral administration of arginine (the natural substrate for synthesis of NO) at a dose of 0.1 g/kg three times daily, reduced high pulmonary blood pressure in 9 out of 9 sickle cell patients [67]. L-carnitine, an analog of the naturally occurring fatty acid carnitine, is thought to stabilize the red cell membrane, and so inhibits haemolysis. Oral L-carnitine, 1 g three times daily, reduced the mean PASP from 40.2 ± 7.2 mm Hg to 32 ± 6.5 in 14 of 18 sickle cell patients age 4–16 years [68]. Oxygen inhalation lowers pulmonary BP in SCD patients with secondary PHT who have steady-state hypoxaemia, or a drop in pulmonary BP following oxygen administration during cardiac catheterisation. Home oxygen therapy may be combined with other treatment modalities for greater benefit.

Primary Stroke Prevention

Stroke prevention has come to be regarded as standard clinical practice since the United States Stroke Prevention Trial in Sickle Cell Anemia (STOP) was terminated ahead of schedule [69]. Interim analysis of the study data showed clearly that regular blood transfusion significantly reduced the incidence of clinically overt stroke in sickle cell patients who have blood velocity ≥ 200 cm/s in the middle cerebral or terminal part of the carotid artery. Such a high blood velocity indicates an increased risk of cerebrovascular accident (CVA) in sickle cell patients [70]. Stroke is a devastating complication of SCD. It adversely affects the life of not only the patient, but also the family, caregivers, and society as a whole. Therefore, every effort ought to be made to prevent stroke. Before the STOP trial, blood transfusion therapy had been effectively used to reduce the risk of recurrent CVA in sickle cell patients [71]. Proactive measures should be taken to prevent CVA in those patients at higher risk. There is a 200–fold increased risk of stroke in the general sickle cell population relative to healthy HbAA controls, and a higher risk in individuals who have carotid or middle cerebral artery blood velocity ≥ 200 cm/s compared with other sickle cell patients. Indeed, current efforts to prevent CVA in SCD have advanced beyond prophylactic transfusions in patients who have blood velocity ≥ 200cm/s. Michael DeBaun and co-workers [72] involved in the Silent Cerebral Infarct Transfusion Trial are addressing the question whether prophylactic blood transfusions can reduce the proportion of sickle cell patients who have silent cerebral infarction (another index of increased risk of CVA in SCD) and blood velocity <200cm/s who develop clinically overt stroke.

Oral Therapy for Iron Overload

Oral therapy for iron overload has been desired for many years by hemoglobinopathy patients and physicians alike because of the daunting challenges of poor compliance and sheer inconvenience associated with long-term infusions of the main iron-chelating drug, desferrioxamine. Whereas compliance with parenteral iron chelation therapy is generally good in young children supported by the highly motivated parents, adherence to the treatment regimen tends to decline (understandably) in adolescents and young adults who are beginning to live independently. Unfortunately, this tends to coincide with the time that sickle cell patients increasingly need chelation therapy, because they have had cumulated iron loading from blood transfusions since childhood. Deferiprone (L1) was the first oral iron chelator that came into clinical use. It was licensed in 1995 in India, and in Europe 4 years later. A bi-dentate ironophore, smaller and more able to diffuse into cells than desferrioxamine, deferiprone has been shown to reduce or prevent increases in liver iron concentration and mean serum ferritin levels in most patients who need regular blood transfusion [73]. Its greater ability to penetrate myocardial cells may account for significantly improved MRI scans, consistent with reduced cardiac iron load and function in patients taking deferiprone, compared with those on desferrioxamine [74]. The side-effects of deferiprone include mild gastrointestinal symptoms of nausea, vomiting, and abdominal discomfort, chelation and loss of zinc from the body leading to deficiency of this trace element, and joint pains. Granulocytopenia is the most important problem from deferiprone encountered in hematology clinics. The incidence is 0.6/100 patient-years [75].

Deferasirox (ICL670 or Exjade) is a new oral iron chelator which, to date, has not been reported to affect granulocyte count [76]. This tridentate bis-hydroxyphenyl-triazole with high specificity for iron showed clinical efficacy comparable to that of desferrioxamine in phase II trials in patients who have transfusion hemosiderosis [77]. The results of a phase III clinical trial in sickle cell patients are awaited. The side effects of deferasirox include mild to moderate nausea and vomiting, mildly increased urinary β_2-microglobulin and, occasionally, skin rash. The absence of agranulocytosis or the deficiencies of zinc, copper, magnesium, and calcium in those on treatment indicate that the safety profile of deferasirox might be promising.

Although a definitive cure is yet to be found for sickle cell disease, its treatment remains the subject of intense research in the public and private sectors. It is hoped that these efforts and the large body of information generated will translate into effective new therapies available to people who have this hemoglobinopathy across the world.

References

[1] Konotey-Ahulu FID. Hereditary qualitative and quantitative erythrocyte defects in Ghana: an historical and geographical survey. Ghana Med J 1968;7:118–9.

[2] Horton JAB. The diseases of tropical climates and their treatment. London: Churchill; 1874.

[3] Herrick JB. Peculiar elongated and sickled red blood corpuscles in a case of severe anaemia. Arch Intern Med 1910;6:517–21.

[4] Steinberg MH, Rodgers GP. Pathophysiology of sickle cell disease: role of genetic and cellular modifiers. Semin Hematol 2001;38:229–306.

[5] Win N, Yeghen T, Needs M, et al. Use of intravenous immunoglobulin and intravenous methylprednisolone in hyperhaemolysis syndrome in sickle cell disease. Hematology 2004; 19:433–6.

[6] Frenette PS. Sickle cell vaso-occlusion: multistep and multicellular paradigm. Curr Opin Hematol 2002;9:101–6.

[7] Okpala I. The intriguing contribution of white blood cells to sickle cell disease—a red cell disorder. Blood Rev 2004;18:65–73.

[8] Pearson HA. The kidney, hepatobiliary system, and spleen in sickle cell anaemia. Ann NY Acad Sci 1989;565:120–5.

[9] Johnston Jr RB, Hewman SL, Struth AC. An abnormality of the alternative pathway of complement activation in sickle cell disease. N Engl J Med 1973;288:803–5.

[10] Anyaegbu CC, Okpala IE, Aken'Ova AY, et al. Complement haemolytic activity, circulating immune complexes and the morbidity of sickle cell anaemia. Acta Pathol Microbiol Scand 1999;107:699–702.

[11] Mollapour E, Porter JB, Kacmarski R, et al. Raised neutrophil phospholipase A2 activity and defective priming of NADPH oxidase and phospholipase A2 in sickle cell disease. Blood 1998;91:3423–9.

[12] Anyaegbu CC, Okpala IE, Aken'Ova AY, et al. Peripheral blood neutrophil count and candidacidal activity correlate with the clinical severity of sickle cell anaemia. Eur J Haematol 1998;60:267–8.

[13] Charache S, Terrin ML, Moore RD, et al. Effect of hydroxyurea on the frequency of painful crises in sickle cell anemia. N Engl J Med 1995;332:1317–22.

[14] Steinberg MH. Management of sickle cell disease. N Engl J Med 1999;340:1021–30.

[15] Shaper AG, Lewis P. Genetic neutropenia in people of African ancestry. Lancet 1971; 2:1021.

[16] Bain BJ. Ethnic and sex differences in the total and differential white cell count and platelet count. J Clin Pathol 1996;49:664–6.

[17] Essien EM. Platelets and platelet disorders in Africa (review). Baillieres Clin Haematol 1992;5:441–56.

[18] Platt OS, Brambilla DJ, Rosse WF, et al. Mortality in sickle cell disease—life expectancy and risk factors for early death. N Engl J Med 1994;330:1639–43.

[19] Ohene-Frempong K, Weiner SJ, Sleeper LA, et al. Cerebrovascular accidents in sickle cell disease: rates and risk factors. Blood 1998;91:288–94.

[20] Kinney TR, Sleeper LA, Wang WC, et al. Silent cerebral infarcts in sickle cell anemia: a risk factor analysis. Paediatrics 1999;103:640–5.

[21] Castro O, Brambilla DJ, Thorington B, et al. The acute chest syndrome of sickle cell disease: incidence and risk factors in the cooperative study of sickle cell disease. Blood 1994; 84:643–9.

[22] Abboud M, Laver J, Blau CA. Granulocytosis causing sickle cell crisis. Lancet 1998; 351:959.

[23] Steinberg MH, Barton F, Castro O, et al. Effect of hydroxyurea on mortality and morbidity in adult sickle cell anemia. JAMA 2003;289:1645–51.

[24] Diav-Citrin O, Hunnisett L, Sher GD, et al. Hydroxyurea use in pregnancy: a case report in sickle cell disease and review of the literature. Am J Hematol 1999;60:148–50.

[25] Byrd DC, Pitts SR, Alexander CK. Hydroxyurea in two pregnant women with sickle cell anemia. Pharmacotherapy 1999;19:1459–62.

[26] De Pass LR, Weaver EV. Comparison of teratogenic effects of aspirin and hydroxyurea in Fischer 344 and Wistar strains. J Toxicol Environ Health 1982;10:297–305.

[27] Okpala IE. Assessment of severity and hydroxyurea therapy in sickle cell disease.

In: Okpala I, editor. Practical management of haemoglobinopathies. Oxford (UK): Blackwell Publishing; 2004. p. 162–8.

[28] Kinney TR, Helms RW, O'Branski EE, et al. Safety of hydroxyurea in children with sickle cell anemia: results of the HUG-KIDS study, a phaseI/II trial. Blood 1999;94:1550–4.

[29] National Institutes of Health (USA). Fetal hemoglobin induction. In: Management of sickle cell disease. 4th edition. Bethesda (MD): National Institutes of Health; 2002. p. 161–5.

[30] Triadou P, Maier-Redelsperger M, Krishnamoorty R, et al. Fetal haemoglobin variations following hydroxyurea treatment in patients with cyanotic congenital heart disease. Nouv Rev Fr Hematol 1994;36:367–72.

[31] Al Jam'a AH, Al Dabbous IA, Al Khatti AA, et al. Are we underestimating the leukemogenic risk of hydroxyurea? Saudi Med J 2002;23:1411–3.

[32] Wilson S. Acute leukaemia in a patient with sickle cell anemia treated with hydroxyurea. Ann Intern Med 2000;133:925–6.

[33] Rauch A, Borromeo M, Ghafoor A. Leukaemogenesis of hydroxyurea in the treatment of sickle cell anemia. Blood 1999;94:415.

[34] Bakanay SM, Dainer E, Clair B, et al. Mortality in sickle cell patients on hydroxyurea therapy. Blood 2005;105:545–7.

[35] Hanft VN, Fruchtman SR, Pickens CV, et al. Acquired DNA mutations associated with in vivo hydroxyurea exposure. Blood 2000;95:3589–93.

[36] Charache S. Mechanisms of action of hydroxyurea in sickle cell anaemia in adults. Semin Hematol 1997;34:15–21.

[37] Cokic VP, Smith RD, Beleslin-Cokic BB, et al. Hydroxyurea induces fetal hemoglobin by nitric-oxide dependent activation of soluble guanylyl cyclase. J Clin Invest 2003;111:231–9.

[38] Okpala IE, Daniel Y, Haynes R, et al. Relationship between the clinical manifestations of sickle cell disease and the expression of adhesion molecules on white blood cells. Eur J Haematol 2002;69:135–44.

[39] Styles LA, Lubin B, Vichinsky E, et al. Decrease of very late activation antigen-4 and CD36 expression on reticulocytes in sickle cell patients treated with hydroxyurea. Blood 1997;89:2554–9.

[40] Atweh GF, Sutton M, Nassif I, et al. Sustained induction of fetal hemoglobin by pulse butyrate therapy in sickle cell disease. Blood 1999;93:1790–7.

[41] Saunthararajah Y, Hillery CA, Lavelle D, et al. Effects of 5-aza-2′-deoxycytidine on fetal hemoglobin levels, red cell adhesion, and hematopoietic diffrentiation in patients with sickle cell disease. Blood 2003;102:3865–70.

[42] Tomer A, Kasey S, Connor WE, et al. Reduction of pain episodes and thrombotic activity in sickle cell disease by dietary n-3 fatty acids. Thromb Haemost 2001;85:966–74.

[43] Ghebremeskel K, Burns L, Costeloe K, et al. Plasma vitamins A and E in preterm babies fed on breast milk or formula milk with or without long-chain polyunsaturated fatty acids. Int J Nutr Res 1999;69:83–91.

[44] Crawford MA, Golfetto I, Ghereeskel K, et al. The potential role for arachidonic and docosahexanoic acids in protection against some central nervous system injuries in preterm infants. Lipids 2003;38:303–15.

[45] Crawford MA, Bloom M, Broadhurst L, et al. Evidence for the function of DHA during the evolution of the modern hominid brain. Lipids 1999;34:S39–47.

[46] Ghebremeskel K, Min Y, Thomas B, et al. The role of essential fatty acids and anti-oxidants in neuro-vascular development and complications of prematurity. In: Kujak A, editor. Textbook of perinatal medicine. 2nd edition. New York: Paphenon Publishers; 2005.

[47] Ren H, Ibegbulam O, Okpala I, et al. Steady state haemoglobin level in sickle cell anaemia increases with the proportion of erythrocyte membrane n-3 fatty acids. Prostaglandins Leukot Essent Fatty Acids 2005;72(6):415–21.

[48] Ren H, Okpala I, Ghebremeskel K, et al. Blood mononuclear cells and platelets have abnormal fatty acid composition in homozygous sickle cell disease. Ann Hematol 2005;84(9):578–83 [Epub 2005 Apr 5].

[49] Okpala I, Ren H, Ibegbulam O, et al. Steady state haemoglobin level in sickle cell anaemia increases with the proportion of erythrocyte membrane n-3 fatty acids. Blood 2004; 104(Suppl):970a.

[50] Van den Berg JJ, de Fouw NJ, Kuypers FA, et al. Increased n-3 polyunsaturated fatty acid content of red blood cells from fish oil-fed rabbits increases in vitro lipid peroxidation, but decreases hemolysis. Free Radic Biol 1991;11:393–9.

[51] Calder PC. N-3 polyunsaturated fatty acids and inflammation: from molecular biology to the clinic. Lipids 2003;38:343–52.

[52] Marcheselli VL, Hong S, Lukiw WJ, et al. Novel docosanoids inhibit brain ischemia-reperfusion-mediated leukocyte infiltration and pro-inflammatory gene expression. J Biochem (Tokyo) 2003;278:43807–17.

[53] Khalfoun B, Thibault G, Bardos P, et al. Docosahexaenoic and eicosapentanoic acids inhibit in vitro human lymphocyte-endothelial cell adhesion. Transplantation 1996;62: 1649–57.

[54] Burr ML, Fehily AM, Gilbert JF, et al. Effects of changes in fat, fish and fibre intakes on death and myocardial infarction: diet and re-infarction trial (DART). Lancet 1989; 2:757–61.

[55] Geusens P, Wouters C, Nijs J, et al. Long-term effect of omega-3 fatty acid supplementation in active rheumatoid arthritis. a 12-month, double-blind, controlled study. Arthritis Rheum 1994;37:824–9.

[56] Belluzi A, Bringola C, Campieri M, et al. Effect of enteric-coated fish-oil preparation on relapses in Crohn's disease. N Engl J Med 1996;334:1557–60.

[57] De Franceschi L, Saadane N, Trudel M, et al. Treatment with oral clotrimazole blocks Ca^{2+}-mediated K^+ transport and reverses erythrocyte dehydration in transgenic SAD mice: a model for therapy of sickle cell disease. J Clin Invest 1994;93:1670–6.

[58] Stocker JW, De Franceschi L, McNaughton-Smith GA, et al. ICA-17043 a novel Gardos channel blocker, prevents sickle red blood cell dehydration in vitro and in vivo in SAD mice. Blood 2003;101:2412–8.

[59] Ataga KI, DeCastro LM, Swerdlow P, et al. Efficacy and safety of the Gardos channel inhibitor, ICA-17043, in paients with sickle cell anemia. Blood 2004;104(Suppl):33a.

[60] Attah AB. The pathophysiology of sickle cell disease. In: Fleming AF, editor. Sickle cell disease: a handbook for the general clinician. Edinburgh (Scotland): Churchill Livingstone; 1982. p. 43–56.

[61] Kaul DK, Fabry ME, Nagel RL. The pathophysiology of vascular obstruction in the sickle syndromes. Blood Rev 1996;10:29–44.

[62] Kaul DK, Tsai HM, Liu XD, et al. Monoclonal antibodies to αVβ3 (7E3 and LM609) inhibit sickle red blood cell-endothelial interactions induced by platelet-activating factor. Blood 2000;95:368–74.

[63] Gray A, Anionwu EN, Davies SC, et al. Patterns of mortality in sickle cell disease in the UK. J Clin Pathol 1994;44:459–63.

[64] Okpala I. Pulmonary hypertension: a complication of haemolytic states. In: Okpala I, editor. Practical management of haemoglobinopathies. Oxford (UK): Blackwell Publishing; 2004. p. 130–3.

[65] Castro O. Systemic fat embolism and pulmonary hypertension in sickle cell disease. Hematol Oncol Clin North Am 1996;10:1289–303.

[66] Coles W, Nicolas JS, Smatlak PK, et al. A clinical study of the efficacy of nitric oxide delivery via portable versus conventional systems to reduce secondary pulmonary hypertension in sickle cell anemia. Abstracts from the National Sickle Cell Conference of USA (Washington [DC], September 17–23, 2002). Washington (DC): Sickle Cell Disease Association of America; 2002. p. 54.

[67] Morris CR, Hagar W, vam Warmerdam J, et al. Arginine therapy improves pulmonary artery pressures in patients with sickle cell disease and pulmonary hypertension. Blood 2002;100(Suppl):452a.

[68] El-Beshlawy A, Abdelaouff E, Bebawy I. Pulmonary hypertension in sickle cell disease.

Abstracts from the 25th Meeting of the International Society of Haematology—African & European Division (Durban [South Africa], September 18–23, 1999). Durban (South Africa): International Society of Haematology; 1999. p. 120.

[69] Adams RJ, McKie VC, Hsu L, et al. Prevention of a first stroke by transfusions in children with sickle cell anemia and abnormal results on transcranial Doppler ultrasonography. N Engl J Med 1998;339:5–11.

[70] Kwiatkowiski J, Ohene-Frempong K. Stroke in sickle cell disease. In: Okpala I, editor. Practical management of haemoglobinopathies. Oxford (UK): Blackwell Publishing; 2004. p. 134–44.

[71] Ohene-Frempong K. Indications for red cell transfusion in sickle cell disease. Semin Hematol 2001;38(Suppl 1):5–13.

[72] DeBaun MR, Mckinstry R, White D, et al. Epidemiology and treatment of silent cerebral infarcts in sickle cell anemia. Education program book from the 46th Annual Meeting of American Society of Hematology (San Diego [CA], December 4–7, 2004). Washington (DC): American Society of Hematology; 2004. p. 35–40.

[73] Hoffbrand AV, Cohen A, Hershko C. Role of deferiprone in chelation therapy for transfusional iron overload. Blood 2003;102:17–22.

[74] Anderson LJ, Wonke B, Prescott E, et al. Comparison of effects of oral deferiprone and subcutaneous desferrioxamine on myocardial iron levels and ventricular function in beta thalassaemia. Lancet 2002;360:516–20.

[75] Cohen AR, Galanello R, Piga A, et al. Safety profile of the oral iron chelator deferiprone: a multicenter study. Br J Haematol 2002;108:305–12.

[76] Galanello R, Piga A, Alberti D, et al. Safety, tolerability, and pharmacokinetics of ICL670, a new orally active iron-chelating agent in patients with transfusion-dependent iron overload due to β-thalassaemia. J Clin Pharmacol 2003;43:565–72.

[77] Piga A, Galanello R, Cappellini MD, et al. Phase II study of oral chelator ICL670 in thalassaemia patients with transfusional iron overload: efficacy, safety, pharmacokinetics and pharmacodynamics after 6 months of therapy. Blood 2002;100(Suppl):5a.

INDEX

Note: Page numbers of article titles are in **boldface** type.